NEW JERSEY:

ENVIRONMENT AND CANCER

NEW JERSEY: ENVIRONMENT & CANCER

by

EUSTACE A. DIXON, Ph.D.

Edited by

V. Eugene Vivian, Ph.D.
Director, Conservation and Environmental
Studies Center, Inc.

Eureka Publications
Mantua, New Jersey

Library of Congress Cataloging in Publication Data

Dixon, Eustace A., 1934-
  New Jersey, environment & cancer.

  Bibliography: p.
  Includes index.
  1. Cancer—New Jersey. 2. Chemical industries—
Hygienic aspects—New Jersey. 3. Environmentally
induced diseases—New Jersey. 4. New Jersey—Statistics
Medical. I. Title. II. Title: New Jersey, environment
and cancer.

RC277.N5D58	616.99'4071	82-1520
		AACR2

ISBN 0-942848-00-4 (paperback)

ISBN 0-942848-01-2 (clothbound)

Cover concept by Lou Palumbo

Cover art by Nina Gaelen

Eureka Publications
PO Box 372, Mantua NJ 08051

DEDICATION

"Praise the Lord", who granted
the lifetime to write this book

This book is dedicated to

"Dardella",

Eustace A. Dixon, Sr., a cancer victim

ACKNOWLEDGEMENTS

Many persons and organizations have helped me in the reading, preparation, document procurement and figure and graph preparation for the various original and final manuscript chapters of this book. In particular, I would like to thank:

Drs., Rita Arditti, V. Eugene Vivian, Royce Haynes, Donald A. Farnelli, Kenneth Rothe, Donald B. Louria, Irving J. Selikoff, Gerard J. McGarrity, Ara Der Maderosian, John J. Thompson, and Diane Graves, Ruth Elson, Esther Slusarski, Dorothy Price, Catherine Harris, Patricia Daniels, Marie Dearlove, and Harry Alsentzer, Robert Slater, Ludi Palumbo, William DeMedio, George Nagorny, and the Library Staff of the New Jersey State Library, Glassboro State College Library, Woodbury Public Library, The American Cancer Society, The Department of Environmental Protection, The Department of Health, The Gloucester County Times, The Review, and various Industries and Federal Agencies.

CONTENTS

PREFACE

Throughout the early 1970's, New Jersey was often referred to as "Cancer Alley." The state occupied a position of first in the production of chemicals in the beginning of that decade, currently yielding to Texas. The cancer mortality rate, which was relatively high compared to the national average, became associated with the heavy concentration of chemical industry. As a resident and life-long student of the environment, I began a literature search for information on cancer in New Jersey in 1976. I quickly realized that no single comprehensive source book existed which was descriptive, historical and experimental. Secondarily, the available sources did not approach the subject holistically. Further, two things disturbed me; that cancer was the second major killer of humankind and as a graduate student in an environmental studies curriculum at that time, no lectures were devoted to the subject. Hence, this first multidisciplinary evaluation of the impact of the New Jersey environment on cancer incidence and mortality in the state, was written.

My target audience are cancer researchers, students of environmental health, science and education and environmental activists. Hopefully, this book will be of interest to the general public and those who make the laws of the state. The value of this book is not limited to New Jersey residents. In many areas New Jersey is only a model for what is or may be happening in other states. Hopefully, this cohesive, personalized presentation of the impact of the environment and life-style on cancer incidence and mortality in New Jersey, will assist in the development of more effective preventive measures against the disease. Extensive references are given throughout the book for the benefit of anyone wishing to retrace the research.

OVERVIEW

The narrative progresses from the period of the most
rapid sensitization to and evaluation of the cancer problem; from 1973 to the present time. The "state reaction"
to certain National Cancer Institute reports along with
the evolution of the cause of cancers and other factors,
are evaluated simultaneously. In chapters 2 and 3, the
reader is given a basic background in cancer biology and
environmental relationships. Chapter 4, the longest
chapter in the book, is an extensive inventory of individual exposure to chemical pollutants and the cancer
risk. This is a resource chapter; the reader is advised
not to attempt to digest it in one sitting. This is
followed by an environmental assessment of the essentially elective exposures to cancer risks, chapter 5 and an
impact statement on New Jersey, in chapter 6. Chapter 7
is a hindsight evaluation of cancer risks in the New
Jersey environment from colonial times up to the pre-
industrial era. This may be called retrospective environmental toxicology with epidemiologic conclusions.
Chapter 8 is a case study of a long-standing confronta-
tion between a South Jersey community and a hazardous
waste disposal facility. The issues of stress as an environmental carcinogen and obtaining detente in environmental problems are both explored. The book concludes
with a synopsis, chapter 9.

LIMITATIONS

The conclusions drawn in this book are based on the
review of public documents, personal involvement, employment in chemical industry, surveys, scientific literature
and inferential reasoning. The reader should bear in
mind, that it is virtually impossible to present material
of this nature and not have some portion be outdated by

the time of publication. The pollutants reviewed in this study are evaluated mainly for their ability to promote or induce cancer. In some instances, toxicity data are also given. Whether all the pollutants described herein may in fact cause all the cancers described, will remain controversial for some time. Without question, all of the substances reviewed as pollutants are in fact *toxic*, that is, at some dose and time in the human life cycle, each will be harmful. I present this book to the reader with all due humility because of the highly complex nature of the cancers.

CHAPTER 1

AN OVERVIEW OF THE "STATE REACTION"
TO THE CANCER INCIDENCE, 1973-1980

"The time has come for
us to do more than bury
our dead-the time has
come for us to fight
back and here in New
Jersey, where this
killer (cancer) is
most prevalent."

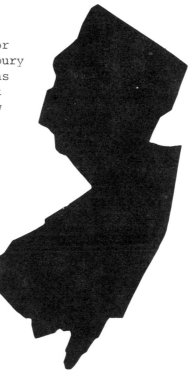

Senator John
Skevin,*
(D.-Bergen),
July 11, 1976

* Chairman of the Senate Commission on the Incidence of
  Cancer in New Jersey.

CHAPTER 1

BACKGROUND

In 1973, researchers T. J. Mason and F. W. McKay of the Epidemiology Branch of the National Cancer Institute (NCI), conducted a statistical study to express national cancer mortality rates by age, sex and race for each county of the contiguous United States.[1] Their study presented alarming statistics about cancer deaths from malignant tumors in New Jersey for the period 1950-1969*:

- highest death rate of nation from malignant tumors in white males
- second highest death rate of nation from malignant tumors in white females
- in the highest twelve percent of states for black cancer patients
- number 1 in ovarian cancers among white women
- number 1 in bladder malignancies among white males
- number 1 in rectal cancer, all females
- nearly the highest rate of intestinal cancers, lung cancers (amongst white males), breast cancer amongst white females

(from a summary by Dr. Donald B. Louria et. al., 1976).[2]

---

* The study also indicated excess bladder, lung, and liver cancer mortality amongst males in 139 counties with a high concentration of chemical industry, throughout the United States.

1

The Mason and McKay Report was a very serious pronouncement, not identifying why New Jersey had these
peculiar cancer incidence characteristics, but citing
them. Did this report from the Federal Government indicate their knowledge of a problem that the state was unaware of? The State of New Jersey maintains its own
public health statistics and with specific regard to
cancer mortality rates, deaths are expressed as total
deaths from all cancers and cancer at specific sites.
In 1975, a 25 year summary of cancer deaths per 100,000
of population showed clearly that cancer was then on the
increase in New Jersey. The presentation of these data
was highly simplistic, not indicating site specific mortality, but anyone could indeed see that New Jersey continued to demonstrate a cancer rate higher than the national average:

New Jersey Public Health Cancer Statistics[3]
1951, 1974, 1975

Cancer Mortality Rate National Average per 100,000 Population		Cancer Mortality Rate New Jersey Average Per 100,000 Estimated Population	Cancer Mortality New Jersey
1951	137 (appx.)	175.9	8,775
1974	169.5	188.8	13,999
1975	174.4	193.4	14,377

The Public Health Department did show statistics listing
the site specific mortality of cancer for the entire
state over the 25 year period, but it was the Mason and
McKay Report that actually contrasted New Jersey site
specific data with the 3,056 counties within the rest of
the contiguous United States.

In February of 1976, Dr. Marvin A. Schneiderman,
Associate Director for Field Studies and Statistics at
NCI, cited New Jersey's highly industralized nature and
exposure to many pollutants by state residents as one
reason for the high incidence of cancer. He added, "And

there are industrial hazards not yet uncovered."[4]

Few of the general public would ever read the original 729 page report by Mason and McKay which listed cancer deaths and rates for 34 types of cancers in each of the nation's 3,056 counties. However, an able press reduced the data to a form readily comprehensible to the average citizen in such stinging news headlines as:

- "N. J. Leads the Nation in Cancer Deaths"
  The Record, Wednesday, May 8, 1974
- "Cancer Rate is Highest in Hudson (County)"
  The Newark Star Ledger, May 9, 1974

In the latter article, Hudson County in northern New Jersey, with the second highest number of manufacturing establishments, was cited as having a cancer mortality rate significantly higher than both state and national averages, per 100,000 population. The statistics were re-manipulated and re-expressed, but what was the basis of the umbilical cord tying them to industry?

Think back to 1970, the Earth Day scene, when there were nationwide protests over pollution which was threatening the environment. The concerned general public was still reverberating to the strains of documented and visible environmental abuse. Stewart Udall's "Quiet Crisis," Barry Commoner's "Closing Circle," and Rachel Carson's "Silent Spring" had all justly sensitized us to air, water and land pollution and abuse.[5, 6, 7] Originally, the protest placards read "Give Earth A Chance," and eventually the fear of poisoning our natural environment was extended to our prime natural resource -- ourselves. The concept of cancer as an environmentally induced disease began taking its place along with the word carcinogen as conversation pieces. The general public -- naive concerning a real understanding of "environment" interpreted that concept in a manner devoid of individual responsibility or control over those personal practises that favored the induction of cancers. Rather, the environment was defined as that which industry pollutes. And in $E=MC^2$ fashion, if industry + pollution = environmental cancer, then New Jersey industrial establishments + pollution = a lot of environmental cancer.

But the dictionary definition of environment is "the aggregate of all external conditions and influences affecting the life and development of an organism." Underscore the word "external" in that definition and bear in mind that there is an internal environment, about which more will be said in chapter 3.

Just before Earth Day, Dr. John Higginson of the International Agency for Research on Cancer, popularized the statistic that as much as 90% of human cancers are caused by environmental factors.[8] Again, environment was interpreted as that which industry pollutes. Dr. Higginson now says, "But when I used the term 'environment' in those days, I was considering the total environment, cultural as well as chemical."[9] But the die was cast; Industry + Pollution = Environmental Cancer became a popular notion. Later, in 1976, Dr. Higginson would make it clear that he attributed a mere 1 - 3% of environmental cancer liability to industry.[10] The major causes he attributed to tobacco and alcohol use, sunlight, diet and behavior.

In July 1974, R. Hoover and J. F. Fraumeni, Jr. of the Epidemiology Center of NCI, in an honest attempt to ferret out other causes for a correlation between cancer incidence and chemical industrialization, re-examined the original data of Mason and McKay.[11] When socioeconomic level (education, income, unemployment) and the location of the industries were established as a base for a correlation, none was found. It began to appear once again that the epidemiological* approach to the incidence of cancer in chemical industry counties was implicating chemicals in the environment as a major cause of the high rate in New Jersey. Specifically, four counties showed a high site specific cancer rate: Middlesex - lung; Gloucester, Salem and Union - bladder. The most important epidemiological finding, however, was the correlation between type of chemical industry and mortality rate by cancer site. A summary is given here:

---

* Determining the cause of a disease by studying its occurrence in relation to occupation, climate, sex, etc.

Bladder Cancer	Manufacture of dyes, dye intermediates, organic pigments, pharmaceutical preparations, perfumes, cosmetics and other toilet preparations
Lung Cancer	Industrial gases, pharmaceutical preparations, soaps and detergents, paints, inorganic pigments and synthetic rubber
Liver Cancer	Organic chemicals, synthetic rubber, soaps and detergents, cosmetics, other toilet preparations and printing ink

It is extremely important that one not draw hasty conclusions because of the correlations resulting from the Hoover-Fraumeni study. Let us review the highlights of their conclusions and their own admitted weakness of the data.

a. If the 10% excesses of bladder, lung and liver cancers amongst men in the chemical industry counties are due to *occupational exposures*, chemical workers stand a 2 - 3 times better chance of contracting cancer.

b. Cancer mortality was not elevated in all chemical industry counties; hence, the above risk may fall on only a small segment of workers.

c. The role of *cigarette smoking* in these correlations has not been defined.

d. Additional work is required by industry, labor and independent investigators to clarify the risk of cancer to chemical industry workers.

In 1975, the Epidemiology Branch of NCI published the Atlas of Cancer Mortality for U.S. Counties: 1950-1969. The original statistical data of the 1973 report (U.S. Cancer Mortality by County) was rendered in

a highly visual map style.[12] Again, New Jersey demonstrated cancer "hot spots"; age adjusted, all site combined rates in the top 10%, identified in the original
by the proverbial danger color -- red, (see Figures 1
through 4). Within minutes after looking at these maps,
the viewer would feel safe or uncomfortable, and for
those in New Jersey, definitely the latter . . . .

The Evolving Role of Diet and Nutrition in the Etiology
of Cancer

    Meantime, across the seas and certainly not primal
in its content, a study correlating dietary factors and
cancer incidence was released. In November 1974, researchers Doll and Armstrong at the Radcliffe Infirmary,
Oxford, England, subjected the incidence and mortality
rates from many countries versus dietary and other variables to an epidemiological study.[13] The results of
their analyses showed "*suggestions* of associations between cancer of the colon, rectum and dietary variables
-- particularly meat (or animal protein) and total fat
consumption." The authors clearly stated the weaknesses
of their data; that some correlations were only suggestions, but that the relationships defined were indeed
impressive. The study was not given much publicity.

The Role of the Media

    Most of us get our daily information from the news
media and this has been proven through survey research.
Dr. Wilbur Schramm of Stanford University has summarized
tenets common to the role of science in the media. One
particularly applicable here is "mass media use is the
second predictor of scientific information; after the
school years, most of the increment of science knowledge
comes from the media."[14] Who of the general public
would make the effort to obtain original documents describing the National Cancer Institute's findings on
chemical industry counties? So, when the Atlantic City
Press or Trenton Times says respectively, "New Jersey
Leads Nation in Bladder Cancer Risks" or "Jersey a Lead-
er in Cancer Deaths" as they did in April and July of
1976, the general public is inclined to accept it. The

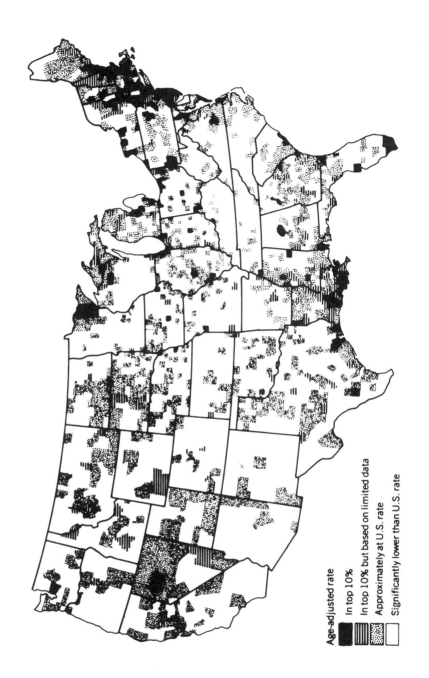

Age-adjusted rate

In top 10%

In top 10% but based on limited data

Approximately at U.S. rate

Significantly lower than U.S. rate

FIGURE 1
Cancer Mortality, 1950-1969, By County,
All States Combined, White Males

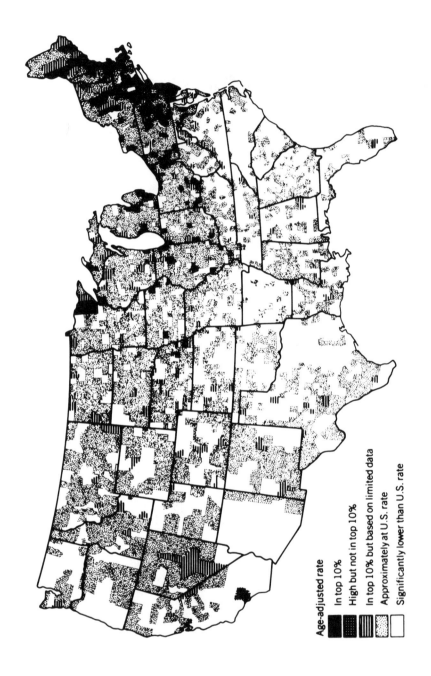

Age-adjusted rate

■ In top 10%

▦ High but not in top 10%

▥ In top 10% but based on limited data

⬚ Approximately at U.S. rate

□ Significantly lower than U.S. rate

FlGURE 2
Cancer Mortality, 1950–1969, By County,
All States Combined, White Females

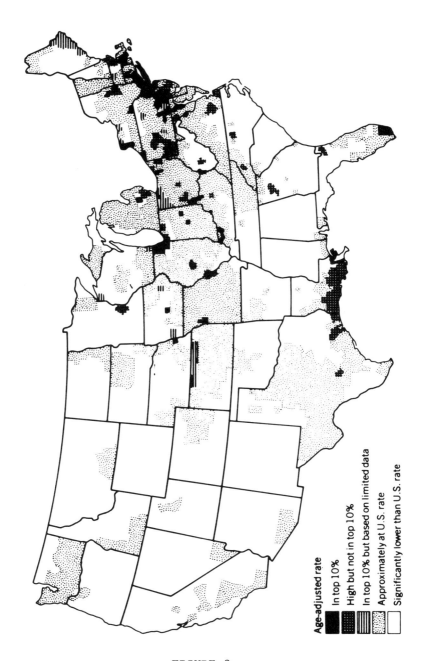

Age-adjusted rate

In top 10%

High but not in top 10%

In top 10% but based on limited data

Approximately at U.S. rate

Significantly lower than U.S. rate

FIGURE 3
Cancer Mortality, 1950-1969, By County,
All States Combined, Non-White Males

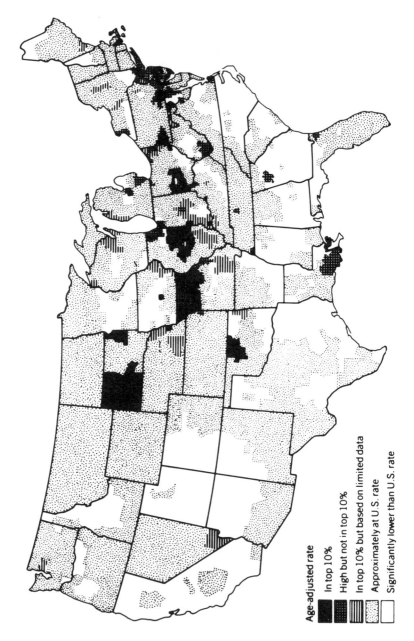

FIGURE 4
Cancer Mortality, 1950–1969, By County,
All States Combined, Non-White Females

Age-adjusted rate
In top 10%
High but not in top 10%
In top 10% but based on limited data
Approximately at U.S. rate
Significantly lower than U.S. rate

media in New Jersey did fulfill their obligation -- to
inform New Jersey residents about the cancer mortality
and what the state would do about it, but the headlines
continued to hammer out conclusions and uncomplimentary
(whether proven or not yet) state titles. This viewpoint is a conviction shared by scientists, that science
reporters sensationalize news. One of the greatest dangers in the field of science writing is the failure to
include the essential, inherent weaknesses in any study.
All scientific studies make assumptions and possess limitations. James Bowman of the University of Wyoming,
writes, "American dailies are key gatekeepers in the
transmission of environmental news to the public. Given
the complexity and profundity of these issues, there is
ample opportunity for public confusion."[15]

Understandably, the media require stimulating headlines to sell papers. If they "water down" data, they
violate freedom of speech and if they exaggerate it,
they violate the tenets of good journalism. An unten-
able position to be in -- but even more so for their au-
diences. On the other hand, however, how well would environmental news articles accomplish the goal of education if they were based on statements from scientists
who often must speak in what I call the "equivocal
tone," i.e., dialogue resounding in uncertainty and in-
conclusivity? For example, consider the following hy-
pothetical newspaper commentary: Dr. X says, "Acid rain
may be detrimental to some species of plants but may
also aid in the dispersion of certain soil nutrients."
Would this be effective reporting? So, newspaper headlines require a mini-content analysis parallel with description of the state reaction to the National Cancer
Institute reports. This will be done as this chapter
progresses.

In recognition of the tremendous responsibility the
media has in conveying the news to the public, other important issues must be addressed. Who decides what environmental news should be brought to the public? The
answer comes, at least partially, from a hypothesis
proffered by Patricia Sutton in a graduate Communications thesis -- environmental news reporting does not
originate from media initiative, but from a response to
public demand.[16] Mrs. Sutton based these findings on a

very recent survey of environmental news reporting
(southern New Jersey versus St. Louis and California)
demonstrating that increased coverage of environmental
news over the years 1970-1979 was based on a response to
public demand as seen by 82% of the media reporters in
the test area (See Appendix). Why, the reader may ask,
am I giving so much consideration to the media? You
simply cannot discuss cancer in New Jersey without talking about the media.

THE "STATE REACTION"

     What is about to be examined is what I term the
"state reaction" to the cancer problem provoked by both
internal concerns and NCI reports. Many professionals
did not agree that there was a cancer problem in New
Jersey, citing a similarly higher than national average
mortality rate in other states:

Age Adjusted Cancer Mortality Per 100,000[17]
U.S. 1950-1969
All Malignant Neoplasms

State	White Male	White Female	Non-White Male	Non-White Female
New Jersey	205	148	230	163
Washington, D.C.	204	142	265	166
Rhode Island	203	143	237	134
New York	199	148	228	153
Connecticut	196	139	232	139
United States	174	130	184	139

But we in New Jersey had a clearly defineable problem.
And on an international basis cancer was and is what I

term pancresic*; that is, worldwide and increasing. But
that did not make us feel any better in New Jersey, no
matter how you juggled the epidemiological data and expressed the results -- our rate was high! Would the
enigmatic pronouncements of the Mason and McKay and
Hoover-Fraumeni reports be a clarion call to the state's
scientific militia? The connotation here is that the
militia was asleep. But, no, the militia was not asleep
and there was mobilization, from the average volunteer
citizen up to the then State Governor, Brendan Byrne.
And the gamut of the array of the militia varied; researchers, physicians, statespersons, environmentalists,
the media and others.

The Cancer Institute of New Jersey

     An organization which would become dormant in a few
years, yet embodied a rather unique concept, came into
being with the founding of the Cancer Institute of New
Jersey in February of 1975.[18] The concept was to form
an agency from the private sector to coordinate all cancer detection, treatment and research in New Jersey.
The founders were members of business organizations,
medical and educational professions. The Chairman of the
Institute, Dr. Celestino Clemente, Vice President of
Medical Affairs of United Hospitals, lead the new organization which was intended to foster statewide cancer
public education, a cancer medical history registry and
utilization of National Cancer Institute funding. Personnel of the Cancer Institute of New Jersey were aware
of the NCI reports linking the state cancer mortality
rate with the conglomerate of chemical industries, but
drew no conclusions, save the need for an independent
study. However benevolent their goals, the Institute
never flourished. Reportedly, the public medical sector
was enthusiastic about any independent studies that
would delineate treatment needs, but not enthusiastic
about anything that would reveal the inadequacies of
such treatments. Further, state medical institutions

_____

* A term coined by the author contrived from "pan" (world) and
   "cresere" (to increase).

wanted privacy in the coordination of the programs.
Bluntly, it appeared (and we now know) that the state
was formulating its own program to unify cancer projects. The Cancer Institute soon became defunct; it
exists today on paper only.

Sierra Club - New Jersey Chapter

     Out of one man's effort to protect the scenic
beauty of the Sierra Nevadas, emerged a crusading organization of naturalists, the Sierra Club in 1892.[19]
John Muir, the founder, could not have possibly conceived of the Sierra Club obtaining national scope. Although they are regarded synonymously with the West
Coast, they are well represented across the nation.
Their goal initially was to explore, enjoy and to protect the nation's scenic resources and eventually they
encompassed our most important natural resource -- humankind. And the NCI reports showed major impact on
this resource, the residents of New Jersey. Diane
Graves, the present and then conservation chairperson,
advised me that she was "tuned in already" prior to the
release of the NCI atlas.[20] The New Jersey Sierra Club
Chapter was aware of the environmental stress in the
state and was already active in air and water pollution
control and solid waste legislation, energy policy,
pinelands protection, land use, and transportation issues just to mention some. They already had at their
command a well-used bag of eco-tactics, not the least of
which was effective journalism.

     The Jersey Sierra Club reaction to the NCI reports
was voiced in the organization's journalistic arm, the
"Jersey Sierran"; "we all know by now that the maps show
New Jersey as having the highest rate of cancer-related
deaths in the nation."[21] The Jersey Sierran did not
pass on to its readers the caveats of the NCI study,
but, impressed with the overall statistics, urged Governor Byrne to launch a study of the state's cancer mortality rate. Members were encouraged to press their
legislators for the passage of a strong toxic substances
control act. Convinced that New Jersey had the highest
cancer death rate in the nation and that it was environmentally induced, the Sierra Club petitioned the Senate

Commission to set up an Emergency Advisory Committee on
Environmental and Occupational Carcinogens in New Jersey. There was a singular emphasis on obtaining the
power to secure information on industrial emissions,
effluents, the nature of the chemicals in use and their
levels in the work place and the outside environment.
By August of 1976, the Sierra Club had gained the support of the Oil, Chemical and Atomic Workers Union, the
American Lung Association, physicians, environmentalists
and academia throughout the state. Utilizing one of
their most vital eco-tactics, social and political action, they advocated prevention as the approach to the
state's cancer problem. In June of 1977, the Club en-
dorsed the attention-getting concepts of the Senate Commission on the Incidence of Cancer in New Jersey. That
Commission had sponsored proposed legislation which
sought to ban 17 known carcinogens used in various manufacturing processes in the state. This bold and unpop-
ular bill (S3035) will be discussed later in this chapter. Although the Sierra Club recognized the holistic
nature of exposure to environmental carcinogens -- "environmental, occupational, food chain, or tobacco," --
it appeared that industry would have to bite the bullet.

The American Lung Association

    The present day American Lung Association (ALA)
came into existence to combat a disease regarded for
centuries as hopeless, tuberculosis.[22] Today, with tuberculosis well under control,* the ALA is combating
lung specific environmental diseases running the gamut
from the harmful and offensive to the fatal; e.g., coal-
workers "black lung," "miner's asthma," asbestosis, be-
rylliosis, byssinosis, emphysema, and chronic bronchitis. They are equally concerned about the problems accompanying hobby and leisure activities; e.g., metal-
working and rock-tumbling. They have fought an enor-
mously frustrating battle to scare smokers into kicking
the habit.

---

* More than 3,000 Americans still die annually from this disease.

The implications of the NCI "Directory," came as no
surprise to the American Lung Association. "The cancer
report (The Directory) caused us to rethink what we kept
saying by rote but hadn't thought through concretely.
Namely, that lung disease, including lung cancer, was
the result of combined assaults of which cigarette smoking was the most distinct," reports Walter Dickinson,
Jr., present Managing Director.*[23] Not only did the
Association develop new environmental allies, but began
to sponsor Occupational Health Conferences, anti-smoking
clinics, health risk seminars and the promotion of on-
site air sampling by both the Department of Labor and
Industry. The Association realized the need for a holistic approach to the state's cancer problem and elected to align itself with other organizations. Particularly, the Association adapted a position expressed in
writing by the Institute for Medical Research, rather
than develop separate testimony of its own.

The American Cancer Society

"People Helping People" aptly describes the American Cancer Society -- an organization that, in my opinion, ranks highly among all concerted efforts to deal
with cancer in New Jersey and nationally. The Society's
goal is to eliminate cancer, save lives and reduce suffering.[24] To some it may seem redundant to even summarize the job the Society does, but my own surveys, discussions and involvement as a public education volunteer
indicate that describing the scope of their outreach
warrants the utilization of every opportunity that presents itself. The purposes and varieties of programs of
this organization are not fully understood. According
to their records, the Society has been instrumental in
raising a once morbid and taboo illness considered to be
utterly fatal, to a now widely discussed disease with a
35% survival rate. At the core of this organization is
the volunteer strength, reportedly numbering some 2.5

---

*   Mr. Dickinson is Managing Director of the Hammonton office.
    There are five other offices throughout the state.

million nationally, with 60,000 in New Jersey.*

If there is one single source of carcinogens over which the literature on epidemiology affords virtually no room for debate, it is tobacco use. This practise in New Jersey will be examined in chapter 4. If one had to pinpoint one aspect of the Society's program deserving of special mention, it would have to be lung cancer "Potential" prevention through tobacco education (and smoking cessation programs). The extent of the Society's program is described further in the appendix and that is an inadequate encapsulation.

My first clue as to the "state reaction" on behalf of the Society's New Jersey Division came from Mr. Kenneth W. Steffan, Director of Public Information, "Historically, the Hoover and Fraumeni reports of 1973 on cancer mortality in the United States had little impact when first issued."[25] Why? The bulky 729 page report just wasn't easy to comprehend. But when a subsequent republication of the data in the form of color-coded maps, delineating site-specific cancers and correlating them with specific counties hit the streets, so to speak, it raised eyebrows. Mr. Steffan continued by describing how the New Jersey Division of ACS organized a medical seminar to explore a possible causal relationship between environmental factors and the statistics.

The medical seminar held May 1-2, 1976, was a veritable cancer expertise think tank. I was able to relive that experience through tapes provided by Mr. Steffan.[26] Among the approximate 200 physicians attending, members of government environmental health agencies and Departments of Health, were Drs. Robert Hoover, Donald B. Louria, Lawrence Garfinkel and Irving Selikoff. A key-

---

* I take this opportunity to present their seven warning signals: (1) Change in bowel or bladder habits, (2) A sore that does not heal, (3) Unusual bleeding or discharge, (4) thickening or lump in breast or elsewhere, (5) indigestion or difficulty in swallowing, (6) obvious change in wart or mole, and (7) nagging cough or hoarseness. If you have a warning signal, see your doctor.

note speaker was Dr. Robert Hoover, one of the originators of the study that precipatated the need for the
seminar. Dr. Hoover described the 729 page study af-
fectionately as the "white elephant." The study generated little interest initially. Later, however, it was
successful in accomplishing Dr. Hoover's goal -- making
people aware of the uniqueness of their own area (not
just New Jersey). However, many caveats were overlooked
as the popular media interpreted the data.

Although the discussion of tobacco usage as a principal cause of lung cancer dominated the seminar, Dr.
Hoover did make reference to the role of diet and nutrition in the etiology of cancers at other sites. Dr.
Donald B. Louria expressed resentment to the NCI data as
represented in the media, depicting New Jersey as "Cancer Alley." Dr. Louria requested that his colleagues
"not leave this conference ascribing cancer in New Jersey to industry." "We have allowed," he continued, "the
public to metamorphosize this (data) into an indictment
of industry." He concluded by stating that our priority
should be to establish a state-wide cancer registry.
However, he felt that the required cooperation between
industry and academia would not be forthcoming. Also
diverting the responsibility for the cancer incidence
away from industry was Dr. Lawrence Garfinkel of the National American Cancer Society's office, who cited tobacco use as a major cause of cancer. Dr. Irving J.
Selikoff, renowned specialist on the effects of human
exposure to asbestos, talked about preventing cancer to
populations of high risk, such as cigarette smokers.

Industry may not have occupied center stage as the
proliferators of the carcinogens responsible for the
cancer incidence in New Jersey at this conference, but
it was certainly no understudy. The roles of asbestos,
b-napthylamine and vinyl chloride, all used in various
manufacturing processes in the state, were also discussed. The environmental impact of these substances are
given special attention in chapter 4. Many recognized
the transient nature of our society and the need to take
into consideration the role of migration into New Jersey
in interpreting the NCI reports. The seminar attendees
concluded that there was a need for more specific data,
post haste, to be followed by immediate counter measures.

The American Cancer Society had been intimately involved in the prevention and cure of cancers in New Jersey and nation-wide before the release of the NCI reports. The organization has no laboratories or research
centers. However, it has provided about 47 million dollars in research grants and fellowships to institutions
in 1979 alone. I believe the Society's critical role as
sponsors of research and providers of seminar formats
demonstrates its inherent ongoing contributions to the
quest of preventing and curing the cancers.

The Institute for Medical Research

What began as a small research laboratory in Camden
to study polio and other contagious diseases in 1949,
became a state chartered, non-profit laboratory, The Institute for Medical Research.[27] Although presently little known to New Jerseyites, The Institute enjoys a distinctive reputation of international scope. Some of
the major projects at the Institute deal with breast
cancer, heritable diseases (e.g., sickle cell anemia),
children's cancer, aging, and the study of chemicals in
the environment that can cause cancer. As a result of
efforts of largely volunteer women's auxiliary groups, a
new environmental research laboratory was added in the
spring of 1977. The Institute not only maintains a substantial library and computerized data base, but also
sponsors postdoctoral courses for physicians and health
professionals, as well as generating numerous scientific
reports. The Institute is a veritable research oasis in
southern New Jersey.

What was the Institutes response to the Mason and
McKay, Hoover-Fraumeni reports as part of the "state reaction?" The Director, Dr. Lewis L. Coriell, states
"long before the reports came out, we suspected but did
not know that the cancer rate in New Jersey was higher
than many other states."[28] Dr. Coriell continued by describing his advocacy that New Jersey should have dedicated more funds to the cancer problem, searched out
more federal aid and sought support for basic and applied cancer research. One basic problem plaguing
southern New Jersey was the absence of both a medical
and dental school. Northern New Jersey could boast of

two: Seton Hall became a state school in 1965 and was later renamed the New Jersey College of Medicine and Dentistry, and Rutgers University at New Brunswick began a medical school in 1966. However, two medical schools could not meet the needs of the then population of approximately 6 million people, neither for cancer patients nor those suffering from any other disease or sickness.

Dr. Coriell has long been an advocate of New Jersey's solving its own health problems, supporting the establishment of a regional medical-dental school in the south Jersey area as far back as the mid-sixties.[29]

The Evolving Role of Diet and Nutrition

Before continuing with the summary review of the New Jersey based organizations' reaction to the NCI, it is again necessary to interject a little more concerning the ascendancy of the importance of diet and nutrition in the etiology of the cancers. Across the Hudson River at the American Health Foundation in New York, Dr. Ernst Wynder and researchers elsewhere were gathering increasing epidemiological evidence concerning the impact of a high intake of dietary fats and overnuitrion on cancers of the colon, pancreas, kidney, breast, ovary, endometrium and prostrate.[30] Although Dr. Wydner graced his findings with the due caveats surrounding causal relationships, he was impressed sufficiently to recommend to a sedentary American society the consumption of a "prudent diet," lower in cholesterol and saturated fats and calories in general. This recommendation matched that of researchers in the field of cardiovascular disease who also advocated diet as an approach to reducing mortality by that number one killer. And what of occupational factors as a cause of cancer? Dr. Wynder relegated their ranking to a "small percentage," posting nutritional factors high on the scale; witness the slow emergence of a school of thought that would place a considerable modicum of control over the body's fate in the hands of the individual.

Federal Government Diet and Nutrition Awareness

A Senate Committee on Nutrition and Human Needs had been in existence since the 1960's. In December of 1977, that committee headed by Senator George McGovern (D. - South Dakota) recommended that Americans reduce their dietary intake of saturated fat while maintaining the same protein intake and increasing dietary carbohydrate and fiber consumption (also while reducing refined and processed sugar consumption).[31] The Senate Agriculture, Nutrition & Forestry Committee which replaced the previous nutrition committee continued the advocacy of diet revision as well as pressing NCI to fund additional diet research. Senator McGovern's efforts and public pressure later resulted in NCI increasing its research spending on nutrition.[32]

The Senate Committee continued to monitor American eating habits and the impact of federal government dietary recommendations is being felt at the state level.

State Government Diet and Nutrition Awareness

A cooperative program exists between the New Jersey Department of Education (DE) and the Food and Nutrition Service of the U.S. Department of Agriculture.[33] DE, in turn, provides funding to subsidiary organizations such as the Educational Improvement Center (EIC) who "provide the training of and technical assistance of food service personnel and administrators." There are four branches of EIC serving New Jersey, providing assistance to public, non-public and residential care institutions in the interpretation of the "new and revised nutritional standards." Although it is difficult to assess the pre-existence of a New Jersey diet, some discussion of that is covered in chapter 5.

THE "STATE REACTION" CONTINUED

The Cabinet Committee on Cancer Control

On May 26, 1976, Governor Brendan T. Byrne signed
Executive Order #40, creating a permanent cabinet level
committee on cancer control.[34] Formed on the basis of
the Governor's personal concern and the advocacy of both
the then Commissioner of Environmental Protection, David
Bardin and the Commissioner of the Department of Health,
Dr. Joanne Finley, the committee would coordinate efforts of the state hierarchy to study, prevent and control cancer. The Committee would command assistance
from all major state departments, including the Departments of Agriculture, Education, Environmental Protection, Health, Higher Education, and Labor and Industry.
Governor Byrne would serve as a chairperson over the
commissioners, secretaries or chancellors of these various departments. The committee's goals were the identification of high-risk populations and areas, reduction
of community exposure to carcinogenic substances and the
development of new programs on smoking prevention and
tobacco education. Ultimately, no single individual may
be given credit for the inception of the Cabinet Committee which has become the state umbrella cancer control
coordinating agency. The committee has been good for
New Jersey; by 1978 it had initiated over twenty state
and federally funded cancer control projects.[35]

State Department of Health

In May 1976, the New Jersey State Department of
Health, headed by Dr. Joanne E. Finley, released a publication entitled, "Controlling Cancer in New Jersey,
Let's Protect Our People."[36] The comment, "the appall-
ing statistics presented (in the report) certainly give
New Jersey the distinction as 'Cancer-State-U.S.A.,'" by
Dr. Finley, provides a state agency interpretation and
reaction to the Mason and McKay and Hoover-Fraumeni reports. The comment also reflects the high level conviction that New Jersey had a "cancer alley" syndrome. The
program outlined in her report actually embodied the
total state approach to the cancer problem delineated by
Governor's Cabinet Committee. It was holistic, interdisciplinary in framework requiring cooperation from
within and outside of the State Department of Health,

and encompassing the Department of Higher Education,
Department of Agriculture, Department of Education,
Occupational Safety and Health Administration (OSHA),
National Institute of Occupational Safety & Health
(NIOSH), and National Cancer Institute (NCI).

The specific tasks of the Department of Health were
to be:

- The institution of a cancer registry, not
  only of deceased, but of new patients (the
  latter providing information on life-style,
  mobility, hobbies, etc.);

- Epidemiologic investigations -- the investigation of environmental relationships --
  considering distribution and cause;

- Identification of high risk areas -- the
  identification and transience and use of
  probably/proven carcinogens throughout New
  Jersey (especially those cited by NIOSH);

- Early detection screening;

- Experimental techniques to develop carcinogenicity and susceptibility testing;

- Follow-up and treatment;

- Laboratory support;

- Health education (tobacco avoidance);

- Delineation of the roles of state agencies.

The Senate Commission on The Incidence of Cancer in
New Jersey

Senator John M. Skevin of the 38th District (D.-
Bergen) was born in Union City, New Jersey on June 14,
1927.[37] Presently an Oradell resident, he has been very
active in charitable, civic and professional societies
including Counsel to the ACS and has worked for legisla-

tive action to abate air pollution and associative
health hazards. Elected to the Senate in 1973 and 1977,
he proposed to utilize the investigative power granted
to the Senate by Congress to establish the Senate Commission on the Incidence of Cancer in New Jersey. This
Commission would become a highly visible platform for
the discussion of issues and the initiation of legislation dealing with the cancer problem in New Jersey. In
fact, Senator Skevin had introduced legislation prior
to the convening of the Commission to require that the
physician filing certificates of death due to cancer,
list critically needed diagnostic and treatment statistics.

I am going to paraphrase some of the dialogue from
the past seven Commission meetings which has been captured in over 300 pages of testimony. The meetings so
well express the reaction of environmentalists, industrialists, state health authorities and politicians to
the state's cancer problem. The dialogue has national
and world-wide implications, wherein environmental abuse
in New Jersey surfaces as a model to be avoided, and our
regulations as models to be emulated. Such a smug
statement should be followed by a knowledgeable, hind-
sighted, contemporary position, from a generation which
knows the real "causes" of cancer -- but many remain
elusive.

All Commission meetings have been held in Trenton,
in the Senate Chamber as was the first one on June 11,
1976.[38] Senator Skevin virtually promised at the onset
that the Commission would "not be a forum for those who
wished to pay lip service in the battle against cancer,
nor will it provide a platform for those simply seeking
to make headlines." In a similar decisive manner, he
proposed a 1¢ tax on cigarette sales to finance scientific research on causes, diagnoses and treatment of
cancer. Next, David J. Bardin, the then Commissioner of
the state's Department of Environmental Protection (DEP),
cited the need to investigate environmental factors including cigarette smoking, exposure to cancer-causing
agents in industries, the air, water, food, and the impact of solar radiation.

These environmental factors, holistic in nature,

were cited as being responsible for the "residual increase in cancer not only in New Jersey but throughout
the United States" as outlined in a study by the New
Jersey Department of Environmental Protection authored
by Drs. Glenn Paulson and Peter W. Preuss. In that
study some of the increase in cancer (in terms of deaths
per year) in the United States between the years 1900-
1960 were explained by the cumulative increase in total
population and life expectancy. However, the actual
number of deaths which exceed that extrapolation, termed
the "residual increase," were attributed to the aforementioned environmental factors; these data are presented in the appendix.

Bardin further commented that statistical techniques tend to show a high incidence of cancer in highly
populated counties and such is the case in most New Jersey counties. However, the overall statistic, that New
Jersey sustained 4% of the country's total cancer deaths
while having only 3.5% of the population could not be
overlooked. Lastly, Bardin elaborated on the DEP approach to minimizing the threat posed by carcinogenic,
toxic and hazardous substances in the New Jersey environment:

    a.   Establish a toxic substances inventory and
         determine the presence and concentration
         of these substances in the air, water and
         wastes throughout the state

    b.   Monitor traditional pollutant emissions
         (i.e., sulfur dioxide, carbon monoxide in
         air and phosphates in water), carcinogenic
         organics, e.g., polynuclear aromatic hydro-
         carbons, chlorinated hydrocarbons, chloro-
         form and landfill leachate in air, water
         and fish and wildlife sediments

    c.   Establish environmentally safe waste treat-
         ment and disposal methods

    d.   Reduce water-borne contamination of drink-
         ing water by toxic substance effluents by
         establishing a monitoring program for pot-
         able water supplies

    e. Reduce air-borne discharges of toxic
        substances

    f. Examine other federal laws/programs;
        avoid duplication

Senator Skevin asked about the statistic that up to
90% of cancer is attributable to environmental factors.
Commissioner Bardin responded saying, certain cancers
had been specifically linked to particular industrial
locations; a correlation exists between cigarette smoking and lung cancer and that a relationship exists between the amount of ultra-violet radiation reaching the
earth in different geographical locations and skin cancer incidence. Comments that Senator Skevin would make
later would reveal that his concept of environmental
factors was equated only with industrial pollution while
Commissioner Bardin's were more holistic.

The Commissioner of Health, Dr. Joanne E. Finley,
praised the quality of the Mason and McKay study for its
ability to describe cancer death rates by counties of
residence of cancer victims and the expression of age-
adjusted rates. Dr. Finley then emphasized that the
most revealing facet of the Mason and McKay study was
that Salem County in New Jersey had an age-adjusted
white male bladder cancer rate of 16.1 per 100,000 population as compared to the national rate of 6.8. Funded
by the National Cancer Institute, the state Health Department was already investigating occupational factors
in bladder cancer incidence. Dr. Finley concurred with
Senator Skevin on the need for a comprehensive cancer
registry, including newly reported cancers, information
on diet, occupation, ethnic origin, education and tobacco use history. Further, she raised a question that
would later serve to crystalize the industrial philosophy toward the worker, the environment and the state
economy, collectively known as socioenvironomics.* Re-

---

* Socioenvironomics: A contraction of the words social, environmental and economics; an evaluatory process where human
   life is placed first, the environment second, and economics
   last.

flecting on the much bandied-about percentage of cancer induced by environmental factors, estimated at 80%, Dr. Finley surmised that no one really knew whether the impact of these factors was pertinent only in "the working place or in the home or in the air breathed around the working place." Could the prospective registry lead to further evidence that chemicals currently used or produced in New Jersey were responsible for the high incidence of cancer? Fourteen chemicals had previously been determined to be carcinogenic or suspect carcinogens in animal research conducted by the National Institute of Occupational Safety and Health.*

Dr. Finley concluded with a suggestion that was supportive of attaining detente over the environmental problems in New Jersey. She recommended that industrial researchers be invited to subsequent hearings because it would be interesting to hear from an industry (DuPont) that everybody is saying probably did cause the bladder cancers in Salem County.

The first Commission meeting closed with testimony from Dr. J. Oliver Lampan, Director of the Institute of Microbiology at Rutgers University's Watson Institute. Dr. Lampan related a summary of the Institute's approach to the cancer problem which consists of basic research into the problems of mutation, blood chemistry changes in leukemia, chemotherapy, molecular biology, virology and immunology. Reflecting over the fact that it took 100 years to control infectious diseases caused by bacteria and fungi, he said that we should not presume the cancer problem will be solved in ten years.

---

* The fourteen known (or probable) carcinogens are: 4-Nitrobiphenyl; Alpha Naphthylamine; 4,4 Methylene bis (2-Chloroaniline); Methyl chloromethyl ether; 3,3 -Dichlorobenzidine; Bis-chloromethyl ether; Beta Napthylamine; Benzidine; 4 Amino diphenyl; Ethyleneimine; Beta Propiolactone; 2-Acetylaminofluorene; 4-Dimethylaminoazobenzene; N-Nitrosodimethylamine. The role of some of these chemicals as carcinogens will be discussed in chapter 4.

Continuing Controversy and Reevaluation of the NCI Reports

The Mason and McKay, and Hoover-Fraumeni reports were to generate much controversy and be subjected to reevaluation over the period 1973-1980. Dr. Donald B. Louria of the New Jersey Medical School, and other researchers collectively conducted one such reevaluation in September, 1976.[39] They re-examined the data from counties with cancer death rates either 50 percent above or less than the national average. Three counties (Hudson, Essex and Passaic) displayed death rates from malignant tumors above the national average for whites and seven counties (Hudson, Bergen, Passaic, Middlesex, Hunterdon, Ocean and Sussex) showed similar results for blacks. Cumulatively, their study concluded that New Jersey ranked first to sixth in death rates among whites and blacks and the northern counties generally showed higher rates than southern counties. The original NCI conclusions were softened further by the statement that only 700 yearly deaths could be attributed to site-specific carcinogens related to industrial exposure (bladder, larynx, leukemia, kidney, stomach and lung), the predominant pattern of cancer mortality in the northern industrialized counties, they concluded, emphasized the role of the industrial introduction of carcinogens into the state's environment.

Concurrently, with others, they advocated that the state institute a mandatory state-wide malignant tumor incidence and mortality register.

The News Media - 1976

Before continuing the account of the Senate Hearings, a brief interjection is required about the ongoing education which the general public had been receiving from the news media about the cancers in New Jersey. For two years the news media had been relaying messages from the National Cancer Institute and from within the state to New Jersey residents; in essence, New Jersey had a monopoly on cancer. The title of an article appearing in February of 1976 seemed almost an attempt at recapturing an emigrating populace:

"Cancer Rate Should Not Lead to Exodus"

Philadelphia Sunday Bulletin, February
1, 1976. Statistics released by the
National Cancer Institute show New Jersey to be the Cancer Capital of the nation. However, Dr. Zinninger, Chief of
Department Radiology-Oncology at Cooper
Hospital and Chairman of the Southern
Regional Planning Committee of the Cancer Institute of New Jersey refutes
that title, concluding our rate is high
presumably because this is a highly industralized state. The victims may
have contacted the disease somewhere
else and lags of 30 years or more between exposure and tumorgenesis make it
impossible to tell where cancer's danger spots may be. Whether cancer is
caused by environmental factors is only
a suspicion; stop smoking and you will
improve your chances against cancer. . .

Throughout 1976 newspapers continued to use headlines
such as "Fight Cancer," "It's War in Cancer Alley,"
"Curb Cancer," "Cancer State," and "Cancer Tax," words
describing the state reaction and condition. However,
the journalists linked industry categorically with the
cancer mortality rate and some industries undeniably
were, as will be shown in chapter 4. Some of the burden
for the reaction to press articles has to be borne by
the individual, but as I said before, only the researchers is likely to read the original NCI reports. In latter years the burden of the responsibility for misinter-
pretation would be served back to the originators, the
federal government; that evolution will be discussed as
this chapter progresses to the 80's.

The Second Senate Commission Meeting

The second meeting was convened on September 10,
1976, and Senator Skevin lost no time in expressing his
dismay over the proliferation of chemical names, carcinogens, in the vocabulary of New Jersey residents.[40]

Once again, he called for a listing of cancer causing
agents, a banning of any products containing dangerous
levels of carcinogens, an implementation of the cigarette tax to fund cancer research, and a bill making
cancer a reportable disease. We all have those virgin
periods in our lives when we undergo the most painful
of all human operations -- having our eyes opened. And
it happened to Senator Skevin; he sincerely and naively
could not believe that his affirmative action legislative proposals could threaten New Jersey's industry to
the point that responsible management would be unrespon-
sive to his recommendations. Senator Skevin suggested
that the fourteen substances listed by the Occupational
Safety and Health Administration as carcinogens, would
be a good starting point in terms of the danger these
chemicals pose to the people of New Jersey. He asked
how might these emissions be controlled without actually
closing the industries involved. His own answer was
quickly forthcoming -- ban the use of all fourteen chemicals!

     Dr. Glenn Paulson, the then Assistant Commissioner
for Science in the DEP, summarized those programs instituted by the National Cancer Institute, The Institute
of Occupational Safety and Health and the International
Agency for Research which held the promise of lowering
the cancer rate in New Jersey.

     With all these coordinated efforts, what could pos-
sibly be lacking? Dr. Paulson concluded that we also
need "information on the incidence, not only death, but
occurrence short of death, or the actual exposure of New
Jersey residents to potential cancer causing agents at
their places of work, residence and play." "These and
other gaps in our knowledge mus be filled as quickly as
possible."

     And so the meeting continued with Commission mem-
bers and attendees enlightening one another with stati
tics that made it difficult to depart without being im
pressed with New Jersey's candidacy for the title "Cancer Alley". . . .

Cancer in the News Media -- The Peak Conflict Quotient
Years, 1976-1977

Throughout the fall of 1976, Delaware Valley newspapers continued to use a style that Clay Schoenfeld described as "conflict quotient" (where stories are based
on a war situation):[41]

> "Attack is Expected on
> DuPont Cancer Report"

> The Philadelphia Sunday Bulletin, Sep-
> tember 19, 1976: Although the E.I.
> DuPont Co. (a major chemical industry)
> denies that the cancer rate at their
> eight New Jersey plants is higher than
> that of the general population, 339
> incidents of bladder tumors were oc-
> cupationally related and traceable to
> chemicals in two plants including the
> Chamber works plant in Deepwater,
> Salem County.

> "State Agencies Stalk
> the Cancer-Causers"

> The Philadelphia Sunday Bulletin, Sep-
> tember 24, 1976: Does living in New
> Jersey heighten your chances of getting
> cancer? Salem County leads the nation
> in per capita deaths from bladder can-
> cer with Gloucester and Union counties
> following close behind. Middlesex
> County is among the top areas of the
> country in lung cancer deaths. On a
> state wide basis, New Jersey leads the
> nation in a range of cancer deaths in-
> cluding rectal, breast, ovarian and
> others. . . .

In preparing this chapter, the content and titles
of numerous newspaper articles were reviewed. On the
basis of that review, I consider 1976-1977 years in
which the "conflict quotient" nature reached its ze-
nith.

Reflecting back, I think most non-environmentally active
New Jerseyans must have experienced what G. D. Wiebe,
Dean of the School of Public Communication at Boston
University, terms "well-informed futility,"[42] living
with what they thought was responsible for the high incidence of cancer, being educated by the dissemination
of readily accessible news, yet being powerless to do
anything about it!

I would even go further to say that there was and
is now a psychological climate conducive to the induction of the cancers in New Jersey. Cancer is a dread
and feared disease and this image and a status of "well-
informed futility" are great sources of psychological
and physical stress. Many have suggested that a certain
personality may be predisposed to cancers, perhaps
brought on by these stress factors. This subject will
be discussed more in chapter 8.

The Third Senate Commission Meeting

At the third meeting of the Commission, held on
October 1, 1976, a number of witnesses from the chemical
and tobacco industry and environmental groups were present.[43] Senator Skevin opened by reiterating his commitment that the economy should never be more important
than human life. The first witness, Mr. Chris A.
Hansen, Vice Chairman of the Chemical Industry Council,
pledged the council's support to the Commission and
categorically denied that industrial working conditions
promoted the incidence of cancer among workers and stated
that industrial emissions were adequately controlled.
Those statistics showing a high incidence of cancer in
New Jersey were not accepted by the council. Mr. Hansen
continued by denying that there was any "clear correlation" between the New Jersey cancer mortality rate and
the presence of chemical industries. The Chemical Industry Council represented 62 member companies in the
State of New Jersey, one of which was DuPont. Ironically, word eating would shortly follow the argument proffered by Mr. Hansen:

"DuPont Assailed on
Employee Cancer Report"

Newark Star Ledger, Tuesday, October 12, 1976. Representative
Andrew Maguire (D.-7th District,
New Jersey) who headed a House
Subcommittee investigating industrial causes of cancer charged
that DuPont had not accurately reported all urinary bladder cancer
cases at their Salem County Plant.
He said DuPont excluded 339 cases
occurring over the period 1929 to
1956 from a 1974 study which cited
226 cases. DuPont responded by
saying the 339 cases were excluded
from the other statistics so they
would 'not obscure any other problem.'

Joseph Katz, New Jersey Public Affairs Counsel for
the Tobacco Tax Council, argued against the proposed
increase in cigarette tax, calling it regressive and
encouraging of buttlegging. Senator Skevin tried many
times to draw him into the well-aired cigarette-lung
cancer debate, but Mr. Katz resisted candidly, saying
the council's concern was the economics, not health aspects, of cigarette smoking. This was followed by an
attempt to dignify and justify tobacco manufacture by
Mr. David Goldfarb of the Tobacco Distributors Association of New Jersey. He argued that in the last twelve
years, the cigarette industry contributed $57 million
towards fighting all causes of cancer in America. He
continued citing the existing loss of cigarette tax dollars through buttlegging and saying that those dollars
would have gone towards financing the state's schools,
health programs and other vital services. He concluded
with an indictment and an enigma for the smoker and the
cigarette industry -- "Why should we, the smallest
really proven cause of cancer incidence bear the cost of
funding the state's research?" A comment tantamount to
the admission of some culpability for mass murder and
surely an affront to the intelligence of all smokers in
attendance and hopefully to those reading this work.

That smallest really proven cause is linked to the death
of more than 3,000 New Jersey residents in that year
alone!

The meeting concluded with an encapsulated overview
on the deterioration of New Jersey's environment with
emphasis on the role of carcinogens by Ms. Diane T.
Graves, Conservation Chairperson of the New Jersey Chapter of the Sierra Club. Concerned with the concurrent
resistance by industry to the passage of the Toxic Substances Control Act, she recommended a merger of the
Governor's Cabinet Committee on Cancer with a proposed
Emergency Task Force on Environmental and Occupational
Carcinogens in New Jersey. In addition, Ms. Graves made
two recommendations that addressed the two components of
a major vicious environmental cycle; she urged the commission to deal with the proper disposal of hazardous
and toxic wastes and that they push EPA to do thorough
groundwater testing in New Jersey. Apparently, no one
could perceive the foresight in Ms. Graves' recommendations; years later, that failure would endanger the
health of many New Jersey residents who would be drinking of chemically polluted water.

The Fourth Senate Commission Meeting

The fourth meeting of the Cancer Commission was
held on November 5, 1976.[44] Senator Skevin immediately
called for a commitment against environmental cancer in
New Jersey to rival the effort to put men on the moon
and to accomplish the Manhattan Project.

Dr. E. Cuyler Hammond of the American Cancer Society
accused the press of using the Cancer Atlas findings as
scare headlines. A perceptive comment, the full extent
of which would reach its maximum effect in the spring of
1977. This will be discussed shortly. However, Hammond
did concede that the scare attitude did force legislators
and private individuals to see the problem. The most
significant testimony of this hearing was provided by Dr.
Harry B. Demoupolus, Director of the New Jersey Cancer
Institute, who prefaced his very comprehensive testimony
with a comment bordering on clairvoyancy: "I think when
these proceedings are finished sometime in the future and

you look back, you will probably find they are among the
most significant events taking place in the war against
cancer." He proceeded to pinpoint cigarette smoking and
alcoholism as being responsible for 20% of the state's
cancer mortality, a statistic he considered extinguish-
able by educational prevention programs. At this time,
industry-related cancers could only account for 600 of
the state's approximate cancer death rate of 14,000. He
did not exonerate environmental pollutants; they should
be evaluated. On being questioned further about where
efforts should be directed on the state's problem, he
responded, apparently seriously, "If this (New Jersey)
were Uganda and I were Idi Amin, fatalities would be reduced 40% to 60% in two years." He apparently forgot
about the period of latency accompanying cancer, but he
must have had a ban on tobacco in mind!

     If so, I share his blunt, unpretentious, prospec-
tive attack on the cancer problem as induced by tobacco
use. Dr. Demoupolus would continue to provide innova-
tive thought on the etiology of cancers. In fact, just
before the Fourth Senate Commission met, he decried the
chemical industry/high cancer incidence link in New Jersey. "The high cancer rate could be attributed to moss
aflatoxins provided by New Jersey's greenery. "The
eastern European countries have done a great deal of research on these oncogenic mosses and fungi (and) those
findings show that New Jersey's warm, moist climate
would favor such plants," he concluded, further recom-
mending that the fledgling Cancer Institute conduct just
such a study as a top priority.[45] The remainder of the
Fourth Commission meeting consisted of discussions about
the many proven and possible cancer causing agents,
those problematic in a worldwide environment; food col-
orings, high fat diets, nitrosamines and those portending specific problems in New Jersey -- automotive emissions, vinyl chloride, asbestos, benzidine and PCB's.

The Resurgence of Dread Disease Insurance

     The extensive publicity which the state's cancer
problem was receiving produced a side effect that may be
interpreted as practical or mercenary. Consider this
insurance ad.

"The same thing that happened to

Babe Ruth, Nat "King" Cole, Walt
Disney, Sophie Tucker, Gary
Cooper, Babe Zaharias, Spike
Jones, Chet Huntley, Jack Benny,
Vince Lombardi, and Gypsy Rose
Lee

Could happen to you

CANCER

This policy is limited to all forms
of Cancer including Hodgkin's disease and Leukemia. See inside for
details."

On March 7, 1977, the above ad appeared in an advertising supplement in the Philadelphia Inquirer. In
fact, it appeared in eight Pennsylvania newspapers
sponsored by the Union Fidelity Life Insurance Company
of Trevose, Pennsylvania. This kind of insurance policy was prohibited from sale in the very state (New Jersey) whose publicity helped to precipatate the renewal
of dread-disease insurance, on the basis of its being
uneconomical. Dread-disease insurance policies were
popular in the pre-polio vaccine 1940's and again in
the mid 1960's, covering such diseases as polio, encephalitis, diptheria, tetanus, small pox and others.

Although the chances of the average American con-
tacting these diseases is reportedly one in 25,568, companies selling dread-disease insurance are doing very
well. Are you recalling the comments of Dr. E. Cuyler
Hammond of the American Cancer Society about "scare headlines?" Pulling out all stops in an attempt to cash in
on the cancer insurance market, the American Family Life
Insurance Company published a full page ad in the
Philadelphia Inquired on March 9, 1977:

"Twenty Years of Stewardship"
"The Truth About Cancer Insurance"

The advertisement was a mini-prospectus additionally
describing how their policy provided the insured "Peace
of Mind." The success of the sales of cancer insurance
would certainly be directly related to the degree of
well-informed futility, the G. D. Weibe concept discussed earlier, engendered in New Jersey residents. Recent
cancer insurance policy evaluations indicate they are of
little value.

The Fifth Commission Meeting

On January 24, 1977, eight months and four commission hearings led to the introduction of Senate Bill No.
3035. The chemicals to be banned now included in addition to those on page 27, asbestos and vinyl chloride.
S.3035 struck at the very core of the priorities expressed by socioenvironomics -- people, the environment,
and lastly, the economy. Towards the end of the 1970s,
socioenvironomical approaches would be described as
risk-benefit and cost-benefit analysis but Galantowitz,
its author and an urban planner, did not place an emphasis on benefits in his terminology. His emphasis was
clearly on *people*.[46]

At the fifth meeting of the commission on February
18, 1977, Senator Skevin pointed out very quickly that
S.3035 was not "politically popular" and witnesses soon
testified concerning the economic impact.[47] The Senator
expressed high hopes that the legislature would not ver-
bally support the commission's recommendations, yet vote
against their proposals. Just how important were the
chemicals to be banned? No one outside the chemical industry knew what quantities were manufactured or used
within or imported into the state, what specific industries were involved or the degree of employee exposure.
Further, what waste disposal problems do they portend?
There was some general knowledge about their use, discernible from technical journals and industrial chemistry texts as indicated in Table 1. But details still
remained to be disclosed by the Toxic Substances Control
and the Resource and Conservation and Recovery Acts.

With the exception of David Moore, Director of the
New Jersey Conservation Foundation, the witnesses given

TABLE 1

KNOWN (OR PROBABLE) CARCINOGENS
AND THEIR USES

Agent	Uses
4-Nitrobiphenyl	Analytical standard
Alpha Naphthylamine	In manufacture of herbicides, dyestuffs, food colors and color film, paint, plastics, rubber and petroleum products
4,4-Methylene bis (2-chloroaniline)	Curing agent for epoxy and other polyurethane resins
3,3-Dichlorobenzidine	In manufacture of printing inks, dyes, plastics and crayons
Bis-chloromethyl ether	In manufacture of ion exchange resins
Beta Naphthylamine	In manufacture of dyes and pesticides, in photography, and as a chemical reagent
Benzidine	In production of dyes, rubber and plastics, printing ink, fire proofing and in medical laboratories
4-Aminodiphenyl	As an antioxidant in rubber manufacture and as an intermediate chemical in dye production
Ethyleneimine	In paper and textile industries in herbicides, resins, drugs, and jet fuel
Beta Propiolactone	In Plastic manufacture

TABLE 1 - Continued

KNOWN (OR PROBABLE) CARCINOGENS
AND THEIR USES

Agent	Uses
2-Acetylaminofluorene	Potentially as a herbicide
4-Dimethylaminozo-benzene	As a dye
N-Nitrosodimethylamine	As an industrial solvent and in synthesis of rocket fuel

Source: Reference 36

below with the fractions they represented, summarily declined to support S.3035:

Charles Marciante	President of the New Jersey State AFL-CIO
George C. McGuinnes	Assistant Commissioner of the Department of Labor and Industry
David Lloyd	New Jersey Business and Industry Association
Anthony Mazzochi	Director of Citizenship Legislative Department, Oil, Chemical and Atomic Workers' International Union
Chris Hansen	Vice Chairman of the Chemical Industry Council
Donald H. Scott	President of the New Jersey State Chamber of Commerce
Dr. Anthony C. Shabica	Chairman of the Research and Development Council of New Jersey and Vice President of Development and Control at the Pharmaceutical Division of CIBA-GEIGY Co.

Some arguments for not supporting S.3035 were re-
sonable.

- That the EPA already had that power, and

- That chemicals were responsible for only
  5 - 10% of New Jersey's cancers.

Other arguments were weak; that the chemicals to be banned were essential for the production of life-saving

pharmaceuticals* and that all environmental risks of
cancers cannot be banned. Unfortunately, Senator Skevin
did not request that industry produce data indicating
the qualitative and quantitative use of the subject chemicals. At least one argument was worthy of a trophy for
inanity --- Dr. Anthony C. Shabica indicated he had been
a chemist for 44 years, living through two 25 year periods where cancers should have developed and did not!
The supposition is that everyone's physiological and
psychological response to the environment is the same;
it is not. Further, that the individual could *yet* manifest cancers.

Mr. Moore introduced Dr. Samuel Epstein, world renowned Professor of Environmental and Occupational Medicine of the University School of Public Health, Chicago,
who spoke on behalf of the Conservation Foundation.
"The majority of human cancers are environmental and occupational in origin and are, hence, preventable," he
offered. Here was the same pronouncement, heard
throughout the hearings from experts, stated a little
differently. He then cited an example of how industry
distorted and manipulated the suggested economic impact
of S.3035. In 1974 the economic impact on the plastic
industry for the reduction of vinyl chloride emissions
to one part per million was estimated to be $68 billion
and a loss of 1.3 million jobs. This estimate was
fraudulent, he continued, because B.F. Goodrich came
into compliance at a cost of $35 million and further
gained profits on the lease of their compliance technology.

Dr. Epstein made several recommendations for
changes in the proposed Cancer Control Act, but ultimately did not support an outright ban. Senator Skevin
closed the Fifth Commission meeting seemingly withdrawn
and not engaging witnesses in rebuttal. On reading the
transcript, one could almost sense the isolation he must
have felt over the almost complete lack of support for
S.3035.

---

* Both the EPA and Dr. Demopoulus indicated there was very
  limited use of these chemicals.

Then it was announced: the defeat of the most direct industrial cancer control recommendation to come out of the Cancer Commission.

Carcinogen Ban Loses to Pressure

> Philadelphia Inquirer, March 25, 1977.
> Faced by widespread opposition and
> threats of economic blackmail, the New
> Jersey Cancer Commission headed by
> Senator John M. Skevin (D.-Bergen) is
> dropping its fight to ban 14 chemicals
> identified as cancer causing agents in
> New Jersey. The ban would have includ-
> ed vinyl chloride and asbestos. Sena-
> tor Skevin added additional reasons for
> dropping the ban fight: lack of sup-
> port from the Byrne Administration and
> some environmental groups.

This was certainly not the first time the issue of socioenvironomics was tested in the state. The DEP once actually relaxed air pollution control regulations in order to accommodate the glass industry.[48] The glass container manufacturers who use a lot of fuel in their processes, complained about the requirement that they use the more expensive low sulfur fuel. The added expense threatened their profit structure and during the period 1974-1976, they reduced their work force from 6400 to 5000. In 1977, the DEP relaxed air pollution regulations pertaining to glass industry emissions. Socioenvironomics, anyone?!

The Sixth Commission Meeting

The sixth meeting of the Senate Commission on the Incidence of Cancer in New Jersey convened on May 20, 1977.[49] With the Commission's efforts now devoted to the possible existence of carcinogenic factors in food and water in the state, Senator Skevin opened by commenting on the timely announcement of a joint underground water supply survey to be undertaken by the DEP and Rutgers, the State University. The Commission had been told by industry repeatedly that more factors than their

air pollution contributed to the cancer problem in New
Jersey and the Commission was now taking an overview of
other important factors such as food and water. Citing
the role of the food eaten in the state as a cause of
environmental cancer, and more specifically, the role
of sodium nitrate in bacon and other pork products as a
cocarcinogen, Senator Skevin announced his plan to ban
"junk" food in state supported or operated schools and
public buildings. The first witness, Dr. John Birdsall,
Scientific Director for the American Meat Institute
(Washington, D. C.) quickly decimated the nitrite-ni-
trate cocarcinogen threat theory. Very succinctly,
he said that we need nitrites to prevent daily spoil-
age: nitrates, which we have eliminated, and the addition of ascorbic acid, which we instituted, prevents
the formation of nitrosamines* on frying. Ninety percent of the nitrates taken into the body are obtained
from vegetables, and lastly, in his opinion, the formation of nitrosamines in the stomach was extremely remote. Senator Skevin seemed to accept these categorical
and controversial pronouncements resignedly.

The next witness, Dr. Peter W. Pruess, then Special
Assistant to the Commissioner of the Department of Environmental Protection, elaborated on the reasons the
DEP was currently planning the aforementioned joint program of underground water survey with Rutgers University. He cited the connection between cancer mortality
and local drinking water quality in New Orleans, where
water analysis indicated the presence of 66 organic
chemicals. A subsequent report on water quality in 80
states by the EPA revealed that some of the same chemicals were present in all of the sources tested including two systems in New Jersey: the Passaic Valley Water
and the Toms River Water Company.

Dr. Pruess went on to outline the comprehensive program yet to be undertaken which included analysis of the
state's surface and ground water to determine the presence of carcinogens, sampling landfill leachate, and

---

* Nitrates and nitrites react with chemicals called amines to form
  a family of carcinogenic compounds called nitrosamines.

determining the effect of chlorination of groundwater.
Dr. Preuss indicated that the DEP was aware of PCB and
kepone contamination in the Hudson River to the north
and the Chesapeake Bay to the south, respectively. He
submitted a report that concluded PCB levels were acceptable. However, and with vision, he considered PCB's
to exemplify the type of problem we may anticipate to
occur again in the future. PCB's have done just this
and this will be further discussed in chapter 4 and
chapter 8. There was an even more basic reason for a
groundwater quality study which was not mentioned by
Dr. Pruess. The DEP knew of many locations where New
Jersey residents were drinking groundwater in areas adjacent to improperly interred chemical wastes! The
meeting ended with the general agreement that although
prospective programs were characterized by inter and
intra-state cooperation, budget resources were limited
and hopes continued for federal relief.

The Seventh Commission Meeting

        I attended the seventh commission meeting which was
held on January 17, 1979.[50] In marked contrast to the
rhetoric of previous meetings, hard data on the water
monitoring program were available. Approximately 5% of
the 400 wells tested representing all 21 state counties
revealed pollution levels sufficient to warrant them
being secured. Those data will be discussed in chapter
4. Dr. Pruess indicated the contaminants could induce
two to three cases of cancer per 100,000 people, based
on National Academy of Sciences estimations. The meeting continued with a summary review of DEP accomplishments; reduction of toxic industrial effluents through
discharge permits, determination of the impact of chemical waste dumping, and the recently released Greenberg
report. That study, "Spatial Distribution of Cancer
Mortality," by Dr. Michael Greenberg, et.al., ultimately created a new wave of controversy by describing the
state's cancer mortality rate as a regional problem
linked to income, employment, and ethnicity.[51] It was
suggested that surface water quality should be evaluated
as a link to the cancer rate in New Jersey. That study
will be discussed further in chapter 4. Dr. Greenberg
would eventually author and co-author several excellent

reports on cancers in New Jersey.

As the hearing approached conclusion, there was an unusual expression of comraderie, a sharing of a common goal, between Senator Skevin and Dr. Paulson. Senator Skevin summarized it well by saying "and what man has done, can be undone." Dr. Paulson responded by saying that those were his sentiments and those of the Governor's Cabinet Committee on Cancer Control. Dr. Paulson attempted to remind us of our environmental blessings by adding that we have at least a dozen chemical dump sites under investigation in New Jersey. He was confident, however, that these sites are nothing like Love Canal and stated that he doesn't "anticipate that we will find any." This comment was an absolute denial of the suffering of over 200 families in Jackson Township who, with the DEP's knowledge, were drinking water polluted with hazardous levels of chemical wastes, leaked from the nearby Legler landfill. Further, Paulson's predictions would prove short-sighted when in the winter of 1980, Gloucester County Times headlines would read:

"County: Another Love Canal?"[52]

These events will be discussed further in chapter 4.

Senator Skevin thanked Dr. Paulson for his cooperation and the presentation of DEP accomplishments, but expressed his disappointment in that the programs contained no sense of emergency. Further, he said, "Enough of the monitoring and mapping. I suggest that to proceed at such a pace when contamination is being found around the state is really to use the people of New Jersey as guinea pigs. . . ." Dr. Pruess responded by saying that DEP reports do not reflect an internal sense of *urgency*.

The Environmental Cancer Liability Game

When one reviews all of the collective approaches to preventing cancer in New Jersey, it appears that considerable effort in most programs was being devoted to proving that industry was responsible for the cancer rate

in New Jersey. And this seemed very plausible. Benzene, for example, commonly used in industry, was now a
recognized carcinogen inducing leukemia, specifically.
Cancer clusters, such as the 32 cases of blood disorder
related leukemias and Hodgkin's diseases identified in
the suburban community of Rutherford in the spring of
1978, brought state and local medical investigators in
search of industrial carcinogens.[53] Although benzene
ranked high on the list of suspect industrial pollutants, air, water and radiation pollution levels in the
southern Bergen County area were later exonerated.
These potential causes will be discussed more in chapter 4. Advocates of virtual industrial innocence in
the incidence of cancers at best yielded to a 1 to 5%
liability.[54] They were not to be supported by a National Cancer Institute study of September 15, 1978 which
indicated that "there is nothing in the gross cancer
statistics for the U.S. population which is inconsistent
with the hypothesis that up to 20 to 40% of all cancers
are (or will be in the next several decades) attributable to occupational factors."[55] Dr. Eula Bingham, Ad-
ministrator of the Occupational Safety and Health Administration, said the study was a "clear call to the nation for action."[56] Industry said the study was without
credibility, erroneous, and indefensible.[57]

     If the best defense is an offense, industry did not
appear to choose this tactic, at least rarely in the
newspapers. Most articles were dominated by an industrial roasting with a rebuttal on the part of the traditional "spokesperson." Their argument was often given
in detail where the general public would not read it;
consider a publication by the Shell Oil Company,
"Ecolibrium." This 1978 winter edition article concluded
that the individual risk of cancer could be decreased
through exercise, self control in personal habits, de-
letion or abatement of tobacco use and alcohol abuse,
over-eating, and reduction of fat intake.[58] Further,
only one to three percent of all cancer was due, according to "Ecolibrium," to occupational exposure. Industry
was serving the ping-pong ball of responsibility for environmental cancer right back to the *individual*.

The New Jersey Cancer Incidence Registry

   With the enactments of Public Laws of 1977, Chapter 266, the much needed and much recommended statewide
Cancer Incidence Registry was established.* Essentially, it is designed to determine:

   .   How different types of cancer vary in in-
       cidence as a function of age, race, sex
       and time lapse,

   .   Where in the state and what groups of re-
       sidents are experiencing a high incidence
       of cancer, and

   .   Whether cancer is increasing or decreasing

I learned of the details of the cancer registry first
hand in a January, 1979 interview with the State Epidemiologist, Dr. Ronald Altman. He advised me that
"the Registry was started on October 1, 1978 and we hope
to get a smattering of data by 1979." He added that the
Department does not expect to get any useful data until
1980. There would be problems with the registry; for
example, when a New Jersey resident receives treatment
out of the state, no data would be reported. However,
the registry had been initiated and it would be mandatory for any diagnosed cancer patient to be listed,
whether treated by a private physician, dentist, or hospital.

   And sometime in the near future, the morbid but essential process of manipulating and evaluating registry
data, with one eye on the cancer incidence and the other
on occupation will begin to provide useful data.

New Jersey: Garden State or Cancer Alley?

   Dr. Elizabeth Whelan, Executive Director of the

---

* The proposed rules on the cancer registry were actually published in the New Jersey Registry Volume 10, Number 6, June 8, 1978.

American Council on Science and Health, and other staff
members, authored a report, "New Jersey: Garden State
or Cancer Alley?" which defended the garden state image
of New Jersey.[59] Categorically, the authors denied:

- That the state displayed a "unique and
  frightening cancer pattern" attributable
  to industry (at least for the period
  1969-1971)

- That there was significance in the
  Rutherford and Palisade cancer clusters
  mentioned earlier

- That these clusters were due to the presence of industry

Furthermore, they were unimpressed with air pollution
as a cause of human cancer. Historically, they cited
the role of the popular media in stigmatizing New
Jersey industry, linking them with air, water and
soil pollution, and ultimately, the cancer incidence
in the state. Further, they cited the well made
observation that environmentally induced cancer was
more commonly interpreted to mean noxious industrial
chemicals rather than the result of personal practises
such as tobacco use and diet. Did the Council concede
to any cancer problem in New Jersey? Yes, in their
opinion, the state's problem was limited to bladder
cancer in white males. And they added that the dye
industry manifesting that site specific cancer incidence, presently posed no occupational hazard because
of the current safety practises. Hence, they concluded
that the state's reaction was much ado about nothing;
there was no need for control or prevention programs --
just stop smoking, consume alcohol in moderation and
avoid overexposure to sunlight. These were the documented means of prevention! The Council's conclusions
would surely earn accolades from industry, excluding
those of tobacco, alcohol, and convertible automobiles.
I was amazed at this learned body's failure to see the
need for a tumor registry and other programs which would
aid in dispelling or proving an industrial factor causa-
tion in the etiology of cancers. The Skevin Committee
received no assistance from this Council.

Carsuicide: A Smoke Screen?

To distinguish externally imposed cancer producing environmental factors such as air and ground water pollution from voluntary life-style activities such as tobacco-alcohol abuse, I coined the term "carsuicide" for the latter.

At a conference on toxic pollutants at Stockton State College in March 1979, Senator Skevin said that the "carsuicide" hypothesis was the most insidious argument against the Commission's conclusions.[60] He did not agree that smoking, lack of exercise and poor nutrition, all factors within the province of the individual's control, result in far more cancer than chemicals. In his opinion, the public was being brainwashed to accept environmental cancer as a way of life, and further, references to non-industrial sources were tantamount to a "smoke screen." Senator Skevin's advocates must have been taken back by his lack of holistic vision. Surely all parameters in the etiology of cancer deserve their due infamy!

The role of New Jersey's industrial chemicals in the etiology of cancer in the state was far from succumbing to carsuicide. In early October 1979, Dr. Joanne Finley, State Health Commissioner, in a report to the Governor's Cabinet Committee, revealed her cumulative frustrations.[61]

Summing up, she said:

- The state has the highest cancer death rate

- That occupational cancers contribute

- New Jersey workers are exposed to hazardous chemicals (aniline dyes, chlordane, plastics and asbestos)

- That the state ranked first in white male bladder cancer mortality

Dr. Finley besought the committee to take steps to protect the 167,000 workers exposed to the aforementioned
hazardous chemicals. This was, no doubt, a difficult
task for a committee that could not come to an agreement
about which substances were most likely to cause cancer
and, further, were afraid of infringing on the province
of the Occupational Safety and Health Administration.

The second appearance of a reported cancer cluster
in Garfield, New Jersey, in October of 1979, would not
serve to precipitate another search for carcinogenic
agents in the environment.[62] The site specific cancer
in this cluster, testicular, of which four cases were
diagnosed over a six month period, was of an uncertain
etiology. At best, New Jersey health professionals relegated the cause of hormonal imbalance to the manifestation of genetic defects.

More NCI Criticism?

"Whoever attempts to lead the nation towards less
cancer, had better be correct because the selection of
the wrong path is the equivalent of leading millions of
Americans to certain death." These were the profound
words of Dr. Harry Demopoulos, addressing the Synthetic
Organic Chemical Manufacturer's Association, October 4,
1969.[63] He pointed out that institute studies were
wrongly interpreted, resulting in the federal government
indicting industry for the cancer mortality rate in New
Jersey. Specifically, he charged that the cancer mortality rate in "dirty cities (cities with heavy industries such as Detroit, Pittsburgh and Birmingham) was
not statistically different from those characterized as
'clean' cities," in the third National Cancer Survey.
Further, he concluded that the pollutant levels in these
"dirty cities" were below the level required to induce
cancers. Summarily, he attributed the bulk of the cancer rate in the state of New Jersey to carsuicide --
tobacco, 35%; diet, 45%; occupation, 5%; background radiation, 3%; and certain preexisting medical disorders,
2%. The balance he attributed to aging. These statistics would surely render Dr. Demopoulus a darling of industry.

The ping-pong ball of the causes of environmental
cancer was again being served back to the individual,
and Dr. Demopoulus lambasted the industrialists in his
audience, saying "I always thought that you fellows were
really hot stuff and would have answered back and I was
surprised that industry was just laying back being beat-
en up." As far as Dr. Demopoulus was concerned, the
verdict was in, the major causes of environmental cancer
were delineated. However, I and surely others, were
still ruminating over his 1976 hypothesis on the potential role of dangerous plant aflatoxins in the state's
high cancer rate.

Contemporary New Jersey - The 1980s

Paralleling a trend in reporting that de-emphasized
the uniqueness of cancer mortality incidence in New Jersey, was one of a series by Dr. Michael Greenberg (F.
McKay and P. White) of the Department of Urban Studies,
Rutgers University.[64] The purpose of the study was to
evaluate the change in cancer mortality rates in the
combined New Jersey, New York, Philadelphia metropolitan
region -- termed REG -- versus the remainder of the nation -- RON. A time-series comparison (type of statistical analysis) on age-adjusted cancer mortality rate
data from NCI acquired over the years 1950-1969, indicated that:

> "The region's rates were almost always
> higher than the RON's, but the gap be-
> tween them had considerably decreased
> by the close of the 1960s."

Further, this study indicated that site specific cancers
in the region were not increasing at a rate exceeding
the RON; rather, that the converse was true, site-specific cancers were increasing more rapidly in the RON compared to the regions. It appears that the overall cancer mortality rate in the United States is catching up
to that of the region. Considering essential caveats,
the study concluded with a recommendation that additional analyses be conducted considering other variables
such as cancer mortality rates for the years 1970-1975
and comparative studies of sub-divisions of the United

States.

New Jersey area newspapers had been printing every variation on the theme of New Jersey as "Cancer Alley" since the early 1970s. When Dr. Greenberg briefed the press on his group's latest report, the headline spoke of a stereotyped image that would be harder to dispel than it was to create in the period of time covered by this chapter: "New Jersey to Lose Reputation as Cancer Alley?"*

SUMMARY AND OBSERVATIONS

An historical and descriptive analysis of the more than seven year period aftermath to 1973-74 NCI reports indicates clearly that there was a unique "state reaction." Many environmentalists were convinced beforehand of a link between New Jersey's cancer incidence and the concentration of chemical industry, with these convictions seemingly being substantiated by NCI reports. As the media performed their role, educating the public at its request, carcinogen became a common vocabulary word and a topic of conversation. Industry surfaced as being principally responsible for environmentally induced cancer, and New Jersey was dubbed "Cancer Alley." The important role of personal habits and life-style, of which there was an emerging body of data, began its ascension, not yet to occupy the media spotlight or significance in public consciousness. Ongoing survey research by the author substantiates this conclusion. Cancer researchers still disagree significantly about the percent cancer incidence attributed to specific environmental factors liability.

The period 1973 and several years after in New Jersey were characterized by marked action, discussion and debate. But what has been accomplished? One could be-

---

* Gloucester County Times, March 18, 1980.

gin to answer the enumerating, for example, the more
than twenty federal and state funded cancer control
projects, a cancer registry, cancer related occupational health programs and numerous monitoring programs.
The NCI reports were good for the state, initiating a
mobilization of cancer prevention and detection machinery not seen in surrounding states.

> . Was there any "state reaction" to the
> 1973-1974 NCI reports in the contiguous
> states?

Two New York counties (Warren and Rockland) were
cited as falling into the high group for bladder cancer
in the Hoover-Fraumeni NCI reports of 1974. Was there a
reaction to NCI reports in contiguous states with a common industrial economic structure, air, water and soil
corridors, to parallel activity in New Jersey? In the
years preceding the NCI reports (1950-1969), the age
adjusted cancer mortality rate per 100,000 population
in New York State was 199 versus 205 for the state of
New Jersey and the rate for New York City for the same
period was 215. It would appear that there should have
been just as much reaction to NCI reports; however,
there was only an increase in public awareness and concern for New York State.[65] A cancer registry had existed there since 1940 and was adopted in New York City by
law in 1973.[66] Although NCI reports did not evoke any
new coordinated state effort to control or prevent cancer, there was a new heavy commitment to epidemiologic
studies to reveal the cause of cancers.[67]

Similarly, Philadelphia County (the city of
Philadelphia) in nearby Pennsylvania demonstrated a cancer mortality higher than the national and New Jersey
rates -- 221 per 100,000. Yet there was no reaction to
the NCI reports there or in the state of Pennsylvania.
Presently, there is no cancer registry in the city of
Philadelphia* or in the state of Pennsylvania and the
need is sorely recognized by both departments of epi-

---

* Available at certain medical institutions and there is a case
  registry for therapy.

demiology that admit to poor cancer control programs.
In the wake of Three Mile Island, Dr. Allan Lipton of
the Hershey Medical Center lamented the inability of
state epidemiologists to determine the cancer incidence
accurately for various counties since there is no registry.[68] Falling into New Jersey's earlier footsteps, a
2¢ per pack cigarette tax to be used for cancer research
was passed by the Pennsylvania House and defeated by the
senate in early 1980.[69]

And what about New Jersey's neighbor to the south,
Delaware? Apparently, no reaction there where there is
a state tumor registry, instituted in 1935, computerized
in 1967.[70]

- Have we in the state ceased to react
  to the superficial impact of the NCI
  reports? No, there was and is an internally, self-sustaining, well-earned
  image of industry and pollutants as the
  major cause of cancer, lasting beyond the
  NCI report evaluation heyday. And again,
  on the basis of my own survey research,
  the image persists today. How can I say
  there is a well-earned image when some
  experts place the percent of occupational cancer liability as low as 1 - 5%?
  Because the impact of industrial pollution is so visual -- fishkills, noxious
  odors, no swimming signs, abandoned
  dumpsites with fires and explosions,
  oil slicks and contaminated and closed
  wells. I could go on and on. But this
  is not necessary for the New Jersey resident.

- How effective have all the federal,
  state, public and private organizational
  efforts been in terms of diminishing the
  cancer incidence and mortality rate in
  the state? We cannot yet know; consider
  cancer latency periods. When you examine
  the incidence of leukemia as a result of
  x-irradiation, from therapy, diagnosis or
  warfare, a seven year latency period is

observed before initial appearance of
disease.[71] On the other extreme, most
occupational carcinogens demonstrate
latency periods of 10 to 50 years before manifestation of tumors.[72] Carsuicide, as tobacco use, requires a
period of at least 20 years before
there is a marked increase in lung cancer.[73] If these data bases are correct,
it will take about 10 years, the late
1980s, before we could begin to experience a diminishing incidence of cancer
in New Jersey and, secondarily, a reduction in the mortality rate, normal-
izing for population growth.

Distressingly, we do know that the cancer mortality
rate in 1973 was 191.0 per 100,000 population, representing 14,077 deaths. 1980 estimates indicate an increase
in rate and total deaths, 206 and 15,400 respectively.[74]
Compared to all other states, we are still unpleasantly
outstanding. Why, depends on who you ask but, without
question, cancer is pancresic.

. Are we over the hill in terms of dis-
covering hidden or unrecognized sources
of carcinogens? Certainly not. For
example, we don't have a Love Canal
"yet" in New Jersey, but the known number of landfills in the state, yielding
toxics to be underground and surface
waters, has mushroomed alarmingly. On
the other hand, during the course of
time of the preparation of this book,
numerous previously unrecognized and
undiscovered personal and industrial
sources of carcinogens have been revealed and many will be discussed in
chapter 3, and 5. Perhaps the only way
we will ever know if the state programs
are effective is to attain a status of
environmental omnipotence. Secondarily,
the population under study is constantly
shifting, with some figures showing the

average family relocating every seven
years.

. What systematic problems afflict those
agencies charged with the responsibility
to cure or prevent cancer? This is the
most controversial area under examination and several authors have amassed
some convincing evidence. Among them
are Dr. Samuel Epstein and Ralph Moss
in "The Politics of Cancer" and "The
Cancer Syndrome," respectively.[75, 76]
Collectively, they have subjected many
organizations whose goals are to cure
or prevent cancer to critical reviews,
demonstrating how they actually stifle
their objective! The charges are made
against ACS, EPA, FDA, NCI, Sloan-
Kettering Institute for Cancer Research, private industry and other
organizations. However, it is those
charges against the ACS, an organization
having a direct influence in the state,
that warrant repetition here.

In Dr. Epstein's exhaustive text, he cites ACS's
refusal to endorse critical legislation designed to
reduce environmental pollution. Specifically, they did
not support the Clean Air Act, FDA ban on DES and saccharin, nor support the Toxic Substance Act. In fact,
rather than support, ACS is "actively hostile to regulatory needs for the prevention of exposure to carcinogenic chemicals in the general environment and workplace." And of the society's target personal priority
pollutant, tobacco, Dr. Epstein says their "efforts to
control smoking have been weak and diffuse" since 1964.

Similarly, it is Moss' hypothesis that the ACS programs of tobacco use cessation are weak, conservative
and "exclusively concerned with education, to the detri-
ment of more effective programs" which he failed to
identify. Further, Moss contends that the Society en-
courages the traditional and statistically unsuccessful
methods of cure (surgery, radiation and chemotherapy)
while squelching non-traditional ("unproven") approaches

(e.g., laetrile, vitamin C, and Cooley's Toxin). The
specter of socioenvironomics is raised high when Moss
speaks of the holding of offices in pharmaceutical corporate structures by individuals also holding leading
positions in the ACS. This conflict of interest has
led to a cure oriented organization which cannot take a
strong position against the broad spectrum of environmental carcinogens, according to Moss.

In summary, Moss suggests that the leaders of organizations whose goal is to cure or prevent cancers are
part of a conspiracy which inhibits the attainment of
the stated goal. Enigmatically, these leaders also fall
victim to the cancers. Moss concludes by saying, "Yet
the evidence points to the fact that it is the system
itself, rather than any particular clique of individuals,
which is really to blame for failure to make progress
against the cancer problem. In particular, the fact
that cancer management is itself a big business means
that it must function according to the rules of profit-
oriented institutions."

It is not the purpose of this book to deal with the
immense complications brought forth by Dr. Epstein, Moss
and others; however, it would be a gross oversight not
to present some of their conclusions. The question becomes, "Can all the agencies and programs working to
prevent or cure cancer overcome the systematic inertia
of a 'cancer establishment' or a 'conspiracy'?" Perhaps
we all stand in the way of progress through greed, carsuicide or reductionism. If so, then we must agree with
Pogo: "We have met the enemy and he is us."

The other organization with the potential to have a
major influence on the preventive aspects of the cancers
in New Jersey is the DEP.

How has that organization fared since its position
paper entitled "Cancer and the Environment" of May 1976,
was issued?[77]

Initially the water monitoring program suffered
from endless delays and the lack of credibility due to
the lack of internal and contractor quality control.

The Toxic Substance Inventory, though not complete, has accumulated valuable information on emissions.[78] However the well water monitoring program is now providing much needed data on the levels of toxic and carcinogenic chemicals in air, water, fish, wildlife and sediments. The treatment and disposal of hazardous wastes remains a major socioenvironomical problem for DEP, industry, and New Jersey residents. Hazardous wastes are excluded from landfills in 1976 after years of the DEP's knowledge of the extent and location of orphan and parented dumps. A case study of a South Jersey community (Logan Township) conflict with a hazardous waste disposal facility (Rollins Environmental Services) and further in-depth evaluation of the DEP is given in chapter 8. The interminably slow response of the DEP to critical pollution, has devastated public confidence and trust in that agency. The department is plagued by insufficient funding and personnel, a poor sense of priority, and management.

A hazardous waste manifest system, however inadequate, has at least been instituted and a strike force has been organized to apprehend and prosecute illegal dumpers. Under the Spill Compensation and Control Act of January 6, 1977, the DEP had a new enforcement tool, the Notice of Violations (NOV).[79] The DEP could levy fines against illegal dumpers. Between the period April 1, 1977, to June 30, 1978, the DEP issued 69 NOVs and collected a paltry sum of $35,000.[80] This average fine of about $507 per "accident" or "error," to the illegal dumper was less than a slap on the wrist. Sometimes it costs as much as $50,000 to clean up a single minor spill. There is little wonder why the fund was virtually depleted in November 1980, leaving New Jersey defenseless!

The DEP did improve the quality of the state's public drinking water through enforcement of the Federal Safe Drinking Water Act. However, it is in the realm of the air, the life support system we are in contact with 24 hours daily, that the DEP made far-reaching changes. Air pollution occupies a major potential role in the transport of environmental carcinogens and the DEP has made significant quantitative reductions through an original program of state-wide automotive emission laws.

DEP reports a 90% industrial emission compliance, 40-
50% carbon monoxide and 70-80% sulfur dioxide reduction.[81] Current research indicates that both industrial and automotive sulfur dioxide emissions have
an impact on cancers incidence and mortality, and that
etiology will be given a descriptive analysis in chapter
4. The Automotive Club of Southern New Jersey has
criticized the DEP's vehicle emission program, saying
the cost outweighs the benefits.[82] New Jersey residents
are still victims of neighboring states' emissions (from
highly industrialized Wilmington, Delaware, and Philadelphia whose emissions effect South Jersey residents)
over which DEP has no control.

      Summarily, the DEP has made significant strides to-
ward the prevention of cancers in the state. How effective is their one program that addresses cancers specifically, The Cancer and Toxic Substances Control Program? The DEP says it is "the most advanced in the
nation, serving as a model."[83] Here again, as with the
ACS, our state's cancer statistics will not yet substantiate their claim until a respectful period of
latency has lapsed and cancer incidence and mortality
data are evaluated.

          .   And what about the Medical School
                for South Jersey? In April of 1980,
                the Medical School drew closer to be-
                coming a reality as Governor Byrne signed
                into law a bill releasing $8.6 million
                for the construction of a new medical
                school in Camden and $1.2 million for
                additional construction at the Rutgers
                medical school, Piscataway Campus.[84]
                In the past, professional jealousy, politi-
                cal and social machinations and funding were
                the principal obstacles. Now, at least
                funding was earmarked. The proposed
                medical school may not exactly be
                seen as a "reaction" to the state's
                cancer problem. A general medical
                care crisis exists; consider the ratio
                of 16 family doctors per 100,000
                population in New Jersey versus the
                ideal 50 per 100,000 suggested by the

American Medical Association.[85]

Hopefully, a new medical school will provide more
family physicians who will stay in the state. A new
medical school could provide a new cancer care and research facility, eliminating the need for South Jersey
cancer patients to journey to Pennsylvania and New York.
Whenever that school does materialize and the oncology*
curriculum designed, hopefully it will be holistic, and
bold enough to encompass the constantly evolving concepts of the contemporary cures for the cancers as well
as the causes. But as of this writing, as we enter the
80s, construction has not yet begun.

.   What of the media as we enter the 80s?
        The concept of New Jersey as "Cancer
        Alley" ascended in the press in 1973-
        1975, peaked in 1976-1977, and then de-
        clined. A popular South Jersey daily,
        The Gloucester County Times, reported
        in March of 1980 "New Jersey to Lose
        Reputation as Cancer Alley?" We have
        not rid ourselves of the "well-informed
        futility" status and the image of our
        uniqueness as a cancer state is not wan-
        ing at the citizen level. In the past,
        the news media characteristically under-
        emphasized the role of disease in the
        cause of death, specifically when due to
        diabetes, emphysema and cancer -- per-
        haps due to their seemingly hopeless
        nature.[86] However, as the role of in-
        dividual responsibility in cancer
        etiology makes its ever evolving effect,
        the media has been making that relation-
        ship manifest.

Visualize, through articles relating the deaths of
two well known personalities, Jessie Owens and John
Wayne:

_____

* The science of tumors.

- (Owens) had adenocarcinoma, a lung cancer that is linked to cigarette smoking. Owens smoked an average of a pack of cigarettes daily for 25 years. . . .[87]

- Then he (Wayne) went into detail about how his habitual six packs of cigarettes a day had resulted in a lung tumor the size of a baseball. . . .[88]

Environmental health news reporting is *changing*!

In August 1981, the New Jersey State Department of Health released a two volume study; the Descriptive Epidemiology of Cancer Mortality in New Jersey: 1949-1976.[89] The report, a collaborative project conducted with the National Cancer Institute, was a refinement and extension of earlier NCI studies, with the coverage of an additional eight year period. Further, that two-volume study provided etiologic clues on the causes of cancer at a smaller geographical unit than previous studies, the municipality. Similar to the earlier NCI studies, volume I was punctuated with demographic maps. Those maps, depicting male/female, all malignant neoplasm mortality rate, by county, are shown in Figures 5 and 6.

Summarily the two-volume study indicated the following trends in New Jersey:

- An overall increase in male cancer mortality

- An overall decrease in female cancer mortality

- A significantly high white male/female cancer mortality in 36 municipalities

- Lung cancer was the major cancer death cause for New Jersey males

- A 200% increase in female lung cancer

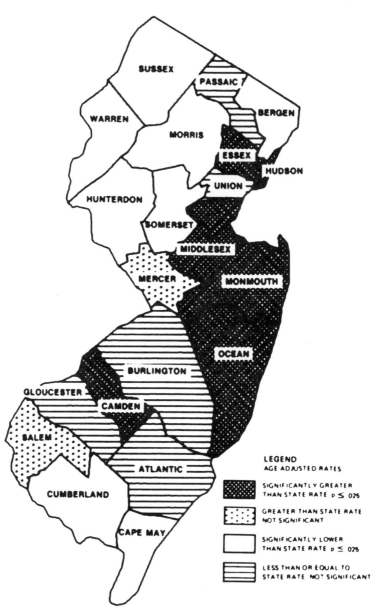

FIGURE 5
New Jersey
All Malignant Neoplasms
Mortality By County, 1962–1976
All Males

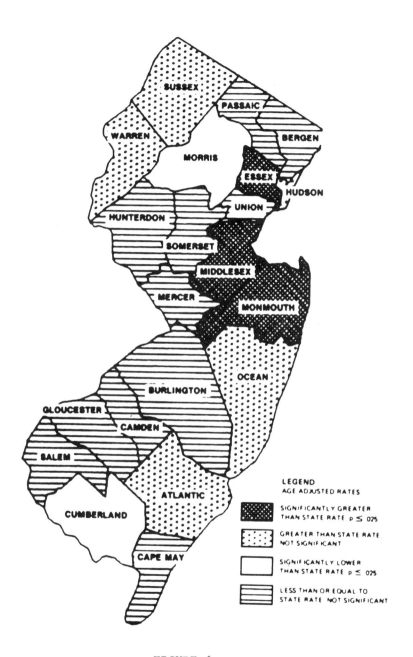

FIGURE 6
New Jersey
All Malignant Neoplasms
Mortality By County, 1962-1976
All Females

The lung cancer increase in women was reportedly attributed to their increase in the practise of smoking, according to the principal author of the two-volume study,
Dr. Annette Stemhagen.[90] The trends in cancer mortality
for all malignant neoplasms over the period 1949 - 1976
are given in the appendix. With specific reference to
non-whites which would reflect cancer mortality prodomi-
nately in blacks, the study showed:

- An increase in cancer of the esophagus
  and Hodgkin's disease in females

- An increase in colon and prostrate cancer in males

The overall tenor of the study was summarized by
State Health Commissioner Joanne Finley, who said, the
state's (cancer) rate has moved closer to the rest of
the nation and no longer deserves the label of "cancer
alley."[91] However, Dr. Finley would have been more accurate had she said, some of the other states had caught
up to and exceeded New Jersey. In fact, the study showed clearly that the national cancer mortality rate was
increasing.

Chapter 1 / REFERENCES

1.   Mason, T. J. and McKay, F. W., U.S. Cancer Mor-
         tality by County: 1950-1969. Department
         of Health, Education, and Welfare Publi-
         cation, No. (NIH) 74-615, Washington, D.C.,
         U.S. Government Printing Office, 1973.

2.   Louria, D. B., M.D., Thind, I., M.D., Najem, G. R.,
         M.D., Lavenhar, M. A., Ph.D., Hamm, R., B.S.,
         and Leming, E., B.A., Cancer in New Jersey:
         An Overview, Journal of the Medical Society
         of New Jersey, Volume 73, No. 9, September
         1976, pp. 749-752.

3.   New Jersey Public Health Statistics, New Jersey
         State Department of Health, 1975.

4.   Golden, Jeff, Cancer Rate Should Not Lead to
         Exodus, Sunday Bulletin, February 1, 1976.

5.   Carson, Rachel L., Silent Spring, Fawcet World Li-
         brary, New York, 1962.

6.   Udall, Stewart L., The Quiet Crisis, Holt Reinhart
         & Winston, New York, 1963.

7.   Commoner, Barry, The Closing Circle, Bantam Books,
         New York, 1971.

8.   Anonymous "Environmental Cancer" is primarily a
         "lifestyle" problem, not a result of indus-
         trialization. . . , American Industrial Hy-
         giene Journal (321), July 1977, pp. A.23-24.

65

9.   Maugh II, Thomas H., Cancer and Environment, (Re-
     print in) Ecolibrium, Volume 9, No. 1, Win-
     ter 1980, pp. 1-3.

10. Ibid.

11. Hoover, R. and Fraumeni, Joseph H. Cancer Mortal-
     ity in U.S. Counties with Chemical Indust-
     ries, Environment Research 9, 1975, pp. 196-
     207.

12. Mason, T. J., McKay, F. W., Hoover, R., Blot, W. J.,
     and Fraumeni, Jr., J. F. Atlas of Cancer
     Mortality for U.S. Counties: 1950-1969,
     Washington, D.C., U.S. Government Printing
     Office, 1975.

13. Armstrong, Bruce and Doll, Richard. Environmental
     Factors and Cancer Incidence and Mortality in
     Different Countries, With Special Reference
     to Dietary Practices, International Journal
     of Cancer, Volume 15, November 1975, pp. 617-
     631.

14. Schramm, Wilbur, Mass Communication, University of
     Illinois Press, Urbana, 1960.

15. Bowman, James, American Daily Newspapers and the
     Environment, Journalism Quarterly, Volume 50,
     221646, 1973, pp. 1-11.

16. Sutton, Patricia Taylor, The Status of Environmen-
     tal Reporting in the Media of New Jersey and
     St. Louis, Master's Thesis, Glassboro State
     College, Glassboro, New Jersey, 1979.

17. Mason, T. J. and McKay, F. W., Op. Cit.

18. Whitlow, Joan, Institute Created to Unify Cancer
     Projects in Jersey, Newark Star Ledger,
     February 25, 1975.

19. Ehrenfeld, David W., Conserving Life on Earth, Ox-
     ford University Press, New York, 1972.

20. Personal Communication, March 11, 1980.

21. Jersey Sierran, Volume 4, No. 1, January-February, 1976, p. 1.

22. American Lung Association, Lung Disease Changes Everything, July, 1977.

23. Personal Communication, May 7, 1980.

24. American Cancer Society, New Jersey Division, People Helping People, 1978 Annual Report.

25. Personal Communication, January 11, 1980.

26. American Cancer Society, "Cancer Highlights," Target: Environmental Cancer, Volume 29, No. 4, 1976.

27. Institute for Medical Research, Twenty Five Years of Progress, Biennial Report to the Community, 1977-1978.

28. Personal Communication, January 4, 1980.

29. Hughes, Frank J., M.D., Coriell, Lewis L., M.D., Ph.D., Keller, Earl B., M.D., Pairfulli, Michael J., Esq., Robbins, Mrs. Arthur W. Shusted, Thomas J., Freeholder, and Zackon, Paul G., D.D.S. A Medical-Dental School in South Jersey, Camden Board of Freeholders, September 1968.

30. Wynder, Ernst L., Nutrition and Cancer Federation Proceedings, Volume 35, No. 6, May 1, 1976, pp. 3109-3115.

31. Select Committee on Nutrition and Human Needs, U.S. Senate, Dietary Goals for the United States, Second Edition, December 1977.

32. Henig, Robin Marantz, Nutrition Research Still Sluggish, But Congress Notes Some Progress, Bioscience, Volume 29, No. 11, November 1979, pp. 699-701.

33. Education Improvement Center-South, "Making the
    Most of Your School Food Service."

34. State of New Jersey, Executive Department, Execu-
    tive Order No. 40, Brendan Byrne, Governor,
    May 26, 1976.

35. Pollock, Stewart G., LLB., Environmentally Related
    Cancer Hazards, Journal of the Medical So-
    ciety of New Jersey, Volume 75, No. 11,
    October 1978, pp. 743-745.

36. Finley, Joanne E., M.D., M.P.H. Controlling Can-
    cer in New Jersey (Let's Protect Our People),
    New Jersey State Department of Health, May
    1976.

37. State of New Jersey, Manual of the Legislature of
    New Jersey, Edward J. Mollin, Editor and
    Publisher, Trenton, New Jersey, 1979, p.
    213.

38. Public Hearing Before the Senate Commission on the
    Incidence of Cancer in New Jersey Senate
    Chamber, State House, Trenton, New Jersey,
    June 11, 1976.

39. Louria, D. B., M.D. Op. Cit.

40. Public Hearings, Op. Cit., September 10, 1976.

41. Schoenfeld, Clay, Environmental Mass Communica-
    tions: Problems and Promises, The Journal
    of Environmental Education, Volume 6, No. 3,
    1975, p. 21.

42. Weibe, G. D., Mass Media and Man's Relationship to
    His Environment, Journalism Quarterly, Au-
    tumn 1973, pp. 426-446.

43. Public Hearings, Op. Cit., October 1, 1976.

44. Ibid. November 5, 1976.

45. Reid, T. R., Expert Links Cancer to Moss, Trenton Evening Times, September 22, 1976.

46. Galantowitz, D., The Process of Environmental Assessments, Part I, New Jersey Federation of Environmental Commissions.

47. Public Hearings, Op. Cit., February 18, 1977.

48. Eisler, Barbara, Air Pollution in New Jersey: Problems, Programs and Progress, American Lung Association, New Jersey Department of Environmental Protection, 1979.

49. Public Hearings, Op. Cit., May 20, 1977.

50. Ibid., January 17, 1979.

51. Greenberg, Michael R., The Spatial Distribution of Cancer Mortality and of High and Low Risk Factors in the New Jersey - New York - Philadelphia Metropolitan Region, 1950-1966, Part I, State of New Jersey Department of Environmental Protection, Program on Environmental Cancer and Toxic Substances, January, 1979.

52. Goldberg, Elliot, County: Another 'Love Canal'?, Gloucester County Times, December 11, 1980.

53. Halpern, William, M.D., Altman, Ronald, M.D., Stemhagen, Annette, M.P.H., Iaci, Alfred W., M.S., Caldwell, Glyn, M.D., Mason, Thomas, Ph.D., Bill, Joanne, B.S.N., Abe, Toshi, M.S.W., Clark, James F., B.S., Journal of The Medical Society of New Jersey, Volume 77, No. 4, April 1980, pp. 267-273.

54. Anonymous. Chemical Week, Workplace Cancer Study Scored, Volume 123, No. 18, October 25, 1978, pp. 87-89.

55. National Cancer Institute, National Institute of Environmental Health Science and National Institute for Occupational Safety and Health.

Estimates of the Fractions of Cancer in the
United States Related to Occupational Factors, September 15, 1978.

56. Chemical Week, Op. Cit.

57. Ibid.

58. Anonymous, The Cancer Problem in Perspective,
        Ecolibrium, Volume 7, No. 4, Fall, 1978.

59. American Council on Science and Health, New Jersey:
        Garden State or Cancer Alley? December,
        1978.

60. Donohue, Joseph, Chemical Industry "Brainwashing"
        Criticized, The Press, Atlantic City, Wednes-
        day, April 4, 1979.

61. Friedman, Alan. Drive Urged on Work-Site Cancer
        Agents, Newark Star Ledger, October 3, 1979.

62. Gloucester County Times (AP), Records Searched in
        Cancer Mystery, October 12, 1979.

63. Demopoulus, Harry. "Environmentally Induced Can-
        cer. . . Separating Truth From Myth," Pre-
        sentation to The Synthetic Organic Chemical
        Manufacturers Association, Inc. Hasbrouck
        Heights, N.J., October 4, 1979.

64. Greenberg, M., McKay, F. and White, P. American
        Journal of Epidemiology, Volume III, No. 2,
        1980.

65. Personal Communication, Burnett, William S., M.D.,
        Assistant Director, Bureau of Cancer Control,
        New York, May 1980.

66. Ibid.

67. New York State Department of Health, Research and
        Development, Bureau of Cancer Control, Pro-
        gram Plan, December, 1973.

68. Lipton, Allan, M.D., Three Mile Island Shows Need
         for Cancer Registry, Patriot, April 28,
         1980.

69. Personal Communication, Witte, Ernest J., V.M.D.,
         M.P.H., Acting Director Division of Epidem-
         iology, Pennsylvania, May 13, 1980.

70. Personal Communication, Finocchraro, Margie, Dela-
         ware Cancer Reporting Service, May 21, 1980.

71. Cairns, John, Cancer: Science and Society, W. H.
         Freeman and Company, San Francisco, 1978,
         Chapter 9.

72. Ibid.

73. Ibid.

74. American Cancer Society, Cancer Facts & Figures,
         1980.

75. Epstein, Samuel S., The Politics of Cancer, Anchor
         Press Edition, New York, 1979.

76. Moss, Ralph W., The Cancer Syndrome, Grove Press,
         New York, 1980.

77. New Jersey Department of Environmental Protection,
         Cancer and The Environment, David J. Bardin,
         Commissioner, May, 1976.

78. A Decade of Progress, New Jersey Department of En-
         vironmental Protection, 10th Anniversary
         Report, 1980.

79. New Jersey Department of Environmental Protection,
         First Report of the Spill Compensation Fund,
         April 3, 1979.

80. Ibid.

81. A Decade of Progress, New Jersey Department of En-
         vironmental Protection, Op. Cit.

82. Goldberg, Elliot, Exhausting Issue, Gloucester
    County Times, August 3, 1979.

83. A Decade of Progress, New Jersey Department of En-
    vironmental Protection, Op. Cit.

84. Gloucester County Times (AP), $8.6 Million is Re-
    leased for Medical School, August 23, 1980.

85. Skowronski, Vic, Family Doctor Shortage Discussed,
    Sunday Bulletin, February 14, 1976.

86. Combs, Barbara and Slovic, Paul. Newspaper Cover-
    age of Causes of Death, Journalism Quarter-
    ly, Winter 1979, pp. 837-849.

87. Gloucester County Times (AP). Life Was Like a Re-
    lay Race to Jessie Owens, December 8, 1979.

88. Bacon, James, The Duke's Back in the Saddle Again,
    Philadelphia Inquirer, Wednesday, June 28,
    1978.

89. Stemhagen, Annette, M.P.H., Mogielnicki, Alexander
    P., M.A., Altman, Ronald, M.D., M.P.H.,
    Mason, Thomas J., Ph.D., Descriptive Epidem-
    iology of Cancer Mortality in New Jersey:
    1949-1976, Ed. by Carolyn, M. Winkler and
    Homer B. Wilcox III, 2 Vols., Cancer Epidem-
    iology Program, Division of Epidemiology and
    Disease Control, New Jersey State Department
    of Health, Trenton, New Jersey, August 1981.

90. Bradley, Bob, N.J. Shedding Image as 'top' cancer
    state, Gloucester County Times, August 9,
    1981, p. 1.

91. Ibid.

CHAPTER 2

CANCERS: THE CUMULATIVE KNOWLEDGE
OF THEIR BIOLOGY AND CHEMISTRY.

"It seems likely that
the major part of
human cancer and gene-
tic defects arises
from damage to DNA
by environmental
mutagens/carcinogens,
which may contribute
in a significant way
to aging and heart
disease as well."

Bruce N. Ames,
Ph.D.*

*   Biochemistry Department, University of California,
    The Co-Evolution Quarterly, Spring 1978.

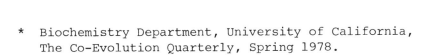

CHAPTER 2

BRIEF OVERVIEW

The purpose of this chapter is to present a brief
overview of the basic biology and chemistry of the cancers. This information is given here as an immediately
available, condensed source on these subjects and is by
no means intended as a substitute for the many excellent sources cited in the references which treat
these subjects in detail.

NORMAL CELL GROWTH AND DEVELOPMENT

Under discussion is a disease that manifests itself at numerous sites in multicellular plants and animals. About 200 separate forms of cancer have been
identified in humans, hence, more properly this disease
should be referred to as the "cancers."[1] In this work
the author will alternate between using "cancer" and
"cancers" because on occasion the attempt to be techni-
cally correct renders some sentences and concepts awk-
ward. Without question, cancers are an abnormal condition of living cells. Within the normal cell is a
structure called the nucleus which enables a cell to
divide and reproduce itself. Also in the cell nucleus
are sub-structures, termed chromosomes, which bear yet
other structures, the genes. It is the gene that pos-
sesses the identity code, dictating what the cell will
reproduce -- hopefully itself. It is the normal process of replication through the agency of genes that
enables bodies to heal when injured or cut, replace
blood losses, grow new nails and hair. Most cells undergo a cyclic process that results in their replication, known as mitosis.[2] There are arrest points in

73

the cell cycle that maintain cell growth and division
in perspective to the total organism.[3] Usually at the
completion of mitosis, the cellular duplication process,
two new daughter cells result. The daughter cells either continue to divide or die and are sloughed off from
the body. The well known ring-around-the-tub after the
bath is more than just dirt or grease; it contains a
good number of your skin cells.

ABNORMAL CELL GROWTH AND DEVELOPMENT

    The word autonomy means to act on one's own behalf.
It also implies self rule and establishing one's own
code of behavior as one sees fit. Regardless of what
causes cancers -- there is one underlying characteristic
displayed by a normal cell transformed into a neoplasm,
a new and abnormal formation of tissue. Its behavior
is autonomous.[4] Autonomy is displayed by both plant and
animal cells. Suddenly a cell behaving according to the
cycle described in the previous section no longer enters
the arresting phase. Instead, the cell continues to perform growth and cell division functions continuously.
Because the cell from which a tumor (an abnormal mass of
tissue) arose, undergoes changes in size and shape (the
new form being termed an anaplasia), a pathologist (one
who studies diseased tissue) specializing in carcinogenesis, is needed to determine the nature of the original
cell.

    All autonomous growths of tissues are defined gen-
erally as neoplasms; however, not all will become malignant. Moles, for example, are benign tumors or neoplasms that are slow growing, not spreading (metastasis-
ing) or displaying abnormal histologic patterns (ana-
plastic), along with other characteristics.[5] Cancer
cells and malignant neoplasms are non-encapsulated, displaying rapid growth and cell division and most charac-
teristically, metastasis. After having given a rather
sharp distinction between a benign and malignant tumor
state, it should be noted that the latter may begin
to behave as the former, in a spontaneous remission.[6]

THE GENESIS OF THE CANCER CELL

There are several theories, hypotheses and conjectures regarding the cause(s) of the cancers. I have
characterized the description in this fashion because
the theories in general acceptance are broad-based models based on numerous observations. Hypotheses are less
complete models based on more limited observations, and
conjectures may be based on a single case history. It
is not the purpose of this work to judge or rank these
various etiologies, but rather to cite them in the name
of holism. The genes of the chromosomes have been determined to consist chemically of DNA (Deoxyribonucleic
acid). Another nucleic acid, RNA (Ribonucleic acid)
which extends over the length of the gene, appears to
be capable of carrying plans for protein synthesis
through the cell nucleus from the DNA, and it is termed
messenger RNA.[7] It is actually the DNA of the gene that
controls messenger RNA which in turn produces the distinctive nature of the organism. Essentially, cancers
are thought to arise from errors in DNA and RNA program-
ming. The errors may be inherent to the cell in that
they are inherited or represent the expression of normally present but repressed genetic information.[8] The
errors are also thought to result from the interaction
of external agents on cellular DNA and RNA, and there
are several categories.[9] The largest category of agents
is represented by inorganic (e.g., certain nickel or
chromium salts, asbestos) and organic chemicals (dyes,
petrochemicals).

Several researchers have observed that the implantation of plastic films into animals (rats and mice)
is followed by tumor formation.[10] The categories of
plastics producing tumorigenesis are extensive and some
examples are:

bakelite	teflon
cellophane	dacron
polyethylene	nylon
polyvinyl chloride	polystyrene
silastic	

polymethymethacrylate (acrylic)

Two schools of thought have arisen to account for tumorigenesis following implantation. One is based on a
chemical reaction occurring between plastic and body
tissue. The other is based on the interference of these
films with normal cellular diffusion. In what practises
would one obtain an implant of any of these substances
previously mentioned? Consider the use of prosthetic
devices (artificial limbs and joints), bust enlargement
and sex change operations, the use of sexodelic contrivances and intra-uterine devices. All of these entail
the implantation into the body of metals and plastics
for periods of time varying from minutes to a lifetime.

The most significant radiation in sunlight are the
ultraviolet rays, but they are non-ionising and do not
penetrate deeply into human tissue. This form of energy
is thought to cause skin cancers by promoting a reaction
between the different nucleotides of which DNA is composed.[11] Ionising radiation, from x-rays and other
radioactive substances, which penetrate deep into human
tissue have the ability to knock electrons from various
molecules in the cell nucleus. When the nucleus of a
cell is irradiated, it is thought that the resulting
ionisation in the aqueous cellular medium produces ions
and free radicals which may react with cellular DNA and
RNA.[12]

Viruses, chemically composed of nucleic acids
(DNA and RNA) may induce cancers in normal cells by
infection and the introduction of new genetic information.[13] Progenitor cryptocides, a micro-organism, has
been isolated and cultivated from human and animal tumors
and may be the cause of some cancers.[14] Stress, as a
psychosomatic carcinogen, has been cited as a common denominator in cancer patients.[15] Personality characteristics such as the denial or repression of feelings and
attitudes, the loss of a loved one or the trauma of
retirement each can cause changes in the normal neurolo-
ogical and hormonal body functions that may induce
cancer. The credibility of the stress hypothesis in humans is being strengthened constantly by the remissions

affected by behavior modification.   Stress is discussed
at greater length in this book in chapter 8, in the
context of a case study of an environmental problem.
Last, but not in the sense of completion, finality or
totality, is the role of diet and nutrition in the etiology of the cancers.[16]   There is a major difference
between the introduction of a carcinogen into the diet
of an organism as an air or water pollutant, and the
post-digestive existence of that carcinogen.   But both
are prima facie hypotheses to account for the causes of
the cancers of the digestive system.[17]   Additionally,
it may be the failure to include in the diet those substances that enhance the inhibition, excretion, or
metabolism of potential carcinogens, that may be
responsible for the cancers of the digestive system.

Chemical Carcinogenesis

    Of all the several distinct etiologic agents re-
sponsible for the cancers, the chemical carcinogens are
probably the most diverse group, and their role warrants
further elaboration.   Many organic and inorganic compounds which have electron-poor atoms react chemically
with electron-rich atoms and the latter are found in
none other than the DNA and RNA of proteins.[18]   This
contemporary concept is most frightening because of the
universality in our environment of chemicals capable of
becoming electron-poor or "proximate carcinogens."   The
reader probably asks how these potentially electron-
poor compounds get that way; the answer: through metabolism.

    When we refer to metabolism in our bodies we might
only think of the process of breaking down food materials (gases, liquids and solids are also metabolised).
But metabolism is also the building up of complex molecules and laboratory studies show that carcinogens undergo metabolism before they can cause normal cells to
become tumor cells.   The process whereby chemicals are
converted by enzymes to effective carcinogens (called
ultimate carcinogens) is called activating metabolism.[19]
When metabolism of a chemical results in a harmless substance, the process is known as detoxifying metabolism.[20]   Whether the particular metabolic process is ac-

tivating or detoxifying, the functional (electron-rich
atom) group is the site at which this biochemical process itself converts one carcinogen into a not so innocuous compound.   Consider the conversion of benzene,
an established leukemogen to phenol, a cocarcinogen.
To sum up this issue, it may be your very own body that
converts an organic chemical, a hydrocarbon or an amine,
into an ultimate carcinogen, which may in turn react
with the nucleic acids and proteins of your particular
genetic code.   Researchers know what chemicals are potential proximate carcinogens and they are legion.
What researchers do not know yet is the full extent of
the micro-cellular components with which an ultimate
carcinogen may react, inasmuch as all of the micro-
cellular components themselves are not known.

However, once the chemical is in the proximate
carcinogen form, it may bond to some structure in the
cells of the body.   Conversion of a normal cell to a
neoplasm may occur in stages and involve more than one
chemical and this may explain the latency period.   For
example, the chemical urethane preconditions the skin
for carcinoma which only occurs after the subsequent
application of croton oil.   Hence, urethane is designated an initiator and croton oil a promotor or cocarcinogen.[21]   In the confines of this work, when the author states that a chemical is carcinogenic, consider
that one of the following has occurred before a malignant neoplasm has occurred:

- the enzymatic process of conversion to the
  ultimate carcinogen
- involvement of the chemical as an initiator
- the action of other chemicals as promotors or
  cocarcinogens

Mutagens and Teratogens

Earlier in this chapter a gene was defined as the
structure in the cell nucleus that possess the identity code, dictating what the cell will reproduce --
hopefully itself.   Environmental agents that affect
the sex cells of a parent organism causing it to reproduce an offspring which is atypical or a variation

of the species, are called mutagens.[22]   This biological process has become the basis of a detection test
for carcinogens, to be described later.   Mutations may
be induced artifically by chemicals, ionising and non-
ionising radiation.   Teratogens are environmental a-
gents which damage the fetus in the uterus, hence in
utero deformations.[23]   These deformations, i.e., birth
defects, may be induced by chemicals, pathogens (e.g.,
German measles) or x-radiation.   The impact of exposure to a teratogen may be confined to the somaplasm
(body cells) of the parents' eggs or sperms, or to the
fertilized egg.   A well known example is the missing
or deformed limbs in human embryos whose mothers were
given the sedative thalidomide during their pregnancies.   On maturity, these children may have normal offspring.   However, when the teratogen affects the em-
bryo's germplasm (ovaries or testes), that damage may
be transmitted to subsequent generations.[24]

The Quantification of Carcinogenic Potency

Is there a minimal dose of a carcinogen that will
induce little or no cancer?   This question, is in essence, the threshold hypothesis.[25]   The other prevailing hypothesis is that the probability of transformation of a normal cell into a cancer cell is directly
related to the dose, which implies that a *single* molecule could cause the transformation.   Hence the latter is termed the "single event" or "one-hit" hypothesis.[26]   There are other hypotheses (e.g., the Probit-
Curve, multiple stage model); however, the "single
event" hypothesis seems to be on the ascendancy.[27]   This
is fortuitous because if regulatory agencies take this
tack, speculative carcinogens will be banned rather
than be allowed to be used by the public with the con-
commitant health risk.

Naturally Occurring Carcinogens

The peculiar distinction that the compounds already discussed, organic, and inorganic substances
have in common is that our modern society produced or
manufactured them.   We are basically responsible for

the presence of most of them in the forms mentioned,
in our environment. Of course, they perform extremely
useful functions, both in contributing to the composition of our bodies and in providing the affluency and
amenities of modern living.

There are exceptions to every rule and there are
organics and inorganics present in our environment over
which we have no control. Let's consider hydrocarbons
--are we totally responsible for removing them from
their comfortable resting place in the ground and in-
troducing them to our atmosphere? No! There are natural seeps into the ocean and in some places on land
where crude oil bubbles to the surface.[28] The raw crude
eventually evaporates into the air and is dispersed by
weather. Benzo(a)pyrene, a well-known tobacco smoke
carcinogen, has been isolated from rural soils along
with fifteen other unsubstituted hydrocarbons. Consider also the many organic chemical compounds produced by
plants and the products of mold metabolism. In 1955,
researchers found that these naturally occurring carcinogens showed the ability to produce tumors in
mice.[29] The following table lists some principle, naturally occurring, carcinogens and their plant sources.

TABLE 2
SOME NATURALLY OCCURRING CARCINOGENS
AND THEIR SOURCES

Safrole	Sassafras (extract of bark or root in cinnamon tree; common in New Jersey)
Capsaicin	Chili peppers
Catechin	Specific vegetable extracts in dyeing and tanning
Turmeric	Spice (currently under inves-tigation)
Bracken ferns and other ferns	(unidentified carcinogenic substances)
Aflatoxin B_1	Metabolite of the yellow mold Aspergillus flavus (one of the most potent carcinogens known)

TABLE 2 - continued

SOME NATURALLY OCCURRING CARCINOGENS
AND THEIR SOURCES

Betel Nuts (Areca)	Fruit of the betel or areca palm
Cycasin	Cycad Nut (dietary constituent of natives of Guam)
Monocrotaline	Senecic shrubbery (medicine tea ingredient, Bantu's South Africa)

Source: Adapted from J. C. Arcos, Tulane Medical
Center[30]

Short-Term Tests

Dr. Bruce M. Ames and co-workers at the University
of California at Berkeley have developed a short-term
mutagen test.[31] It is based on the ability of a mutant
bacterial strain (Salmonella typhimurium) which normally cannot synthesize the amino acid histidine, to repair its own DNA in the presence of certain chemicals
(mutagens), and synthesize that amino acid. Ninety
percent of those chemicals yielding a positive Ames
test have also been demonstrated to be carcinogens.
The Ames test is much less costly than bioassays and
gives results in a few days to a week. It is a major
step forward in carcinogen detection. Although Ames
is quoted as saying "Most animal cancer studies are
models of non-thoroughness," at the other end of the
spectrum he says (of the Ames test) "It's never going
to be 100% diagnostic."*[32] Why? Certain chemicals
causing mutations such as diethylstilbesterol (DES)
once used to fatten cattle will not cause bacteria to
undergo mutation. One unique facet of the Ames test
is its ability to diagnose the mutagenicity of mix-

---

* Metals cannot be tested.

tures.   Several other short-term tests are also under
evaluation.[33, 34]

The Institute for Medical Research in Camden,
New Jersey, is currently conducting an air and water
monitoring program under contract to the DEP.[35]
The Ames test is being used there to determine the
presence of environmental mutagens.   Studies at other
laboratories, showing smokers' urine to be mutagenic,
have been confirmed at the Institute.   Several major
manufacturers of chemicals with laboratories in New
Jersey conduct their own research to determine if a
raw material or product is carcinogenic.   E.I. DuPont,
with installations in South Jersey (Salem, and Deepwater), was one of the first industrial toxicological
laboratories to use the Ames Test.[36]   These screening
tests along with animal studies conducted at the
Haskell Laboratory in Wilmington, Delware, have resulted in the identification of 24 carcinogens.   Among
those chemicals that have been classified as carcinogenic are carbon tetrachloride and hexamethylphos-
phoramide.

Federal Guidelines on Carcinogens in the Workplace
Environment

The Department of Labor (DOL) issues regulations
on chemicals in the workplace environment and they
have established a widely used classification system.[37]
Substances in Category I are confirmed carcinogens, in
Category II, suspect, and there are inadequate data to
classify those in Category III.   These criteria for
rating carcinogens are used principally in chapter 7.

Chapter 2 / REFERENCES

1.   International Union Against Cancer. Illustrated
          Tumor Nomenclature. Springer-Verlag,
          Berlin, 1965.

2.   Patten, Bradley M., Ph.D., and Carlson, Bruce
          M., M.D., Ph.D. Foundations of
          Embryology, McGraw-Hill Book Company,
          New York, 1974.

3.   Braun, Armin C., The Story of Cancer, Addison-
          Wesley Publishing Company, London, 1977,
          p. 66.

4.   Pitot, Henry C., Fundamentals of Oncology,
          Marcel Dekker, Inc., New York and Basel,
          1978, p. 16.

5.   Cairns, John, Cancer: Science and Society,
          W.H. Freeman and Company, San Francisco,
          1978, pp. 16, 27, 30.

6.   Braun, Armin C., Op. Cit.

7.   Pitot, Henry C., Op. Cit.

8.   Braun, Armin C., Op. Cit., Chapter IV.

9.   Pitot, Henry C., Op. Cit., Chapter 3.

10.   Eckardt, Robert E., M.D., Ph.D., and Hindin,
          Richard, The Health Hazards of Plastics,
          Journal of Medicine, Vol. 15. No. 10,
          October 1973, pp. 808-818.

11. Cairns, John, Op. Cit., pp. 85, 103.

12. Winchester, A.M., Heredity: An Introduction to
        Genetics, Barnes & Noble, Inc., New York,
        1966, p. 242.

13. Todaro, George J., and Huebner, Robert J., "The
        Viral Oncogene Hypothesis: New Evidence,"
        National Academy of Sciences Proceedings
        U.S.A.   Vol. 69, No. 4, April 1972,
        pp. 1009-1051.

14. Alexander-Jackson, Eleanor, Ph.D., FAAAS, Pro-
        genitor Cryptocides: The Specific Micro-
        organism of Malignancy, Abstract, Cancer
        Dialogue '80, October 18, 1980.

15. McQuerter, Gregory, Cancer: Clues in the Mind,
        Science News, Vol. 113, No. 3, January
        21, 1978, pp. 44-45.

16. Proceedings of the American Cancer Society and
        National Cancer Institute, National
        Conference on Nutrition in Cancer, June
        29-July 1, 1978, Seattle, Washington.

17. Gori, Gio Batta, Ph.D., Ibid, pp. 2151-2161.

18. Miller, James A., and Miller, Elizabeth C., Chemi-
        cal Carcinogenesis: Mechanism and
        Approaches to Its Control, Journal of the
        National Cancer Institute, Vol. 47, No. 3,
        September, 1971, pp. V-XIII.

19. Arcos, Joseph C. Cancer: Chemical Factors in the
        Environment, An Overview, Part II, American
        Laboratory, Volume No. 10, July 1978,
        pp. 29-41.

20. Ibid.

21. Pitot, Henry C., Op. Cit., p. 84.

22. Waldbott, George L., M.D., Health Effects of
         Environmental Pollutants, C.V. Mosby
         Co, Saint Louis, 1973., Ch. 17.

23. Dox, Ida; Melloni, John Biagio, Ph.D., Candi-
         date) and Eisner, Gilbert M., M.D.,
         F.A.C.P., Melloni's Illustrated Medical
         Dictionary, The Williams and Wilkins
         Co., Baltimore, 1979.

24. Josephson, Julian, The Workplace Reproductive
         Hazards, Environmental Science & Tech-
         nology, Vol. 14, No. 12., December 1980,
         pp. 1418-1429.

25. Maugh II, Thomas H., Chemical Carcinogens:
         How Dangerous are Low Doses? Science,
         Vol. 202, 6 October 1978, pp. 37-41.

26. Ibid.

27. Ibid.

28. Blumer, Max, Polycyclic Aromatic Compounds in
         Nature, Scientific American, Vol. 234,
         No. 3, March 1976. pp. 34-45.

29. Arcos, Joseph C., Op. Cit.

30. Pitot, Henry C., Op. Cit., p. 34.

31. Ames, Bruce M., Environmental Mutagens/Carcino-
         gens, The CoEvolution Quarterly, Spring
         1978., pp. 27-28.

32. Fox, Jeffrey L., Ames Test Success Paves Way for
         Short-Term Cancer Testing, Chemical &
         Engineering News, Vol. 55, No. 50,
         December 1977.

33. Anon. Short-term Tests for Cancer Not Yet Per-
         fected. Chemical Week. Vol. 124,
         No. 24, June 13, 1979., pp. 31-32.

34. Fox, Jeffrey L., Op. Cit.

35. Institute for Medical Research "Twenty Five
         Years of Progress," Biennial Report
         to the Community, 1977-1978.

36. Occupational Safety and Health: A DuPont Company
         View. Rev. September 1, 1977, pp. 1-58.

37. Regulatory Analysis of A Proposed Policy for the
         Identification, Classification and Regula-
         tion of Toxic Substances Posing a Potential
         Occupational Carcinogenic Risk, U.S.
         Department of Labor, Occupational Safety
         and Health Administration, Washington,
         D.C., October 17, 1978.

CHAPTER 3

ENVIRONMENT, PHYSIOLOGY
AND ECOLOGY

"I am a part of all
 that I have met."

Alfred Lord Tennyson,
Ulysses (1842)

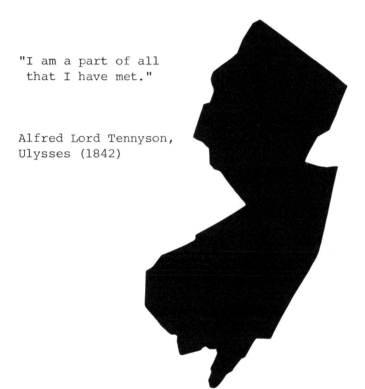

CHAPTER 3

DEFINING THE ENVIRONMENT

The evolution of the definitional concept of the "environment" was discussed briefly in chapter 1. Although it is a definition which is constantly evolving, it must encompass the impact of life-style as well as natural and urban communities and industrial pollution. However, defining the environment really defies the confines of a single sentence. The human race not having attained eco-omnipotence cannot really define it. But environmental interaction, which is really ecology, may be explored, to obtain a better understanding of the complexity of the environment and its impact on our health. And that is the purpose of this chapter; to explore typical and atypical environmental relationships with an emphasis on the holistic etiologies of the induction of cancers.

When we try to envision the environment, our image may be a static one. Yet the environment has vertical and horizontal dimensions in time and space. Consider that a water molecule in your next sneeze aerosol may become a drop in tomorrow's rain or at the least one molecule in your next glass of water may have likewise satisfied the thirst of Christ Himself some 2,000 years ago!

What then, is the environment and some of its intricate interrelationships? To a tapeworm, the environment could be the intestines of a human being, to a fish the ocean, and to a bluejay, tree limbs and air. Simplistically, the environment is everything that an organism comes in contact with, and usually coincides with the states of matter; gas, liquids, solids and radiation. There is a psychological environmental contact; however, that concept will be discussed

in chapter 8. An organism's contact with any one of
these media is not the same, however. For example,
our predominant contact with the environment is through
the air we breathe involuntarily throughout the course
of our lives. Considerable quantities are taken into
the lungs: 10,000 to 20,000 liters (21,134 quarts)
daily.[1]

The Lungs -- The Principal Entry Route to the Inner
Environment

The breathing of less than pure air, such as that
found at sea, containing even low levels of pollutants
or carcinogens, represents a potential environmental
hazard. Fortunately, our respiratory system is provided with protective mechanisms. The Creator has
given us an extremely efficient first line contaminant detector, the nose. Fortunately, many toxic and
carcinogenic chemicals are sensed by the nose at very
low concentrations.

The very toxic hydrogen sulfide, capable of producing respiratory failure within seconds after inhalation has a well known rotten egg odor. This flammable
gas may be detected in air by the nose at concentrations as low as 0.002 mg/l (0.0000002%).[2] Before
the era of sophisticated contaminant gas detectors,
miners used canary birds to alert them to the presence
of toxic gases. Today, in most homes or commercial
establishments there are "human canaries," those with
a keen sense of small. Be thankful for the presence
of them amongst you for they serve to *alert* those of
lesser sensitivity to the presence of air pollutants.

Nose hairs serve to remove large particulate
matter (about 95% of those particles larger than 4
microns)* and the mucous-coating of the respiratory
tract absorbs undesireable gases.[3] Particulate matter
smaller than 4 microns is cleared from the lungs by

---

* Essentially those particles less than 1.2 microns are not
   removed.

entrapment in secreted mucous which is projected upward
by the undulating wave motion of hairlike structures
in the upper lung airways. This clean-out process is
called mucociliary transport.[4] These processes prevent entry of undesireable environmental agents into
the tiny air pockets of the lungs called alveoli. It
is in these alveoli that oxygen and carbon dioxide are
exchanged, along with adverse environmental agents not
removed by nose hair and mucous. Particulate matter
successful in reaching the alveolar space are absorbed
by body scavenger cells; the alveolar macrophages.[5]
You can appreciate the concept of an internal environment on considering the total surface area of the
alveoli in a pair of lungs, some 1,000 square feet![6]

Coughing, choking, sneezing and swallowing also
assist in the removal of extraneous environmental agents
from the respiratory tract. Environmental agents not
removed by these processes either react with lung tissue, become permanent residents there or are absorbed
by another dynamic internal environment, the circulatory system. The latter is actually a very special
function of the lymphatic system which serves as a
make-up network for returning materials from the body
tissues to the blood.[7] In this manner surplus tissue
fluid and protein are returned to the blood. Lymph
also removes dead cells and invading bacteria from the
body. Who has not experienced a swelling of these
lymph nodes accompanying the body's natural defense
against bacterial infection? They are located under
the jaw, the arm pits, in the groin and in many other
locations.

The ability of an air pollution episode to have
far reaching and immediate deleterious effects has been
demonstrated in New Jersey and is described below.

The Piscataway Inversion

An inversion is a peculiar air pattern in which
a cool air layer near the ground possibly containing
high levels of pollutants, is trapped by an overlaying
strata of warmer air, preventing its normal dispersal
into the upper atmosphere. This phenomenon occurred

in the highly industrialized area of Piscataway,
northern New Jersey, on September 15, 1971.[8] The
oxidant count, the probable principal contaminant being ozone, resulting from the reaction between fuel
combustion vapors, oxides of nitrogen, sunlight and
chemicals, attained levels ranging from 0.022* to
0.096 ppm. Lacrimation (tearing from the eyes),
irritated throats, chest pains and respiratory diffi-
culties were experienced by students at several area
high schools who were engaged in outdoor sports in a
10 by 25 mile area affected by the smog, trapped by
the inversion. No explanation is available to account
for some students becoming ill at some schools, and not
at others, but it is probably related to individual
sensitivity and respiration rate.

The Piscataway inversion was not a new or unique
phenomenon. However, attention is drawn to the un-
common combination of environmental factors required to
produce that episode: pollutants, temperature, baro-
metric pressure, dispersion, sunlight and other factors.
Similarly, other toxins and carcinogens may be dispersed
for many miles beyond their point of origin.

The next phase of environmental contact is through
liquids. Since humans, unlike creatures of the sea,
do not live in the water, our most extensive external
contact with this medium is by bathing for hygienic or
recreational purposes. Our principal daily internal
contact is through what we drink and eat; soups,
beverages, vegetables, meats, pastries, since just about
every edible food contains water.

It may be easily understood that the digestive
system has limited defense mechanisms and anything not
rendered neutral by digestive tract acidity or alkalinity or rejected by regurgitation will have a major
impact on every body tissue during its active life or
residence time before it is excreted, whether it be an
aged pizza, intestinal virus or contaminated well water.

---

* 0.02 ppm is the normal ozone concentration in unpolluted dry air.

Masonville Well Water Contamination

The consumption of drinking water with elevated nitrate levels may cause a condition known as methemoglobinemia; a decrease in the body's blood oxygen-bear-
ing capacity, and concomitant fatigue and depression.
Nitrates are actually responsible for methemoglobinemia;
however, nitrites, when present, are metabolised to
nitrates. Masonville (Burlington County), New Jersey
residents consuming water containing up to 140 parts per
million of nitrates (federal limit 10, New Jersey 6.8),
experienced headaches, stomach cramps and sluggishness.[9]
However, the more serious chronic problem may be the
conversion of the amines present in the digestive tract
to very potent carcinogens -- nitrosamines. And
there are many other toxic and carcinogenic substances
in New Jersey residents' drinking water (especially
ground water) to be discussed in chapter 4. At Masonville, the origin of the nitrates was from leachate of
high nitrate soil, contaminated by septic systems and
plant fertilizers. More than 70% of the nitrates taken
orally are absorbed by the blood circulatory system,
pass through the liver and kidneys and are ultimately
excreted in the urine.[10]

We also make contact with the environment through
solids. The human body is covered with epidermal cells
which are for the most part small and microscopic in
size. Present theory indicates that each cell has some
sort of membrane or layer surrounding it which regulates
the flux of materials from the environment or from cell
to cell.[11] The solids of the environment may pass through
the cell wall but they must obviously become soluble
first by dissolving on wet skin or be absorbed by fatty
or aqueous cellular components. A number of external
topical factors may influence the skin permeability to
an environmental agent. Obviously, if the skin is
moist, the permeability to water soluble compounds is
enhanced; if it is oily, passage of organic compounds
will be enhanced. In addition, other factors such as
molecular size, pH (alkalinity or acidity) and ionisation regulate the transfer of environmental agents.
Consider the following environmental interactions
involving ingestion, inhalation and irradiation
simultaneously.

Luminous Dial Painters

In the 1920's, radium watch dial painters at a
northern New Jersey factory indulged in the functional
but deadly practise of "pointing"; putting small
brush tips in between the lips in order to get dis-
orderly hairs arranged into a nice point.[12] As a
result of this practise, several female workers
developed fatigue, pallor, weight loss, anemia and
jaw degeneration. The paint formulation consisted
of luminous zinc sulphide, copper, radium bromide
and sulphate. Epidemiologists of that era, familiar
with the effects of gamma-rays, which when used to
treat tongue cancer, could produce necrosis of the
jaw, identified radium in the paint as the adverse
environmental agent. The radium in the paint literally irradiated the dial painters, specifically,
their jaw-bones. Like asbestos, contamination by
radium was not limited to the practise of "pointing".
The very clothes of workers were said to be luminous
in the dark along with hair, faces, hands, arms,
underclothes, nasal discharges and handkerchiefs.
And the complex cycle of dispersal of an adverse
occupational carcinogen continued *beyond* the factory
confines by workers acting as vectors. Under
these circumstances it is plausible to envision the
transfer of a carcinogen from one person to another,
for example, during intimate contact.

The Parenteral Introduction of Environmental Agents

There is at least one further route of entry of
environmental agents into an organism and it may be
intentional or accidental; the parenteral route. Inadvertently, even the intentional parenteral route
(injection) may be accompanied by an unwanted environmental agent, e.g., infectious hepatitis. However,
we do inadvertently stick ourselves with pins, nails
and needles, and even insect pests (e.g., mosquitoes
and green-head flies) effect parenteral injections.
The mosquito occupies a rather distintive role in
disease transmission which will be discussed shortly.

Reflecting for a moment comprehensively on all

the possible routes of entry into the human body by
carcinogens, one point may be obvious but must be
stated. In few instances are the environmental
contacts discretely singular. For example, the
cigarette smoker absorbs most of the carcinogens present in burning tobacco through his or her lungs.
However, particulate matter deposited on the ciliated
mucous membrane elutes to the pharnyx and there mucous
entraps the particulates and some of this mixture
along with salivary secretions is swallowed. Hence,
carcinogens (mutagens and teratogens) enter the
stomach similarly. If the smoker is a nail-biter
as many adults are, additional tobacco carcinogens
absorbed on and about the fingertips are transferred
to mouth mucous membranes.

Biotransformation, Translocation and Storage Sites

     The principal routes of entry of environmental
agents into the body have just been described. Once
in the body the environmental agent must be utilized
through metabolism or eliminated. Gases may be
released through delivery to the lungs, by the
circulatory system; liquids may be excreted by the
kidneys or perspiration or respiration. However,
before any of this takes place, the environmental
agent must enter the individual cell. For this purpose there are at least two modes of transport.[13]
The mammalian cell membrane is composed of lipid
(fat-like) materials, bound on both sides by protein.
Carrier molecules that are fat soluble, bind to water
soluble substances and carry them through the cell
membrane. The "piggy back" water soluble molecule
may be a good environmental agent such as ascorbic
acid (vitamin C) or a water soluble economic poison
(i.e., a pesticide). Low molecular weight organic
acids may also simply diffuse through the cell wall.

     Now that the modes of transport through the cell
wall have been described, the role of the liver and
kidneys should be mentioned again. Although attention
has been drawn in this chapter to the entry of pollutants into the body, the major portion of solids, and
liquids enter the stomach as foodstuffs. Once in the

stomach, the products of digestion enter the capi-
llaries of the intestinal villi and thus into the
circulatory system. Blood from the intestine and
stomach is then shunted through the liver where
carbohydrates, fats, proteins, minerals, etc., are
metabolised. Blood leaving the liver returns to the
heart, the brain and the rest of the systemic circula-
tion where it is ultimately filtered by the kidneys,
with the waste products becoming urine. This extremely simplied bit of human physiology quickly demonstrates
how environmental agents may be hepatoxic (poisoning
the liver), nephrotoxic (poisoning the kidneys), cardio-
toxic and also affect the brain. Because of the specific affinity which toxic substances demonstrate for the
latter organs, they are known as target organs.

Once inside the cell, the environmental agent
may be altered (biotransformed) by enzymes, moved to
different sites (translocated) or deposited in tissues,
with these latter called storage sites.[14] It may
be the release of toxic or carcinogenic environmental
agents from storage sites in the presence of newly
arrived pollutants that accounts for the synergistic
effect of some chemicals in an organism.[15]

Thus far in this chapter, the multi-faceted concept of environment has been expressed in the interrelationship between humans, the air, water, solid
masses and irradiation. The animal kingdom is certainly not to be overlooked.

ZOONOSES

Documents from the beginning of recorded history
verify the long standing close relationship the human
race has held with the animal kingdom. Diseases,
however, may be transferred from animals to humans
and vice versus. Public health researchers call these
diseases zoonoses and of the more than one hundred
types , some are given below.[16, 17]

Disease:	Transmitted by:	Animal vector or causative agent:
Scabies	Arthropods	Mites
Salmonellosis	Bacteria	Turtles(feces)
Malaria	Protozoa(trypanasomes)	Mosquitoes
Rabies	Viruses	Dogs, Bats, Foxes, Skunks
Trichinosis	Pork tapeworm (Helminths)	Carnivorous mammals

The point is that the smallest animal, a microscopic protozoan, or a horse may carry or be a vector in the zoonotic cycle. That wildlife and domestic animals may harbor disease organisms highlights their negative aspects. New Jersey, which is a mixture of rural and urban life, has experienced health problems as a result of its close contact with the animal kingdom. Of particular concern in New Jersey has been rabies, encephalitis, Rocky Mountain Spotted Fever, tularemia and leptospirosis.[18] The actual microorganism responsible for zoonoses are in some cases viruses, invertebrates or bacteria.

Zoonoses in Cancer Etiology

Gastric Cancers

Researchers Pfeiffer and Threlfal have been studying the high incidence of gastric cancer in Newfoundland fisherman.[19] Their findings indicate the possibility of a chemical or viral carcinogen being present in the triad of seabirds, fish packing plants and fishermen.

Burkitt's Lymphoma

The most significant research in the real world demonstrating the role of zoonoses in human environmental cancers, has been conducted by Dr. Dennis Burkitt, currently the senior research fellow at the St. Thomas' Hospital Medical School in London, England. Dr. Burkitt observed that a high incidence of tumors of the reticuloendothelial system* (RES) in Central Africa, accompanied chronic malaria.[20] Further, he observed that lymphoma (malignancies of the lymph nodes) was endemic to those areas where malaria is holoendemic (prevalent in unusual numbers but limited to a region), that chronic malaria damages the RES and that malarial pigmentations were identified in the autopsied victims. Collectively, he reasoned that the vectored parasite is probably malaria, responsible for the lymphoma. Although Burkitt's Lymphoma is an evolving etiology, it serves notice on the research community of the danger in not approaching the causes of cancers holistically.

Bladder Cancers

Snails infected with schistosomes, a trematode parasite, may release the larvae of this organism in water. The microscopic water-borne larvae called cercariae may penetrate the skin of a wader or swimmer and invade the circulatory system. Once there, the larvae proceed to infect other organs: lungs, liver, colon, kidney, depending on their species. Dr. Cheever of the Laboratory of Parasitic Diseases, National Institute of Health, has observed a frequent association of schistosome infections and bladder cancer, and a high prevalence of bladder cancers in schisto-somiasis endemic areas.[21] Additionally, there is an association between lymphoma and leukemia and schistosomiasis. Although these parasitic infesta-

---

* A cell system present in the thymus glands, spleen and lymph nodes concerned with engulfing bacteria and other foreign bodies.

tions are normally associated with the inhabitants of
China, Japan, Phillipines, the Nile Valley, Africa,
Brazil, parts of the West Indies and other tropical
countries, they have been seen with increasing frequency in the United States. Considering the influx
of immigrants from Southeast Asia, in recent years,
an increased incidence can be anticipated.

     Dr. Cheever's review cites the many futher
research needs in establishing a proven relationship;
rigorous statistical proof, possibility of carcinogenic substances in schistosome eggs and the interaction of urine with excreted chemicals (e.g., nitrosamines) just to mention a few. Cancer of several organs
has been attributed to schistosomiasis but conclusive
evidence is not extant.

Esophageal Cancers

     There is a good body of data to indicate that the
nematode* Spirocerca lupi may be responsible for malignant esophageal lesions in man's best friend, the
dog.[22] After ingestion of the larvae, they migrate from
the stomach, invade the wall of the esophagus and this
is followed by the development of malignant lesions.
The spirocerca larvae are also found in the kidney,
bladder, trachea, lung and elsewhere. Eventually, the
larvae reach maturity within the host and the cycle is
repeated. The death of the host as a result of larval
migrations occurs following the formation of an abcess,
sudden rupture of the aorta and other complications.
As with human forms of cancer it is not always the
malignancy itself that brings on death. The potential
scope of the well-travelled internal Spirocerca environment is displayed in the number and nature of hosts:

dragon-flies, hedgehogs, ducks, chickens, rabbits,
rodents, beetles, lizards, and roaches.

---

* A nematode is a small parasitic worm found in soil and water.

The adult worm, the spirurid, has been found in other
animals: fox, wolf, jackal, lynx, jaguar, snow leopard
and cat. The larvae of Spirocerca, (free and encysted)
that initiate the infection, may be transmitted by
dung, beetles, chickens, lizards, and animals
that the dog consumes. In a rural area near Auburn,
Alabama, where the disease has been more prevalent than
in the general southeastern United States, chickens
were cited as the principal vector. Spirocerca infections appear to have increased over the last ten years.

Viral Leukemia in Cats

    Plants and animals manifest cancers and we live
in close association with both. On the basis of pet
mobility and our tendency to smother them with affec-
tion, zoonoses and cancers warrant more research than
is being conducted currently. Our most environmentally
sound mouse-trap, the cat, plays a somewhat disturbing
role in the transmission of feline leukemia. Young
and adult cats, innoculated with feline leukemia virus
(FeLV) may infect other cats housed together, with FeLV,
within a month of exposure. The mode of transmission
is by salivary excretions from the trachea, oral area
or the urine. These studies conducted by Jarret and
Essex and others demonstrate that viruses may be transmitted horizontally; from one unrelated animal to
another.[23, 24]

    Some scientists disregard horizontal transmission
of cancers, preferring to perceive of the transmission
as restricted to the vertical mode; through the genetic
code. The work of Jarret and Essex strengthens the
former hypothesis, however, the latter mode also exists.
In one study, seven out of ten test animals manifested
viral leukemia which became terminal within eighteen
months.[25]

    One more disturbing piece of evidence stems from
research indicating that cats infected with FeLV
(subgroups B and C) and FeSV (Feline Sarcoma virus)

may transmit the same viruses to human fibroblasts*, at least in the laboratory.[26] However, these cells show no change in morphology or general health subsequent to infection.

The Cockroach -- A Willing Vector?

Continuing in this vein, consider our most ancient of pests, the cockroach. Although long considered an obnoxious uninvited guest and an adjunct to unsanitary conditions, it was not determined to be a vector in any significant disease cycle. In other words, the cockroach would have been preferred compared to the housefly, tick, flea or mosquito in terms of disease transmission. However, it has now been demonstrated that the cockroach may transmit microorganisms via mouth parts, legs and body parts. The microorganisms carried reflect the "environment" through which it sojourned, in an "I am a part of all that I have met" fashion. Some of the microorganisms transported may cause such intestinal disorders as food poisoning. Roaches also carry coliform bacteria which as fecal bacteria have been associated with dysentery, typhoid fever, cholera and polio.[27] And what of virus transport by the cockroach? Research is not presently being conducted to my knowledge, and yet the environmental cancer implications are obvious. Having travelled over considerable segments of the world, this author will attest to the ubiquitous occurrence of the cockroach and the need to discuss it in the context of zoonoses. The same authors conducting the research noted herein, cite the ability of subterranean termites to transport bacteria from one sanitary landfill to another. What may be substituted for "bacteria" in those findings, in time?

---

* A common cell type found growing in human connective tissue.

MISCELLANEOUS INTERRELATIONSHIPS

We now arrive at a concept of the environment
that involves an interrelationship with microorganisms and animals as well as humans, the air, water,
solid masses and irradiation. And we have only
scratched the surface in understanding the complexi-
ties of environmental relationships and especially
those portending cancers.

Consider the following unrecognized and
unevaluated, potentially hazardous exposures to
environmental carcinogens, not just peculiar to New
Jersey, but of global concern.

Landfill Operations

The more traditionally recognized environmental
hazards stemming from landfill operations are ground
water pollution by leachate, venting of methane gas
and failure to maintain a daily soil cover. However,
the extent of exposure of landfill operators to toxic
or carcinogenic agents resulting from decomposition
or in-situ chemical reactions, has not been evaluated.
The more gross known evolutions of methane no doubt
bring to the surface other gases.

There is at least one more potential hazard
posed by landfills in addition to operator exposure
by toxins and carcinogens. In the past few years
there has been considerable apprehension and resistance to the approval of research on recombinant DNA
from both the public and scientific sectors. This
very practical concern is based on the potential
creation of new and deadly bacterial or viral strains
capable of annihilating animals and plant life. Recombinant DNA technology under controlled laboratory
conditions may bring society low cost interferon,
which has been proven capable of controlling some
cancers. However, landfill chemistry and kinetics
provide an incomprehensible, in-situ beehive for

unrestrained recombinant DNA accidents, with no physical and biological containment systems. I would suggest that some of the research budgets devoted to deliberate recombinant DNA research be diverted to assess the accidental.

Lost, Stolen and Recycled Radiation Sources

During the author's years in the Delaware Valley area, a number of small quantities of radiation sources, industrial, research, and medical in nature have "disappeared" from trucks, cars and institutions as reported by the news media.[28, 29] Some, undoubtedly, have fallen into the hands of children, possibly have been incorporated into building structures and wound up in landfills. There is no way of even estimating the possible leukemia cases (or other cancers) resulting from these incidents. On a national basis, the inability of the nuclear facilities in the United States to account for some 8,000 pounds of highly enriched uranium and plutonium,[30] is more disturbing.

Radon seeds (containing radioactive gold), used to treat cancerous tumors during the period 1930-1940, may have been recycled into jewelry such, as rings.[31] Thus far, contaminated jewelry has been found only in New York and Pennsylvania. The New York State Health Department has surveyed 100,000 pieces of jewelry, finding 100 contaminated pieces. This jewelry has already produced a variety of adverse health effects; superficial irritation, skin cancer and subsequent finger and hand amputation. The New Jersey Bureau of Radiation Protection is aware of this situation and has 21 stations ready to check jewelry in the state. Apparently they are waiting for public alarm or a body count before activating the monitoring stations.

Trihalomethane (THM)

The practise of chlorinating drinking water may result in the formation of parts per billion (ppb) quantities of THM's.[32] The most simple form is chloroform ($CHCL_3$). THM's produce kidney and liver

tumors in mice and rats.[33] Several studies have shown
a statistical relationship and association between the
ingestion of chlorinated drinking water and cancers
of the brain, respiratory and gastrointestinal system,
kidney, bladder and rectum.[34, 35, 36, 37] The Environmental Protection Agency takes the position that the
benefits of chlorination (the destruction of disease-
causing organisms) outweighs the cancer risk.* Municipal well systems in Mantua, New Jersey, have given test
results of 250 ppb THM's.**[38]

The hazard presented by THM's is ostensibly confined to ingestion of drinking water so contaminated.
However, it is quite plausible to consider inhalation
of THM vapors, released during the practise of taking
hot baths, showers, and especially about the air at
the typically overly chlorinated public swimming pool.

Incense Combustion

The burning of incense, a mixture of perfumes
and spices, is an historical part of religious services and other practises. It is during at least
one specific use that the author has observed considerable discomfort accompanying that practise --
during the Episcopal Choral Eucharist where priest,
acolytes and parishioners may be left red-eyed and
coughing as a result of the copious quantities of
smoke generated.

Typically, incense contains an oriental gum
obtained from the trunk of the European, North or
Central American storax tree. Chemically, it is a
complex mixture of esters and organic acids. Of
particular importance here is the 5 - 15% free cinnamic acid and styrene moiety.[39] Styrene, also called
vinylbenzene is a contemporary plastic monomer (used
to synthesize polystyrene) and a suspect carcinogen.

------

* Final Regulation, November 29, 1979.

** Limit 100 ppb, the results were not duplicated.

The intact and degraded monomer (possibly benzene) would be present in the aerosol produced by incense combustion. The other cyclic organic compounds present, such as cinnamic acid, may polymerize on combustion forming polycyclic aromatic hydrocarbons (PAH's) which are carcinogenic. Several PAH's will be discussed in chapter 4. The inhalation of vapors from styrene produces eye and mucous membrane irritation and in high concentrations is a narcotic. Incense combustion products and their impact on those in proximity require evaluation. There is a significant risk population in New Jersey as elsewhere.

Boiler Descaling Operations

The practise of boiling water to generate steam eventually results in the building up of scale (calcium carbonate and rust) in the pressure vessel. To continue the effective exchange of heat, that scale is removed periodically by acid cleaning. Chelates are also added to the descalant mixture to bind any copper present in solution and one of the chemicals used for this purpose is 1,3 diethyl thiourea (DETU).

In 1978, ethylene thiourea, a structurally-related compound, was determined to be an animal carcinogen.[40] DETU was still given a clean bill of health and chemical descalers continued to use it throughout New Jersey and elsewhere. In 1979, DETU was determined to be an animal carcinogen. A close examination of the actual use of DETU reveals the user exposure hazard. Operators and any personnel in the vicinity of the trucks where these chemicals are mixed (hot), are all exposed to vapors from the descalant mixture, only one of which is DETU. The boiler water-sides of steam generators require periodic scale removal with a nominal 10% hydrochloric acid solution containing DETU. The author has conducted and monitored these operations many times in previous years. Since becoming aware of the carcinogenicity of ethylene thiourea, some operators have eliminated DETU, and others continue its use. Operators still using DETU may wear face shields to avoid splashing liquids,

but none wear respirators for protection from vapors.
They very often stand on the trucks with a lengthy 2" x
4", gazing into manholes, to check tank liquid levels.

SUMMARY

    All of the practises described above may result
in the exposure of small groups of persons to potential carcinogenic environmental agents. Hopefully,
the discussion will engender an appreciation of the
complexity of the environment, and how much our health
is a function of it. And further, why any approach
to environmental problems must be taken with a
holistic viewpoint. Bernard Glemser in his comprehensive book, "Man Against Cancer" said, "Clearly, the
environment -- the total environment, the sum of all
the elements surrounding the individual human being --
plays a significant part in the induction of cancer."[41]
Throughout this chapter some *liberty* has been taken
in suggesting or opening new avenues of investigation
for environmentally-induced cancers. Hopefully,
epidemiologists at the state and national level are
keeping an even more open mind. It is the observation
of the sometimes ridiculous or seemingly unrelated
event by a researcher that has helped to bring this
country to triumph over many once highly fatal diseases.
No environmental fact of life in New Jersey or elsewhere is too ridiculous or remote to be considered in
the etiology of the cancers, whether it be zoonoses or
weather patterns.

    Dr. Dennis Burkitt, whose research in Africa was
discussed earlier, said, "From these observations
(cited in his article) one wonders whether cancer research is to 'blinkered' in that it tends to be
focused only on malignant lesions to the exclusion
of other conditions, the investigation of which might
point the way to better understanding certain forms
of cancer."[42] Perhaps we are entering an era when
the scientific community is becoming willing to

admit more to having been "too blinkered." Consider
the comment made by Dr. H. David Lyons on visiting an
alternative cancer treatment clinic, "I knew that this
experience would challenge my established belief
systems, and I looked forward to this opportunity
to talk with doctors and patients for whom alternative methods of treatment are working."[43]

Most researchers whose studies are pertinent to
cancer are working on a highly specific phase of
the problem. Given all the essential funding, one
person could not garner in a single lifetime enough
expertise to be more than an "expert" in a limited
area. Some of the more esoteric and seemingly highly
specific forms of cancer research such as the "high
electron conductivity" of Dr. Albert Szent-Gyorgyi,
is really interdisciplinary.[44] The point is that
recognizing that one can really only be effective in
one area, it is all the more essential to remain in
touch with other disciplines at least academically.
The scientific community is forced by sheer economics
to work on a single problem -- a sort of de facto
reductionism. There is another reason, Dr. Commoner
calls "intellectual independence" and cautions that
it not be translated into a kind of mandatory avoidance of all problems that do not arise in their own
minds -- "an approach that may cut them off from the
real and urgent needs of society, and from their
students as well."[45] Even in the framework of
intellectual independency, the scientist must remain
in touch with other disciplines, sifting, sorting and
retaining those ideas that strengthen their particular interests.

Dr. John Higginson, of the 90% environmentally
induced cancer hypothesis fame, spoke at a September,
1980, American Cancer Society symposium.[46] He
lamented the unwillingness to conduct certain basic
life-style studies instead of costly animal studies.
There already is a great body of recently evolved data
on life-style in relation to cancers etiology. In
October, 1980, the Omega Institute sponsored a monumental holistic forum (Cancer Dialogue '80) for explor-
ing the interface between the pathological, psychological and sociological implications of cancers.[47]

The recognition of life-style and its importance in
cancer treatment modalities was highlighted at this
symposium. To my knowledge, no other symposium has
brought together such specialists and experts in
such diverse fields as surgery, immunotherapy, psycho-
logy, metabology, chemotherapy, nutrition and radiation therapy. Truly this symposium approached that
concept of holism as defined by its author, Johann
Christian Smuts (1870-1950) wherein the human race
is viewed as but a component of a comprehensive
system.[48] Perhaps Cancer Dialogue '80 will precipitate a period of scientific ecumenism in the search
for the cause of cancers and prevention.

Chapter 3 / REFERENCES

1. Brain, Joseph D., The Respiratory Tract and the
    Environment, Environmental Health
    Perspectives, Vol. 20, October 1977,
    pp. 113-126.

2. The Merck Index of Chemicals and Drugs,
    Merck & Co., Inc., Rahway, N.J., 1977.

3. Hesketh, H.H., Ph.D., Understanding and Con-
    trolling Air Pollution, Ann Arbor
    Science Publishers, Ann Arbor, Mich.,
    1974.

4. Brain, Joseph D., Op. Cit.

5. Ibid.

6. Keeton, William T., Elements of Biological
    Science, W. W. Norton & Company, Inc.
    New York, 1973, p. 123.

7. Ibid., pp. 145-146.

8. Jackson, D., The Cloud Comes to Quibbletown,
    Life 71: 72-75, 79-82, 1971.

9. Carney, Art, Danger Seeps in One Town's
    Water, Philadelphia Inquirer, November
    12, 1977.

10. Altman, Phillip L. and Dittmer, Dorothy S.,
    Metabolism, Biological Handbooks
    Bethesda, Maryland, 1968, pp. 418-421.

11. Loomis, Ted A., Ph.D., M.D., Essentials of
        Toxicology, Lea & Febiger, Philadelphia,
        Pennsylvania, Chapter 3.

12. Castle, William B., M.D., Drinker, Katherine R.,
        M.D.,and Drinker, Cecil K., M.D., Necrosis
        of the Jaw in Workers Employed in Apply-
        ing A Luminous Paint Containing Radium,
        Journal of Industrial Hygiene, Vol. 7,
        No. 8, August 1925, pp. 371-382.

13. Loomis, Ted A., Op. Cit.

14. Ibid.

15. Arcos, Joseph C., Cancer: Chemical Factors in
        the Environment: An Overview, Part II,
        American Laboratory, July, 1978,
        pp. 29-41.

16. Schnurrenberger, Paul R., and Hubbert, William T.,
        Reporting of Zoonotic Diseases, American
        Journal of Epidemiology, Vol. 112, No. 1,
        1980, pp. 23-31.

17. Steele, James H., Zoonoses of Domestic Animals,
        In Critical Reviews in Environmental
        Control, Vol. 2, 2nd Issue, Ed. Bond, R.G.
        and Straub, C.P. CRC Press, Cleveland,
        Ohio, 1971, pp. 243-292.

18. Applegate, James E., The Wildlife Reserves of New
        Jersey, Chapter 19 in New Jersey Trends,
        Norman, Thomas P., Esq. (Ed.), Rutgers
        University, New Brunswick, N.J., 1974.

19. Pfeiffer, Carl J.,and Threlfall, W., Seabirds:
        A Possible environmental Factor In Gastric
        Cancer in Newfoundland, Digestion 16
        (1/21) pp. 1-9, 1977.

20. Burkitt, Dennis P., M.D., F.R. C.S. Ed.,
         Etiology of Burkitt's Lymphoma: An
         Alternative Hypothesis to a Vectored
         Virus, Journal of the National Cancer
         Institute 42: 19-28, 1969, pp. 19-26.

21. Cheever, Allen W., M.D., Schistosomiasis and
         Neoplasia, Journal of the National
         Cancer Institute, Vol. 61, July 1978,
         pp. 13-18.

22. Bailey, W.S., Parasites and Cancer: Sarcoma
         in Dogs Associated with Spirocerca
         Lupi, New York Academy of Science.
         Annals. 108, 1963, pp. 890-923.

23. Azocar, A. and Essex, M., Susceptibility of
         Human Cell Lines to Feline Leukemia
         Virus and Feline Sarcoma Virus,
         Journal of the National Cancer Insti-
         tute, Vol. 63, No. 5, November 1979,
         pp. 1179-1184.

24. Jarrett, William, Jarrett, Oswald, Mackey,
         Lindsay, Laird, Helen, Hardy, William,
         Jr., and Essex, Myron, Horizontal Trans-
         mission of Leukemia Virus and Leukemia
         in the Cat., Journal of the National
         Cancer Institute, Vol. 51, 1973,
         pp. 263-266.

25. Azocar, A. and Essex, M., Op. Cit.

26. Ibid.

27. Alcamo, Edward I., Ph.D. and Frishman, Austin M.,
         The Microbial Flora of Field-Collected
         Cockroaches and Other Arthropods,
         Journal of Environmental Health, Vol. 42,
         No. 5, March/April, 1980, pp. 263-266.

28. Clancy, John F., Radioactive Cancer Device Lost
         at HUP, Philadelphia Inquirer, September
         12, 1978.

29. The Gloucester County Times, November 30, 1979,
        p. A-7.

30. Burnham, David, The Case of the Missing Uranium,
        The Atlantic Monthly, Vol. 243, No. 4,
        April 1979, pp. 78-82.

31. Sachs, Linda, New Hazard Appears: Radioactive
        Jewelry, Hazardous Waste News, Vol. I,
        No. 8, November 1981.

32. Youssefi, M. and Zenchelsky, S.T., and Faust,
        S.D., Chlorination of Naturally
        Occurring Organic Compounds in Water,
        Journal of Environmental Science and
        Health, A13 (8), 1978, pp. 629-637.

33. Proctor, M.H., Ph.D., and Hughes, James P.,M.D.,
        Chemical Hazards of The Workplace,
        J. B. Lippincott Company, Philadelphia,
        1978

34. Environmental Protection Agency, Epidemiological
        Studies of Cancer Frequency and Certain
        Organic Constituents of Drinking Water,
        National Academy of Sciences, Washington,
        D.C., September 1978.

35. Council on Environmental Quality, Drinking Water
        and Cancer, December 1980.

36. Cancer Study Reports Firmer Link of Chlorinated
        Water to Tumors, (AP) New York Times,
        October 17, 1980

37. Cantor, Kenneth P., Hoover, Robert, Mason, Thomas
        J. and McCabe, Leland J., Associations
        of Cancer Mortality with Trihalomethanes
        in Drinking Water, Journal of the National
        Cancer Institute, Vol. 61, No. 4, October
        1978. pp 979-985.

38. Lucas, Charlotte-Ann, High Toxin Levels Found
         in N.J. Town's Drinking Water,
         Philadelphia Inquirer, July 30, 1980.

39. The Merk Index, Op. Cit.

40. Letter from Penwalt Corporation, December 1,
         1978.

41. Glemser, Bernard, Man Against Cancer, Funk and
         Wagnals, New York, 1969, p. 94.

42. Burkitt, Dennis P., Guest Editorial, Journal
         of the National Cancer Institute, Vol.
         47, No. 5, November 1971.

43. Lyons, David H., The Alternative Clinics: A
         Doctor's Reaction, Holistic Living
         News, Vol 3, Issue 2, October - November,
         1980, p. 16.

44. Szent-Gyorgyi, Albert, The Living State and
         Cancer, Marcel Dekker, New York, 1978.

45. Commoner, Barry, The Closing Circle, Alfred
         A. Knopf, Inc., New York, 1971, p. 191.

46. Anon., Wanted: A Sharper Focus for Research on
         Cancer, Chemical Week, Vol. 127, No. 13,
         September 24, 1980. p. 43.

47. Omega Institute, Cancer Dialogue '80, New York
         City, October 16-19, 1980.

48. World Book Encyclopedia, Field Enterprises Educa-
         tional Corporation, Chicago, 1971.

CHAPTER 4

OCCUPATIONAL, INDUSTRIAL AND
INSTITUTIONALLY SPONSORED EXPOSURE
TO CARCINOGENS, MUTAGENS, AND TERATOGENS

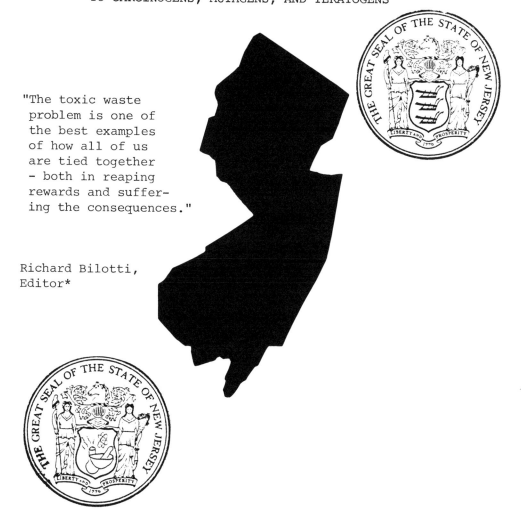

"The toxic waste
problem is one of
the best examples
of how all of us
are tied together
- both in reaping
rewards and suffer-
ing the consequences."

Richard Bilotti,
Editor*

* Gloucester County Times Publisher, September 29, 1980

CHAPTER 4

BACKGROUND

The early New Jersey colonialists symbolized their independence from England by displaying a specially designed seal. [1] This practise, denoting the authority of a new government, dates back many centuries. The New Jersey state seal shown on the chapter frontispiece shows Ceres the goddess of vegetation, a horse's head, and three plows. Various mottos have been placed on the scroll under the plows and currently the state's motto is "Liberty and Prosperity." With the past emphasis on agriculture as the foundation of the state's economy, the cognomen, "The Garden State" seemed very appropriate in yesteryear. [2] However, since then the state has undergone several transitions; agriculture initially, then encompassing a short-lived Merino sheep raising mania, a "silk fever" and a swine and cattle industry era. [3]

John T. Cunningham, noted New Jersey historian, said in his preface to "Made in New Jersey", "few people have to be told that New Jersey is an industrial state, of course, sight, sound and smell proclaim that fact. . . ." [4] He was referring to odors that represented the emissions from about 1200* various manufacturing plants. [5] More specifically, New Jersey, the 46th state in size, is second only to Texas in the production of chemicals. [6] Figure 7 indicates how well New Jersey has done in several areas of manufacture (during the early 70's). Table 3 shows the state's major sources of income and employment distribution

---

* In 1978 the number of chemical facilities was estimated at "more than 900." (See reference 6).

113

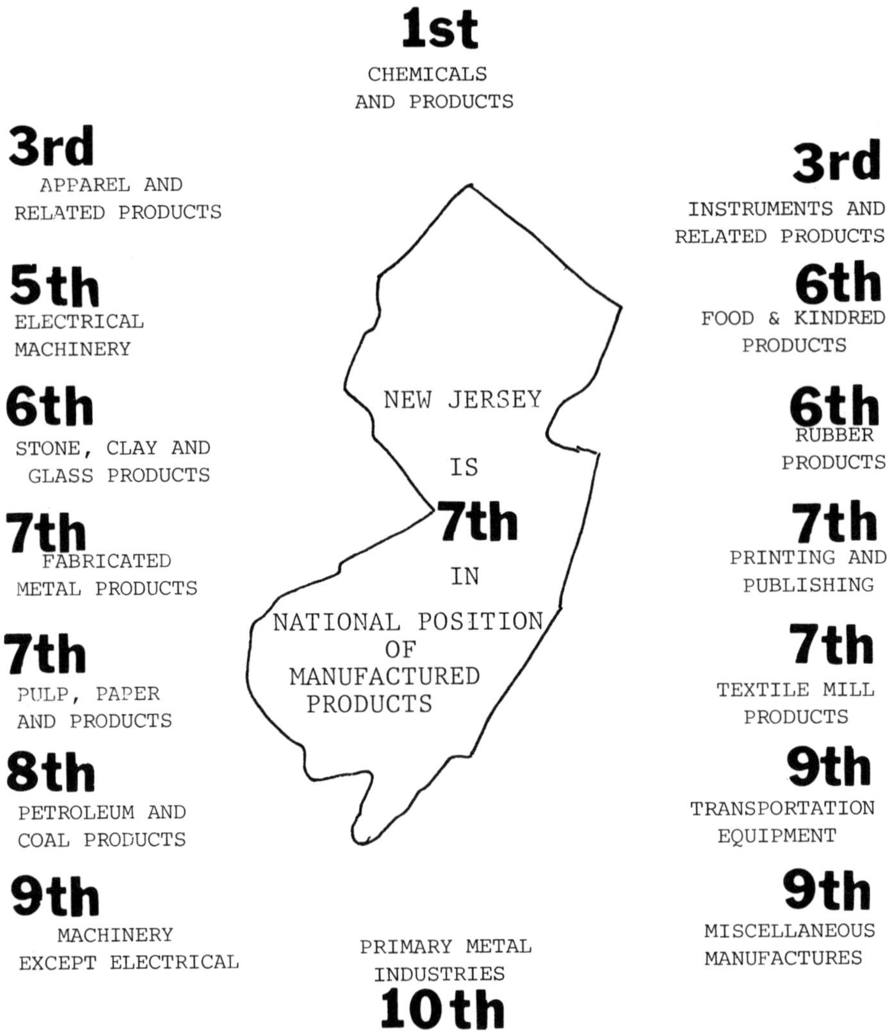

1st
CHEMICALS
AND PRODUCTS

3rd
APPAREL AND
RELATED PRODUCTS

5th
ELECTRICAL
MACHINERY

6th
STONE, CLAY AND
GLASS PRODUCTS

7th
FABRICATED
METAL PRODUCTS

7th
PULP, PAPER
AND PRODUCTS

8th
PETROLEUM AND
COAL PRODUCTS

9th
MACHINERY
EXCEPT ELECTRICAL

3rd
INSTRUMENTS AND
RELATED PRODUCTS

6th
FOOD & KINDRED
PRODUCTS

6th
RUBBER
PRODUCTS

7th
PRINTING AND
PUBLISHING

7th
TEXTILE MILL
PRODUCTS

9th
TRANSPORTATION
EQUIPMENT

9th
MISCELLANEOUS
MANUFACTURES

NEW JERSEY

IS

7th

IN

NATIONAL POSITION
OF
MANUFACTURED
PRODUCTS

PRIMARY METAL
INDUSTRIES
10th

FIGURE 7

SOURCE: New Jersey, Land of Industrial Advantages,
N.J. Department of Labor & Industry, Division of
Economic Development, Trenton, N.J., circa 1976.

by major occupation.   Perhaps now in the 20th century
the seal shown in the lower left hand corner of the
chapter frontispiece would be far more *appropriate*.
However, New Jersey is much more than industry. What,
if any peculiar characteristics, could be used to
describe New Jersey and its nearly 7.3 million residents? You may begin with the remarkably high average
population density -- 957 persons per square mile, the
highest of all the states.* The actual range spans a
low of 147 for Sussex County to a high of 13,094 for
Hudson County.[7]

New Jersey has been the subject of humor because
of the pig farm odors of Deptford Township, the flat-
lands of south Jersey and the tear inducing odors of
the industrial complex around exit 13 on the turnpike.

However, New Jersey is also a real fun place, a tour-
ist attraction, from which we have derived an income
just second to that provided by the chemical industry.
Pennsylvanians, lacking a marine coast line, flock to
the extensive New Jersey coast by the thousands yearly
and join residents at the recently opened gambling
casinos. The more than 800 lakes, fresh water fishing
and associated activities are also very popular attrac-
tions. The Delaware Bay attracts hosts of fishermen
and crabbers who can always tell tales about the
green-head flies if they come home empty handed. The
slowly recovering New York Shipbuilding Corporation
in south Jersey's Camden, once boasted of the construction of the revolutionary 1959 nuclear powered mer-
chant fleetship, the Savannah, and the aircraft
carrier Kitty Hawk.[8] On the academic side we boast
of 24 universities and colleges and some Nobel prize
winners.[9] Our environmental legislation protects
an area of some 970,000 acres with a distinctive pristine ecology, the "Pinelands." Similarly, our wet-
lands, seemingly worthless, swampy areas, provide important buffers of tidal energy and serve as marine
nurseries.

----

* Total area: 7,495.73 square miles

In the spring of 1976, the New Jersey coast was a
front page item as the public was given an opportunity
to approve or disapprove of offshore drilling for oil
and gas.[10] This activity helped to popularize another
little known east coast geographical feature, "the
Baltimore Canyon," a potentially oil and gas rich area.

Are we no longer the "Garden State"? In 1979 the
average dollar value of agricultural products sold per
acre was $373, four times the national average.[11] The
fruits of the labor of migrant workers, residents and
farmers brings in a dollar value equal to 2% of all
goods produced in the state. About 1/3 of our farm income comes from the raising of vegetables and they require a lot of hands at harvest time. We are still a
"gardening state." For more explicit, verbal pictures,
read John Cunningham's works and better yet -- come and
visit a diverse sociological, topological and ecologi-
cal environment yourself.

What has just been given is an encapsulated description of the New Jersey environment. Given that
cancers are environmental diseases, an examination of
the environment peculiar to New Jersey should ferret
out some causes. That is the purpose of this chapter,
to conduct an overview environmental assessment of the
state and to cite the types of cancers that could result from the exposure to the environment. Secondarily, this assessment is purposely separated into two
chapters: the occupational, industrial and institutional moiety, chapter 4, versus the personal, chapter
5. The latter, representing those instances where the
individual exercises considerable control over the
exposure; i.e., "carsuicide". This scheme is not
perfect and surely some will disagree in areas. Another
limitation is that the author certainly cannot out-do
the hopefully far more thorough analysis being conducted by those in the state responsible for this
immense project. At best, only an overview of the
potential impact of the New Jersey environment on the
state's cancer incidence and mortality rate can be
covered here.

TABLE 3

New Jersey - Income Sources

Industry	Income
Chemical Industry	$2,825,000,000
Tourism	2,500,000,000
Electrical Machinery Manufacturing	1,738,000
Food Processing	1,249,000,000
Agriculture	281,200,000
Industrial Research	200,000,000
Green House and Nursery Products	32,000,000
Mining	73,000,000
Fishing Industry	10,716,000

New Jersey Employment Distribution by Occupation

Trade	Number of Employees
Manufacturing	876,000
Wholesale and Retail	481,100
Services	358,300
Government	324,100
Transportation and Public Utilities	166,700
Construction	120,700
Finance, Insurance and Real Estate	107,700
Agriculture and Mining	36,600

SOURCE: World Book Encyclopedia, Field Enterprises Educational Co., Chicago, 1971.*

---

* 1980 statistics are not yet available. 1971 statistics are cited intentionally to reflect New Jersey income sources and occupation-distribution at that time.

117

In the disciplines of environmental science and epidemiology it is possible to present only the data favorable to the particular authors' or organization's viewpoint. Oft times there are minority viewpoints and contradictory data. Further, the evaluation of the carcinogenic nature of chemicals is an ongoing process and occasionally a considerable body of previously acceptable data are refuted due to improper test procedures or the use of impure test materials.[12, 13] For this purpose I have attempted to include some controversial test studies, at the risk of seeming equivocal. The reader is sternly advised that the strength of the data on the carcinogenicity, mutagenicity or tetratogenicity of a substance in humans or animals in vitro or in vivo does vary. And those qualifying adjectives must not be skipped over. For example:

- Who knows? We're not sure?
- It is suspected that x is linked to or associated with y.
- There is a suggestion that x is linked to or associated with y.
- x is linked to y.
- x is correlated to y.
- x is causally related to y!

Air Pollutants

In 1978 an estimated 5.6 million tons of the major air pollutants were released from sources within the state to the air.[14] The major air pollutants, particulate matter, oxides of sulfur, oxides of nitrogen and hydrocarbons, are currently recognized as potential carcinogens or cocarcinogens. These emissions have been quantified by the EPA. The area (ground level) and point (released from elevated sources) source emissions are summarized in Table 4. Any quantitative statements made about these emissions in this section exclude the concentration of carbon monoxide. The emissions in Table 4 represent those pollutants to

TABLE 4
NEW JERSEY AREA/POINT POLLUTANT EMISSIONS TONS PER YEAR

Emission Category		Particulates	Sulfur oxides	Oxides of Nitrogen	Hydrocarbons
Fuel Combustion (internal, external, combustion, power generation, space heating)	A	10,184	51,999	48,898	2,423
	P	15,185	180,355	100,918	1,996
Industrial Processes (chemicals, petrochemicals, metals, minerals)	P	38,294	59,428	30,243	281,002
Solid Waste Disposal (industrial, municipal, residential, commercial)	A	24,609	4,142	5,117	41,542
	P	1,050	295	336	563
Transportation (industrial, commercial privately owned vehicles)	A	225,540	20,973	273,110	388,012
Miscellaneous (fires, solvent evaporation)	A	87,989	11?	512?	336,289?
TOTAL	A/P	402,851	317,203	459,134	1,051,827

A=area source, P=point source. The arrows indicate the trend of change in the last two years.

SOURCE: 1975 National Emissions Report, EPA, Research Triangle Park, N.C., May 1978.

119

TABLE 5

NEW JERSEY STATE AIR POLLUTANT STANDARDS (CONDENSED)

Total Hydrocarbons	A non-criteria pollutant; typical annual average at Camden Laboratory 2ppm, 1968-1977.
Nitrogen Dioxide	The 12 consecutive month arithmetic mean concentration shall not exceed 100 micrograms/cu.m. or 0.05 ppm, primary and secondary standard. Typical annual average at Camden Laboratory was less than 0.05 ppm during 1975-1979.
Oxides of Nitrogen	A non-criteria pollutant. Typical annual average at Camden Laboratory ranged from 0.056-0.082 ppm, 1968-1978.
Sulfur Dioxide	Primary[2]. Twelve consecutive month arithmetic mean concentration not to exceed 80 micrograms/cu.m. or 0.03 ppm.
	Secondary[3]. Twelve consecutive month arithmetic mean not to exceed 60 micrograms/cu.m. or 0.02 ppm. Typical annual range at Camden Laboratory 0.017-0.038 (1975), 0.007-0.022 (1979).
Suspended Particulate matter	Primary. Twelve consecutive month geometric mean value of all 24 hour averages not to exceed 75 micrograms/cu.m.
	Secondary. Twelve consecutive month geometric mean value of all 24 hour averages not to exceed 60 micrograms per cubic meter. Typical South Jersey municipality (e.g., Salem, Camden, Woodbury and Cherry Hill) suspended particulate matter value was less than the primary standard. (Camden was less than the primary standard. Camden exceeded the primary limit almost throughout 1977.)

Notes:
1. Non-criteria pollutants do not have ambient air limits.
2. Primary air quality standards intend to protect public health.
3. Secondary air quality standards intend to protect public welfare.

SOURCE: New Jersey State Air Pollution Code

120

which virtually every state resident is exposed. Further they represent the largest categories of emissions to be quantified. Ambient air quality standards
have been set for these pollutants and those levels
are given in Table 5. For these reasons the evaluation of air in New Jersey begins with these "criteria
pollutants."

Hydrocarbons

    In the strictest sense of the definition, a hydro-
carbon is a chemical which contains only carbon and
hydrogen. In this section, a wide variety of organic
chemicals are also discussed in the context of hydrocarbons. Hydrocarbons represent the largest single
category of air pollutants released in the state of
New Jersey (see Table 4). Most of these emissions are
derived from the combustion of fossil fuels used for
private transportation and therefore, more properly,
will be discussed under "Personal Pollutants", in
chapter 5. However, a large quantity of hydrocarbons
are also released from industrial combustion processes.
The combustion of fossil fuels releases or forms a
class of compounds called polycyclic aromatic hydrocarbons (PAH), many of which are known animal carcinogens. Some of the PAH type constituents identified
in combustion products are:[15]

        Benzo[a]anthracene
        dibenzo (a,j)anthracene
        Benzo[b] fluoranthene
        Benzo(a)pyrene
        dibenzo [e,l]pyrene
        Indeno[1,2,3-cd]pyrene

Suggestive relationships have been made between communities with measureable quantities of benzo[a]pyrene
in the air and an increased incidence of lung
cancer.[16, 17] The DEP has conducted a preliminary
evaluation of PAH levels in Newark, Elizabeth, Rutherford and Camden. However, no conclusions have been
drawn on that limited data. In the context of occupational exposure to PAH's, petroleum refinery coke,

asphalt, coal-tar and pitch workers are examples of cohorts that have an increased risk for skin and bladder cancers. New Jersey petroleum refinery workers representing a rather large group at risk of cancers at many sites, will be discussed separately later on in this section. Another major source of hydrocarbons is from chemical and manufacturing processes; e.g., distillation, evaporation, degreasing, filtration, digestion and extraction procedures. Evaporation contributes a major portion of the hydrocarbons released from all of the industrial procedures just mentioned, particularly during degreasing operations. Workers have been exposed to some very toxic and carcinogenic vapors during degreasing operations; e.g., tetrachloroethylene, trichloroethylene, methyl chloride, benzene, and carbon tetrachloride. Based on the author's observations, certain degreasing operations in New Jersey such as dry cleaning, and auto body repairing, and printing shops, place workers and patrons alike to a risk of cancers due to exposure to solvent vapors. Retrospective epidemiological studies suggest an elevated risk for cancers of the liver, kidney, genitals, bladder and skin in dry cleaning workers.[18]

Priority Pollutants

In 1978 the EPA entered into a consent decree with several environmentalist organizations. As a result, 129 priority pollutants were listed, of which regulations would be established for 65 on discharge into national waterways. Many of these "priority pollutants" are toxic and carcinogenic chlorinated hydrocarbons. The volatility of some and the entrance of vapors into the air also render them a threat to acceptable air quality. Their impact on the state waterways will be discussed later on in this chapter. Volatile priority pollutants released from industrial processes are:

> haloethers
> acrylonitrile
> benzene

carbon tetrachloride
1,1,1 trichloroethane
chloroalkyl ethers
chloroform
dichlorobenzenes
diphenylhydrazine
trichloroethylene
nitrobenzene
nitrosamines
pentachlorophenols
phenol
phthalate esters
vinyl chloride

Priority Pollutant Analysis

The DEP (Office of Cancer and Toxic Substances
Research) has conducted a preliminary analysis of the
concentration of eleven of these priority pollutants
in selected northern New Jersey areas. Those data are
given in Table 6 and a table correlating the county
where measured may be found in the appendix. The DEP
does not consider these data as providing conclusive
answers about carcinogens in New Jersey's air. Although
these volatile substances are present at only trace
levels, qualitatively, they have the potential to
initiate tumors at many sites in the human body as indicated in Table 6. Of 20 volatile organic substances,
(vos), analyzed in a second DEP air monitoring program,
the following three were determined to be present at
average levels exceeding one ppb (part per billion by
volume):

benzene   - 2.63
toluene   - 4.64
O,M,P-xylene   - 4.35

Although the DEP considered the concentrations of
all 20 vos' to be below levels known to be toxic or
carcinogenic, they regarded their widespread presence
as *a cause for concern.*

Solid Waste Disposal

Most of the hydrocarbon emissions under solid waste are derived from residential burning and incineration and are more properly "personal pollutants." Industrial, municipal and commercial waste disposal does contribute carcinogens to the ambient air. Plastics, on incineration generate carcinogenic halogenated compounds. Rubber, more likely to be present in commercial and industrial wastes, generates PAH's on incineration. Flue-fed municipal incinerators contribute formaldehyde, an animal carcinogen*, to the ambient air, especially when not operating at optimum efficiency. Hazardous waste disposal facilities contribute the most toxic and carcinogenic emissions of all the solid waste disposal sources. These emissions are discussed separately later on in this chapter.

Miscellaneous Area Sources

Hydrocarbons from miscellaneous area sources are derived mainly from solvent evaporation accompanying industrial processes. Here again they represent the priority pollutants. Gasoline station evaporative losses in New Jersey amount to 33,851 tons yearly. American gasolines contain at least 1% (liquid volume) benzene; hence, a lot of these vapors contain benzene, a toxic, leukemogen.[20] Ambient benzene measurements at bulk marketing terminals indicated an overall average operating personnel exposure of 0.35 parts per million (ppm) and occasionally as high as 100-250 ppm.[21] Gasoline service station exposure levels have been determined to range about 0.3-3.2 ppm, nationally.[22] The U.S. Occupational Safety and Health exposure

---

* Formaldehyde is also a controversial human carcinogen.

TABLE 6

Summary of the Office of Cancer and Toxic Substances Research Volatile Substances Evaluation in Northern New Jersey Counties

Compound	Use	Site Specific Cancer, Other Hazard	Concentration PPbV
Benzene (benzol)	Major industrial intermediate Primary solvent, Gasoline additive, Pesticide ingredient	Confirmed leukemogen (mouse, Man) Liver, Kidney, lung damage Extremely toxic, Primary irritant (skin, eye, nose) Narcotic (CNS depressant)	3.21
Carbon Tetrachloride (tetrachloromethane)	Fire extinguisher, Drycleaning agent, Major solvent Grain fumigant/pesticide, Industrial intermediate	Liver cancer (mouse, hamster, rat) Mutagen, Very toxic, Kidney damage, Dermatitis, Visual disturbances	0.22
Chloroform (trichloromethane)	Anesthetic, Major solvent, Fire extinguisher ingredient Pesticide, Veterinary medicine	Liver cancer (mouse, hamster, rat) Moderately toxic, Dermatitis Irritant (eye, nose), Hypotension/myocardial depression, Central nervous system, paralysis after prolonged exposure, Releases phosgene gas when heated	0.69
ortho-Dichlorobenzene (1,2-dichlorobenzene) (1,4-DCB)	Major solvent, Insecticide, Degreaser (metal, leather, wool), Metal polisher ingredient, Dye, agrichemical intermediate	Liver, kidney injury, Moderately toxic, Primary irritant (skin, nose), Central nervous system depressant, Leukemia link cited, but based on insufficient evidence	0.46

125

TABLE 6 - continued

Summary of the Office of Cancer and Toxic Substances Research Volatile Substances Evaluation in Northern New Jersey Counties

Compound	Use	Site Specific Cancer, Other Hazard	Concentration PPbV
para-Dichlorobenzene (1,4-dichlorobenzene) (1,4-DCB)	Moth repellent, Space deoderizer, Dye, insecticide, pharmaceutical intermediate	Liver, bladder damage, Moderately toxic, Primary irritant (skin, eye, throat), Central nervous system depressant, Leukemia link cited, but based on insufficient evidence	0.36
1,2-Dichloroethane (ethylene dichloride) (EDC)	Chemical intermediate largely for vinyl chloride monomer), Solvent/degreaser Anti-knock gasoline additive Fumigant/insecticide	Stomach, breast, lung cancer (rat, mouse) Mutagen, Liver, kidney damage, Moderately toxic, Primary irritant (skin, eye, nose) Dermatitis, Narcotic	0.50
Nitrobenzene (nitrobenzol)	Manufacture of aniline, soap, shoe polish, Refining lubricating oils	Heart, liver, kidney damage, Extremely toxic, Primary irritant (skin), Central nervous system effects, Allergic reactions/sensitization	0.30
Tetrachloroethylene (perchloroethylene) (ethylene tetrachloride)	Drycleaning agent, Metal degreaser, Major solvent, Chemical intermediate Fumigant	Liver cancer (mouse) Moderately toxic, Dermatitis, Irritant (skin, eye, throat) Narcotic (CNS depressant)	0.88

126

TABLE 6 - continued

Summary of the Office of Cancer and Toxic Substances Research Volatile Substances Evaluation in Northern New Jersey Counties

Compound	Use	Site Specific Cancer, Other Hazard	Concentration PPbV
1,1,1-Tri-chloroethane (methylchloroform)	Cold type-metal, plastic mold cleaner, Chemical intermediate	Liver, kidney, lung damage, Reduced Growth, Irritant (eye, nose), Narcotic	0.24
Trichloro-ethylene (ethylene trichloride) (TCE) (tri)	Degreasing agent, Cleaning fluid ingredient, Medicine, food process, Paint, printing ink ingredient, Chemical, pharmaceutical intermediate, Grain fumigant Anesthetic	Liver, lung cancer (mouse) Mutagen, Kidney, liver, spleen damage, Toxic to central nervous system, Irritant (skin, eye, respiratory), Dermatitis, Narcosis	1.07
Vinyl Chloride (chloroethylene) (VCM) (VCI)	Intermediate for polyvinyl chloride and other resin Refrigerant, Additive to specialty coatings	Liver, brain, lung cancer (in Man) Lung, breast, liver cancer (mouse) Skin, lung, liver, kidney cancer (rat) Suspected mutagen, teratogen (Man), Cardiovascular effects Irritant (skin), Narcotic, Releases phosgene gas upon thermal decomposition	3.11

SOURCE: New Jersey DEP, Program on Environmental Cancer and Toxic Substances, Initial Report on Selected Volatile Organic Substances in Air, October 1979.

limit is 10 ppm, TWA** for an eight hour workday   forty
hour work week.

Fires

Fires and their resultant emissions could have
been discussed here. However, fires contribute more
particulates than hydrocarbons to the air as well and
will be discussed later on in this chapter.

Oxides of Nitrogen (NO_x)

Examination of Table 4 indicates that oxides of
nitrogen are the state's second major pollutant
emission category. More than 70% of the state's NO_x
emissions are derived from such activities as electric
energy generation, commercial, institutional and
industrial operations and solid waste disposal.
Transportation sources account for most of the balance
of the oxides of nitrogen emissions, with about half
of the NO_x being derived from private vehicles. Oxides
of nitrogen (NO_x) consist predominantly of nitric
oxide (99.5%) and are a well recognized air pollutant. On inhalation into moist lung alveoli, nitric
oxide is converted into the very irritating and corro-
sive nitrous and nitric acid.

Of concern here, however, is the reaction between
nitrous acid and amines to form compounds called
nitrosamines which are potent liver carcinogens. This
reaction is known to occur in the air in industrialized areas.[23] Further, nitrosamines as such are used
in several industries; e.g., organic chemical synthesis, rocket fuel manufacture and rubber processing.
It should be recalled that n-nitrosodimethylamine
(DMN), a potent carcinogen, was one of the chemicals
to be banned by S.3035. Mice fed a diet containing
only 50 ppm of DMN for a week developed lung and

** TWA = Time Weighted Average

kidney tumors. [24]

Nitrosamines are also found in foods, water, alcoholic beverages, consumer products and tobacco smoke. There are no data on the levels of concentration of this group of chemicals in the New Jersey environment and the acquisition of their data should be included in the DEP's Office of Cancer and Toxic Substances Research (OCTSR) program.* Until these data are available, the cancer risk to the public from nitrosamines in industrialized areas remains unqualified.

Particulate Emissions

Examination of Table 4 indicates that the state's particulate emissions are the third largest category of air pollutants. Approximately 57% of these emissions are derived from fuel combustion, industrial processes, and solid waste disposal. Transportation particulates are derived mainly from private vehicle use. They are discussed further in chapter 5. Particulate matter portends a dual environmental cancer hazard in that the particles may be comprised of an inorganic (i.e., metallic) and organic (e.g., a PAH) moiety. Another factor that enhances their adverse nature is that airborne PAH's occur in a particle size range not efficiently removed by the respiratory system defense mechanisms (discussed in chapter 3). The EPA list of 129 priority pollutants cites 13 metals as toxic pollutants. Several, as indicated earlier, are known or suspect carcinogens. Under the New Jersey state DEP program (OCTSR), an initial evaluation of airborne particulate emissions has been conducted in selected northern state counties. Table 7 summarizes those data and a complete table indicating the specific counties is given in the appendix.

---

* Preliminary attempts by the DEP to measure N,N-Dimethyl-nitrosamine were unsuccessful.

TABLE 7
SUMMARY OF OCTSR DATA, SELECTED HEAVY METALS IN NORTHERN NEW JERSEY COUNTIES

Use/Source	Cite Specific Cancer Other Hazard	Concentration, ug/m³ in New Jersey Avg.	Max.	Concentration ug/m³ in a Typical City	OSHA Permissible Exposure Limit ug/m³
Arsenic — Coal combustion, pesticide and fungicide manufacture, glass manufacture, shale oil production, copper smelting, cigarette smoke	Skin, lung, lymphatic cancer (Humans) Teratogen (hamsters)	0.28	6.03	0.02-1.4	10 (inorganic) 0.5ug/m³ (organic)
Cadmium — Zinc smelting, sewage sludge, phosphate fertilizers, fungicides, plastics incineration, electroplating operations, storage batteries, cigarette smoke	Suspected cause of prostate cancer (Humans) Bone disease, kidney dysfunction, anemia	0.005	0.079	rural 0.01 urban 0.05	200 dust 100 fume
Lead — Automotive exhaust emissions, lead smelting, refining, brass manufacture, paint manufacture, paint formulations, plastics incineration	Anemia, learning and memory impairment, neuromuscular disorders, visual and auditory impairment, irritability (Limited data on adenomas and carcinomas in rats.)A	0.75	11.30	urban avg. 1-3, up to 44 in tunnels	50,000

TABLE 7 - continued

SUMMARY OF OCTSR DATA, SELECTED HEAVY METALS IN
NORTHERN NEW JERSEY COUNTIES

	Use/Source	Cite Specific Cancer Other Hazard	Concentration, μg/m³ in New Jersey Avg.	Max.	Concentration μg/m³ in a Typical City	OSHA Permissible Exposure Limit μg/m³
Manganese	Automotive exhaust emissions, fossil fuel combustion, dry-cell battery manufacture	Central nervous system deterioration, lethargy (Limited date on lympho-sarcomas in mice.)B	0.30	0.289	---	5,000
Mercury	Mining, refining processes, chloralkali plants, agricultural practices, fossil fuel combustion, paper, pulp, plastics, electronics industry	Linked to cerebral palsy, mental retardation, central nervous system disorders in humans.	0.003	0.011	---	100
Nickel	Fossil fuel combustion, nickel production, storage battery production, asbestos processing	Linked to cancer of the lung, nasal, sinus cavities and larynx in humans	0.16	3.81	0.03-0.12	1,000 (inorganic) 7 (organic as carbonyl)

131

TABLE 7 - continued
SUMMARY OF OCTSR DATA, SELECTED HEAVY METALS IN NORTHERN NEW JERSEY COUNTIES

Use/Source	Cite Specific Cancer Other Hazard	Concentration, $\mu g/m^3$ in New Jersey Avg.	Max.	Concentration $\mu g/m^3$ in a Typical City	OSHA Permissible Exposure Limit $\mu g/m^3$
zinc Biocide applications, dry cell battery production, galvanized iron, paint, rubber, glass and paper manufacture	Respiratory irritant, fever producing agent in humans.	0.31	1.29	up 0.08	1,000 zinc chloride 5,000 zinc oxide

A. Kraybill, H.F. and Mehlman, Myron A., Advances in Modern Toxicology, Vol. 3, Environmental Cancer, John Wiley & Sons, New York, 1977

B. Shottenfeld, David, M.D. and Haas, Joanna F., M.D., Carcinogens in the Workplace, CA-A Cancer Journal for Clinicians, Vol. 29, No. 3, May/June 1979. American Cancer Soc., Inc.

SOURCES: Adapted mainly from N.J. DEP Program on Environmental Cancer and Toxic Substances, Initial Report on Selected Heavy Metals in Air, October 1979, and other miscellaneous sources. See references to Kraybill/Mehlman and Shottenfeld/Haas.

The DEP has well selected the metals listed in Table 7 as they represent some of the most important and potentially hazardous airborne pollutants. The study indicates, as suspected, that lead is the most ubiquitous particulate in urban areas of northern New Jersey. The only pollutant subject to a National Ambient Air Quality Standard in this study is lead, and that limit is 1.5 $\mu g/m^3$.* The maximum value found in this study, 11.30 is 7.5 times greater than the recommended level. Based on the ubiquitous nature of this environmental pollutant, the high levels found in the preliminary study and also the number of facilities producing lead chemicals in New Jersey, the DEP should continue to evaluate lead levels in the environment. Emphasis should be placed on determining lead levels in the communities (and inside houses) adjacent to the facilities listed in Table 8, representative of lead related industries in New Jersey.

TABLE 8
LEAD CHEMICAL MANUFACTURERS IN NEW JERSEY

Chemical	Company/Location in N.J.	Uses
Lead emissions	National Lead Industries**, Pedricktown	Automobile battery salvage
Lead alkyls	E.I., Dupont de Nemours & Co., Inc., Deepwater	Fuel anti-knock additives

---

* quarterly average

** National Lead Industries has been cited many times by the DEP for air and water pollution. Hundreds of residents have been tested for lead poisoning; however, no cases have been detected yet.

TABLE 8 - continued
LEAD CHEMICAL MANUFACTURERS IN NEW JERSEY

Chemical	Company/Location in N.J.	Uses
Lead arsenate	Dimensional Pigments, Inc. Rond Pearl, Inc., Bayonne	Insecticides/ herbicides
Lead benzoate	City Chemical Corp., Jersey City	Insecticides/ herbicides
Lead dioxide	Hummel Chemical Co., Inc. South Plainfield	Batteries, curing agents, textile mordants
Lead naphthanate	Troy Chemical Corp., Newark	Wood preservatives, lube oil additives
Lead oleate	The Norac Co., Inc./Mathe Division, Lodi	Varnishes

SOURCE: Status Assessment of Toxic Chemicals - Lead, EPA - 600/2-79-210h, Dec. 1979

The data on the concentrations of the known carcinogens, arsenic, cadmium and nickel (in specific chemical states) are most significant; however, little are known about their long-term health effects. Hence, there are no recommended ambient levels to compare these emissions against. When compared against OSHA standards, i.e., the workplace, a confined or defined environment, none of these three carcinogens exceeds safe limits. However, toxicity is not translatable to carcinogenicity.

The role of particle site in the inhalation of
particulate matter was discussed in chapter 3. The
average percent metals, described in Table 7, which
fall within the range which is not readily removed
by lung filtration systems, are summarized below:

Average Percent Metals in 1.1-0 micron
size range

Lead	49
Zinc	21
Cadmium	28
Arsenic	28
Manganese	37
Nickel	41
Mercury	10

Again, it is lead, the most ubiquitous airborne metal
particulate, that poses the major threat to the
respiratory system (on a quantitative basis). The DEP
(Office of Cancer and Toxic Substances Research) conducted a second heavy metals analyses and the highest
overall microgram concentrations (found in that study)
are summarized below:

Lead	0.976
Arsenic	0.186
Manganese	0.035
Nickel	0.235
Cadmium	0.007
Mercury	0.0008

Overall ambient lead levels in the Camden, Elizabeth,
Linden, Newark and Rutherford areas did not exceed
the national ambient air quality standard. However,
the DEP regards the continued presence of all six
heavy metals with their potential long-term, chronic
health effects, as *a cause for concern*.

Sulfur Oxides

Sulfur oxides emissions represent the state's
smallest emission category of the principal quantifi-

able air pollutants. Fuel combustion, industrial processes and solid waste disposal account for 87% of
these sulfur dioxide emissions. This ancient pollutant
is an eye and upper respiratory irritant that may
also cause cough, lung edema and pneumonia. Of
specific importance here is the cilatoxic action of
sulfur dioxide. The cumulative effect of cilatoxic
agents such as sulfur dioxide is an interference with
mucocilliary transport -- a condition which favors
lung neoplasia.[25]

Hazardous Waste Disposal

    There appears to be no valid documentation for
the number of hazardous waste generators in the state
of New Jersey. As of November 1979, the DEP could
account for 813 through the manifest system, but
indicates there may be as many as 10,000.[26] At least
720,000 "documented tons" of hazardous or special
wastes result from industrial operations in New
Jersey each year.[27] Although some generators of
these wastes treat them on-site, most ship them off-
site. There are 20 commercial off-site and 24 on-site
waste treatment facilities in New Jersey.[28] According
to the DEP, "virtually all of these New Jersey facilities have experienced operational mishaps and violations of environmental standards at one time or
another."[29] When a resource recovery strategy is not
practical, hazardous wastes are treated as indicated
in Table 9.

    The use of these technologies at waste treatment
facilities has resulted in varying degrees of human
exposure to toxic and carcinogenic chemicals. Plant
personnel are exposed to toxic and carcinogenic substances as a result of the use of all four methods
cited in Table 9. Community residents are exposed to
toxins and carcinogens directly and indirectly as a
result of biological degradation, landfilling/compost-
ing and incineration. Landfilling and subsequent
leaching of toxic and carcinogenic chemicals are a
serious problem in New Jersey. These water-related
problems are discussed later on in this chapter.

Incineration is recognized as the "technology of choice" for the degradation of extremely stable organic compounds.[30] Although incineration efficiencies of 99.5-99.9%* have been cited under experimental and ideal conditions, there is great public and scientific concern over possible incinerator malfunction.[31] Further, there is great need for on-site qualitative and quantitative identification of the fraction of chemicals leaving incinerator stacks intact.

TABLE 9
HAZARDOUS WASTE TREATMENT

Method	Treatment	Environmental Impact
Chemical/physical	neutralization, precipitation, oxidation, reduction, carbon sorption sedimentation, evaporation	localized air pollution at facility
Biological degradation	Anerobic/aerobic lagoons, stabilization basins, trickling filters	Local and community air pollution
Landfilling/composting	soil absorption	local and community air, soil water pollution fires

---

* At 1200 degrees celsius and an incinerator residence time of at least two seconds.

TABLE 9 - continued
HAZARDOUS WASTE TREATMENT

Method	Treatment	Environmental Impact
Incineration	high temperature combustion (more than 1200 degrees celsius)	local and community air pollution, chemical fallout

The Rollins Environmental Services (Logan Township Branch), the major hazardous waste treatment facility in the state, has applied for a permit to incinerate a class of compounds called polychlorinated biphenyls (PCB's).*[32] These extremely stable chemicals have served many useful purposes since their initial synthesis by the Monsanto Company in 1930; capacitor and transformer dielectrics, heat exchangers, hydraulic fluids, and carbonless copy paper. However, as a result of numerous accidental environmental contamination episodes and laboratory studies, PCB's have been determined to cause the following effects:[33, 34]

Effects of PCB Poisoning

In Humans		In Animals
Chloracne	Headaches	Topical application results in death in guinea pigs, liver degeneration and hepatomas in mice
Increased skin pigmentation	Liver dysfunction	
Increased eye discharge	Anorexia	
Lethargy		
Numbness		

---

* Monsanto trademark is Arclor (e.g., Arclor 1254 contains 54% chlorine).

There is also evidence to demonstrate a "possible link" between exposure to PCB's and cancers (melanoma, sarcoma and myeloma).[35] All PCB's contain trace quantities of another extremely toxic chemical, dioxin.[36]

Further, dioxin has been demonstrated to be a photodecomposition product of PCB's. Hence, anyone in the vicinity of an incinerator "degrading" PCB's will be exposed to a "fractional" quantity of PCB's and dioxin. Another product of the incomplete degradation of PCB's is hexachlorobenzene (lindane) which causes liver and capillary tumors in hamsters.[37, 38]

Just how much PCB would you be exposed to if you lived in the vicinity of an incinerator? Studies show that the dispersion from a 100 meter stack incinerating PCB's would result in an ambient ground level concentration range of 39 to 164 ng/m^3, within a 1.5 to 15 kilometer range of the stack. Average urban/metropolitan air concentrations of PCB's typically do not exceed 39 ng/m^3.[40] Are we free from PCB's in New Jersey without incineration? No, they constantly degas from landfills and capacitor manufacturer establishments. The subject of bioaccumulation in local flora and fauna of PCB's, which is not well understood, is a dissertation topic in itself.

PCB's are only being used here as a model for the environmental problem that incineration presents. Literally, thousands of organic compounds almost as stable and more toxic than PCB's are being incinerated at four sites (including Rollins) in New Jersey:[41]

> DuPont Corp., Chambers Works,
> Deepwater, Salem County
> American Cyanamid, Linden, Union County
> Hercules, Inc., Parlin, Middlesex County
> Rollins Environmental Services, Logan Township Branch, Bridgeport

The societal and psychological aspects and long-term environmental impacts of a hazardous waste disposal facility are discussed at length in chapter 8.

Hazardous Waste Chemical and Petrochemical Spills

The dual terms of hazardous waste chemical and petrochemical spills really form a hybrid category. These substances may vary from very non-volatile solids and pressurized gases to extremely volatile liquids. When these materials are present, there may be vaporization and a concomitant air pollution impact, absorption in soil and depending on the volume of the spill and soil permeability, surface or ground water pollution. Further, all these events may continue to occur as a function of time, e.g., rain may release soil bound pollutants or pollute a waterway due to run-off. During the first 15 months* activity of the DEP's Office of Hazardous Waste Substances Control (OHSC), there were 1642 verified spills.[42] Twenty-nine percent required OHSC assistance and about 189,000 gallons of an estimated 1.6 million gallons were cleaned up. May it be assumed that the remaining 1.4 million gallons distributed itself in the various places in the environment described above? Some of the more toxic and carcinogenic spill chemicals were benzene, formaldehyde, PCB's, styrene, trichloroethylene and pesticides. However, petroleum and petroleum products made up the greatest spill volume. There is no way to assess the cancer risk to those coming in contact with these spilled materials whose volumes and concentrations are ill-defined. Nonetheless, in total they represent an identifiable category of environmental carcinogens constituting a cancer risk in New Jersey.

Fires

Background

The major direct and immediate loss of life in fire situations is due to asphyxiation by carbon monoxide, oxygen depression and tissue damage due to

---

* April 1, 1977 through June 30, 1978.

the heat.   Of concern here are the combustion products of materials other than the ubiquitous paper
and wood of the environment that represent a cancer
risk for the survivors of fires, fire fighters and
community residents.   This is not to say that wood
or paper form no carcinogens on combustion; e.g.,
wood combustion releases about 80 ppm of the suspect
carcinogen formaldehyde.[43]   However, in the residential and industrial fire it is plastics combustion,
particularly of polyethylene, polystyrene, and polyvinyl chloride that generate carcinogenic decomposition products.   Polyethylene and related plastics,
used in the manufacture of rugs, bedding and furniture, form paraffinic hydrocarbons on decomposition.[44]   Polystyrene, used in many household goods
including toys, refrigerators and packaging materials,
degrades to the suspect carcinogen monomer styrene.[45]
Polystyrene also forms the leukemogen benzene upon
decomposition.   Polyvinyl chloride, a major commercial plastic used in electrical insulation, furniture
manufacture, flooring materials and packaging, releases the carcinogenic monomer vinyl chloride on
decomposition.[46]   Formaldehyde, which causes cancer
in rats, "offgases" from urea formaldehyde foams
(UFF) at room temperature.   Under fire conditions,
this reaction is enhanced.

In addition to the carcinogens discussed above
formed during residential fires, the fire fighter is
exposed to the decomposition products formed during
fuel oil and chemical industry type fires.   As discussed earlier, the combustion of any fossil fuel
generally results in the formation of certain recognized carcinogens (e.g., benzo[a]pyrene).   Studies
on the chemical analysis of the soot formed in the
breathing zone of fire school instructors as a result
of diesel oil number 2 combustion, indicated the presence of several polycyclic aromatic hydrocarbons.[47]
In that same study, benzene, styrene and naphthalene
were also found in atmospheric grab samples.   Eighty
percent of the soot particles measured were less than
one micron in size, indicating their degree of potential entrapment in the lungs.

Fires in New Jersey

The combustion products formed in residential fires in New Jersey probably do not differ from fires elsewhere. State-wide, it is likely that more lead particulate is formed in some of the older homes of high density urban areas. It is the institutional, chemical and petroleum industry type fire peculiar to New Jersey because of their great numbers, that results in the dispersion of carcinogens, both intact and rearranged structurally by the intense heat. Civil defense and DEP authorities are usually aware of the possible formation of toxic and carcinogenic compounds formed in the smoke by these fires -- when they know what's burning. And that's the problem -- they are not always advised by plant owners, who themselves are frequently not available!

One of two contrasting fire episodes was a Weehawken pier fire, March 1980, where thousands of curiosity seekers watched and were exposed to concomitant emissions of an unknown nature.[48] In like manner, a Perth Amboy industrial park fire in July of 1980 fueled by 2,000 drums of hazardous solvents resulted in the early dismissal of 2,000 area workers.[49] However, fire chief Rick Kharman reportedly sat on the sidewalk eating a sandwich commenting "You take your chances and do what you gotta do." Area residents vied for risk honors along with Kharman, declining to evacuate the area. One of the most spectacular fires in recent times in New Jersey occurred at the now well-known Chemical Control Corporation in Elizabeth, New Jersey in April, 1980.[50] The fire at this three acre site, a controversial hazardous waste disposal facility, created smoke and fumes that threatened residents of Elizabeth as well as those of Staten Island and New York. Some of the reported 50,000 barrels of hazardous wastes stored there contained acids, bases, nitroglycerine, azides, perchlorates, picric acid, nitrocellulose and drums of sodium metal.

The gases formed in these fires usually dissipate in a few hours to a few days depending on weather

conditions.   The DEP conducted a particulate analysis
of ambient air during a Newark warehouse fire in
January of 1979.[51]   In this instance no unusually
high levels of metals were determined to be present.
However, according to the literature, particulates
are usually present in high concentration at fires.[52]
Further, particulates may bear absorbed polycyclic
aromatic hydrocarbons.   With the heavy concentration
of chemical industry in the state, especially in
northern New Jersey, fire emissions analysis require
further evaluation.   Fire emissions also quickly become
indoor pollutants and those kinetics are also worthy
of study.

    Due to the more recent knowledge of the air
contaminants fire fighters are exposed to and the use
of self-contained breathing apparatus, smoke inhalation incidents are being greatly reduced.[53]   The
cancer risk to firefighters is probably past its peak
(assuming they elect to take advantage of all available safety equipment).   However, many firefighters
in New Jersey have not yet exhibited the symptoms
which may ultimately result from previous exposures.

Asbestos

    Background

    The well-known properties of asbestos; i.e.,
ability to withstand friction, acid attack, heat,
flexibility and exceptional textile strength, have
well been exploited by science and technology.
Chemically, asbestos is a calcium, magnesium silicate
mineral occurring in two groups:[54]

            serpentine (chrysotile), the most widely
            used form, and amphibole which contains
            the minerals anthophyllite, amosite,
            crocidolite, tremolite and actinolite.

The irony of the use of asbestos is that a material
which has been synonymous with safety and protection

has now been determined to cause site-diverse cancers;
lung, pleural (lung cavity lining) and peritoneal*
mesothelioma, and gastro-intestinal.

The routes of absorption have been established
to be by ingestion** or inhalation.[55], [56], [57] The
time for manifestation of symptoms varies from fifteen
to fifty years. All types of asbestos fibers have
produced malignant tumors in animals by many routes
of administration. Asbestos has been determined to
be contaminated with trace quantities of hydrocarbons,
nickel and chromium and the converse is somewhat
true.[58] For example, asbestos has been found to con-
taminate talc coated rice, marketed on the west coast
of the United States.[59] In 1976 a TLV for exposure to
asbestos of two fibers/cc was established.[60] NIOSH
has recommended a lowering of the workplace standard
to 0.1 fibers per cubic centimeter of air.

Asbestos - Distribution and Diseases in New Jersey

In 1941, U.S. Navy requirements for asbestos
insulation led to the establishment of the Union
Asbestos and Rubber Company in Paterson, New Jersey.
933 men employed between 1941-1945 have become an
unfortunate but important epidemiological study group.
Dr. Selikoff and associates at the Mount Sinai School
of Medicine have been monitoring the health of 582
former plant workers since the period 1961-1965.[61], [62]
These workers had completed a twenty year lapse since
employment. In 1971, Dr. Selikoff and associates
concluded that based on the study of this cohort:

> "Occupational exposure to amosite asbestos
> can be associated with serious hazard of
> lung cancer, pleural and peritoneal
> mesothelioma, pulmonary asbestos and

---

* Abdominal and pelvic cavity lining

** Currently regarded as a risk and related with statistical
significance, but not causally related.

perhaps cancer of the stomach, colon and
rectum."

Dr. Selikoff and associates continued their
observation of the original 582 workers and by 1971,
304 additional deaths had occurred. Dr. Selikoff
and his associates concluded that the combination of
tobacco use and asbestos exposure increased the lung
cancer incidence by a factor of 80! Further, asbestos
employment of *one* month results in a clear excess
cancer risk, and the longer the exposure, the greater
the risk.

One of several prospective studies being conducted by Dr. Selikoff and associates is sponsored
by the International Chemical Workers Union. X-ray
examination of plant maintenance employees of American
Cyanamid's Bound Brook, New Jersey, facility indicated a high incidence of asbestos-related lung
diseases.[63] Dr. Selikoff reported that 48% of the
more than 20 year employee and 16% of less than 20
year employee population had asbestosis. Bound
Brook plant employees handle asbestos treated pipe
insulation material and the study indicated the need
for evaluation of all asbestos containing products.
In April 1980, the Occupational Safety and Health
Administration investigated and cited two south
Jersey DuPont plants (Repaupo and Deepwater) for
several employee asbestos exposure offences:[64, 65]

- willful violation of the OSHA asbestos
  exposure limit
- failing to report worker job-related
  asbestosis to OSHA
- failure to provide OSHA with employee
  records
- failure to notify employees who worked
  with asbestos about the results of
  plant medical tests
- failure to keep accurate records
- failure to provide protective clothing
  or install air purifiers

The DuPont Company does not manufacture asbes-

tos; however, employees did use asbestos tank and
pipe insulation.

The cancer risk due to asbestos exposure certainly does not end at the periphery of the manufacturing plant. Workers transport asbestos home
via their clothes, hair, and lunch boxes. Anderson
and associates demonstrated the viability of "household contact" in the etiology of asbestos induced
cancers.[66] These researchers concluded that of a
study group of 326 "healthy household contacts of
amosite asbestos workers examined 25-30 years after
the onset of presumed household contamination with
amosite asbestos, 35% had chest x-ray abnormalities
(pleural and/or parenchyma) characteristic of
asbestos exposure."

Former asbestos plant workers and spouses continue to file massive class action suits against
asbestos manufacturers and users. The Raybestos-
Manhattan, Inc., Passaic, New Jersey plant closed in
1973, after nearly 120 years of operation.[67] They
manufactured a wide range of asbestos containing products. That they employed 2,000 workers at the peak
of their operation clearly demonstrates the amount of
asbestos their operations must have distributed
throughout northern New Jersey.

In June 1975, about 307 former plant workers and
spouses entered into a class action suit against
Raybestos-Manhattan, Inc. They claimed they were not
advised of the danger of asbestos exposure which
resulted in their contracting asbestosis and lung
cancers. By the fall of 1980 there were about 1,100
asbestos damage suits filed by shipyard, insulation,
construction, and auto workers alone in New Jersey
federal courts.[68] Johns-Manville and Raybestos-Manhattan, Inc. were the principal defendants; however,
Owens-Corning Fiberglass (Berlin, New Jersey) and
Research Cottrell, Inc. (Bridgewater, New Jersey)
are also involved in litigation.

Navy Oriented Exposure/Sources

Asbestos has a long history of use in or near
New Jersey in conjunction with the shipbuilding
industry. For example, workers at the Philadelphia
Navy Yard have been crossing the Delaware River since
1804. However, asbestos use dates back to 1929.
Direct exposure and "household contact" for south
Jersey yard workers and families may be said to have
begun at that time. Subsequent construction of the
several bridges linking New Jersey with New York,
Pennsylvania and Delaware only enhanced the asbestos
transport.

Public Buildings

The search for asbestos in schools and other
public places in New Jersey began in 1977, when a
physician diagnosed an elementary school student's
respiratory illness as asbestos poisoning.[69] Over-
night, an asbestos ceiling hunt began and still continues. Asbestos was used as an insulation in public
schools and buildings constructed in New Jersey
between the years 1950 and 1973. Ultimately, some of
the ceilings in the state's 2,500 public schools would
be removed or sealed, straining the financial structure of some school budgets. Asbestos installed as
tiles and insulation does not pose a health hazard as
when asbestos is sprayed on. This latter process
does not encapsulate the fibers which may become
airborne on flaking and fraying. However, Johns-
Manville says "the facts are that the use of asbestos spray materials in the construction of schools or
other public buildings has not been shown to be
hazardous."[70]

Housing

Although federal regulations banned the use of
applied asbestos in 1973, a decorative use loophole
persists. For example, "K-spray", a ceiling texture
paint, containing asbestos, was used in the Winston
Towers Apartments in Palisades, New Jersey.[71] Although EPA tests indicated dangerous amounts of asbestos

in the air of those apartments, in late 1976 the
decorative use loophole prevented them from taking
any action, short of attempting to halt sales at the
condominium. Again, asbestos litigation is in process by tenants against the condominium developers
and the asbestos texture paint manufacturers.

Landfilling and Transport

Of the 720 metric tons of asbestos processed for
domestic use in the U.S. (1972), 182 metric tons
were disposed of principally by solid waste landfilling and incineration.[72] Both processes result in
some dispersion of asbestos into both air and water.
Take a brief glimpse at first quarter 1979 excerpts
of the New Jersey hazardous waste disposal manifest
log for asbestos:

Facility	Quantity, Pounds
Marvin Jonas (Sewell)	142,344
(a transfer station)	
Modern Transportation	45,000
(Kearney)	(all in 1978)
Kinsley Landfill	20,000
(Deptford)	
Unknown (exactly as listed)	156,080
Rollins Environmental	7,430
Services (Bridgeport)	

Community Cancer Risk

Clearly, a lot of asbestos has been moving through
the New Jersey environment. Couple the exposures
discussed with the state's extensive highway system,
normal brakelining disintegration, contact with asbestos containing consumer products (lawn furniture, hair
dryers), and what is the conclusion? Airborne asbestos ranked highly, up to about the late 1970's, as
a major environmental carcinogen in New Jersey. Even
into the '80's, industrial exposure to asbestos continues.

Studies show that average urban asbestos levels

exceed those of non-urban areas (29 ng/m^3 vs. 1 ng/m^3).
Further, since there has been a higher concentration
of asbestos industries in northern New Jersey, the
cancer risk due to asbestos exposure both occupationally and communally would be higher in those areas. The
ability of waterborne asbestos fibers to induce cancers
has been a subject of controversy. However, at least
one recent epidemiological study shows a significant
relationship between waterborne chrysotile asbestos
consumption and white male lung/white female gall-
bladder and pancreas and peritoneal cancers in both
sexes. With so much attention being given deservedly
to chlorinated hydrocarbon and heavy metal water
pollution in New Jersey, little has been given to
asbestos leachate.

The determination of asbestos in certain select
areas should be a top priority for the DEP, namely;

> groundwater supplies adjacent to landfills
> urban/suburban communities adjacent to
> asbestos industries

Amines, Dyes and Related Compounds

Organic chemicals consisting of an amino (NH_2)
group bound to a cyclic or straight chain hydrocarbon are called amines. An entire industry is
based on their ability to couple with other organic
compounds, e.g., diazotisation, forming several types
of dyes. There is a long history of both laboratory
and epidemiological studies demonstrating the ability
of these compounds to cause bladder cancers:[73, 74]

> 1895 - bladder tumors associated with the
> industrial use of benzidine type dyes
> 1906 - dyes determined to induce animal
> tumors (Fisher)
> 1906 - dyes determined to induce animal
> tumors (Kinosita)
> 1928 - B-naphthylamine causes high
> bladder cancer incidence in

                    rubber industry, tire and electric
                    cable workers
        1949 - epidemiological study of 186
                    workmen demonstrates benzidine
                    and B-naphthylamine are potent
                    carcinogens

In spite of this growing body of data, B-naphthylamine
use continued up until 1972. Benzidine is used in
the manufacture of numerous organic chemicals, as a
rubber compounding agent, an azo dye intermediate,
and a reagent in analytical and clinical laboratories.[75] Similar to the biochemical properties of
other amines, benzidine induces the formation of
malignancies, specifically in the bladder. And the
mean survival time after diagnosis of the malignancy
is only three years in humans.[76] Derivatives of
benzidine, which contain names such as azoic, disperse and direct dyes are degraded by enzymes, intestinal bacteria and the liver to the parent compound --
benzidine. Hence, the derivatives are just as carcinogenic.[77]

    In addition to manufacturing, forensic, clinical
and waste water exposure risks, benzidine exists as a
contaminant in many benzidine derived azo dyes.*[78]
It is estimated that these dyes are used by over 300
manufacturers of textiles, papers, clothing, leather
goods and consumer dye packets. Another potent bladder
specific carcinogen, 4-aminodiphenyl, was formerly used
as a rubber anti-oxidant and dye intermediate.
Current usage is limited to research.[79] Two other
carcinogenic dyes whose target organ is the bladder,
are auramine (yellow) and magenta (red). Many hair
dyes have been determined to cause cancer in laboratory rats and mice.[80] Their cancer risk could have
been discussed later on under "consumer products" in
chapter 5; however, their use is probably not inordi-
nate in New Jersey.

----

* Actual limit 20 ppm, in practice less than 10 ppm.

Bladder Cancer in New Jersey

Several bladder cancer epidemiological studies
in the United States have demonstrated clearly that
New Jersey has a pronounced bladder cancer problem.[81, 82] During the period 1950-1969, eighteen of
twenty-one counties manifested bladder cancer mortality rates in the highest 10% of all U.S. counties.
Further, the bladder cancer mortality rate in Salem
County, 16.1% (per 100,000 white male population),
was highest among all U.S. counties with a white population of at least 10,000. The heavy concentration
of chemical industry in the state "may account" for
these elevated bladder cancer rates.[83] Figure 8 shows
the Salem County bladder cancer mortality rate versus the rest of the state from 1950-1969.[84] Particularly suspect is the DuPont Company which employs
nearly 25% of Salem County's population. The DuPont
Company concedes to "upwards of 300 cases" of bladder
tumor among DuPont employees exposed to B-naphthylamine.[85] The unit producing this dye was shut down
in 1955. DuPont continued to synthesize dyes from
B-naphthylamine utilizing a closed manufacturing system and claims no employee who worked with this new
unit has developed a bladder tumor. Twenty-four other
carcinogens that present occupational hazards at
various sites have been identified by the DuPont
Haskell Laboratories.[86] That the company conducted
this research indicates that at least some of these
chemicals are in use or were in their New Jersey
operations.

The 1981 New Jersey epidemiology study, cited at
the end of chapter 1, indicates that bladder cancer
continues to be a major cause of cancer mortality for
New Jersey males over the period 1949-1975. However,
both male and female age-adjusted bladder cancer
mortality rates show a significant decline over that
same period. On a county basis, Salem continued to
express a bladder cancer mortality rate in excess of
the state rate (15.70/100,000), for the period 1962-
1975.

FIGURE 8
RATIOS OF NEW JERSEY COUNTY MORTALITY RATES TO THE U.S.
MORTALITY RATE: CANCER OF THE BLADDER 1950 - 1969
white males - U.S. rate

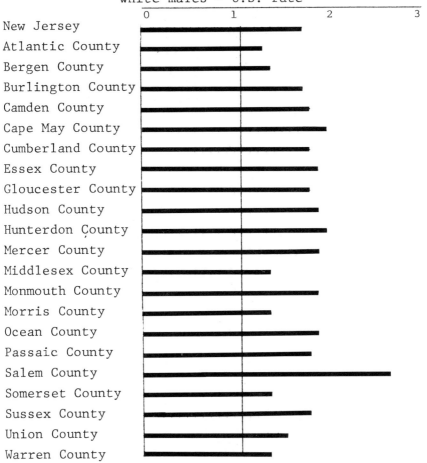

Key: Relative ratio of 1=no difference between
N.J. rates & U.S. average rates.
Prepared by the Public Health Statistics Program
New Jersey State Department of Health

Another recent Department of Health, state bladder cancer survey (1979) indicates that bladder cancer deaths for white and non-white males, and white and non-white females during the period 1972-75, were again above the national average.[87] Additionally, bladder cancer deaths in white males continued to be prevalent in Salem, Gloucester, Cumberland, Ocean, Burlington, Warren, Morris and Hunterdon Counties. Unlike previous studies, several non-chemical indus- tries occupations also had a high bladder cancer death rate: bank officers, inspectors, postal clerks, welders, taxi drivers, bartenders, educational ser- vices employees, and printing industry employees.

This observance could be due to the impact of other less site specific environmental carcinogens which also impact on the bladder. For example, trihalomethanes (cited in chapter 3,) and alcohol/ tobacco/coffee use, which will be discussed in chapter 5.

Blot and Fraumeni indicated that "cigarette smoking is not likely to be responsible for the elevated mortality in the northeast, inasmuch as the available national surveys show only small region- al differences in smoking practices."[88]

Manufacturers, Users

It is not easy to trace or recognize the manu- facturer of benzidines due to the use of trade names. C.I. Direct Red 2, which chemically is 3,3'-dimethyl benzidine, is manufactured by several companies under various names:[89]

Dye	Manufacturer
benzopurine 4B ex. conc. 4b special	Atlantic Chemical Corp., Nutley, New Jersey
Direct purpurine 4B	Fabricolor Inc., Paterson, N.J.

The Toms River Chemical Company (TRC) uses about 60
chemicals regarded as suspect carcinogens. Two are
benzidine congoners*; o-tolidine (3,3 -dimethyl
benzidine) and o-dianisidine (3,3'-dimethyloxybenzi-
dine). TRC does not *believe* that all of the chemicals are carcinogenic, saying, "However, only time
and further testing will clear their [the chemical]
name."[90] Two other New Jersey based benzidine dye
and similar dyestuff manufacturers are the American
Cyanamid Company in Wayne, and BASF Wyandotte in
Parsippany. The health hazards of benzidine type dye
extends also to other industries; textile, leather
and paper dyeing workers.

Community Cancer Risk

The EPA has cited three counties in New Jersey
as benzidine risk areas, as shown below:[91]

Companies and Locations of Potential Benzidine
Risk Areas in New Jersey

Company	City	Population Density People/ Km	County	Population
Fabricolor Chemical Corporation	Paterson	913	Bergen Passaic	874,660 456,200
E.I. DuPont de Nemours and Co., Inc.	Salem	345	Salem	61,700

One potential route of environmental transport is
through plant waste water discharge. Industrial activities report that daily benzidine discharges do not exceed 0.454 kg/day (about a pound daily). Neither the
DEP nor EPA has assessed these releases in New Jersey.

---

* of similar chemical structure

There are hazards associated with the use of consumer
products containing benzidine dyes that should be
discussed here rather than under "consumer products"
because of their sale without due caveats. Consumers
are exposed to a cancer risk due to the use of
stationary, paper towels, tissues and colored dia-
pers.[92] Forty percent of the benzidine dyes produced
are used in these products. Further, ingestion or
absorption of mutagenic dyes results from blanket-suck-
ing, thread and yarn pointing, clothes washing and
bleaching, perspiration transport and ironing.

The Plastics Industry

    Background

    Vinyl chloride (VC) is polymerized to form poly-
vinyl chloride (PVC) which is used to fabricate several
plastic products; pipes, films, flooring, furniture,
electrical insulation, packaging materials and other
products.[94] Vinylidene chloride (VDC), is another
chemical monomer which is polymerized to form barrier
resins, packaging materials and to synthesize 1,1,1-
trichloroethane.[95] Both VC and VDC are toxic, causing
skin and eye irritation, central nervous system depression and altered liver function. In 1972 the ability
of VDC to induce cancers of the liver (angiosarcomas),
lung, kidney, skin and other sites was demonstrated in
animal studies.[96] In that same year, prospective
epidemiological studies by Tabershaw and Gaffey suggested that VC was a multipotent carcinogen in humans.[97]
The multipotent carcinogenicity phenomenon was confirmed
in 1980 as a result of cumulative animal studies at the
Instituto di Oncologia in Italy.[98] Under the leadership
of Ceasare Maltoni, VC was determined to induce tumors
at concentrations as low as 10ppm.

    Production and Risk of Cancers

    In addition to the established toxicity and
carcinogenicity of VC and PVC, VDC is now a suspect
carcinogen.[99] Twenty-seven of forty six VDC workers

at the BASF Wyandotte, South Kearny polymerization
plant, manifested at least a 50% liver function impair-
ment. [100] The current knowledge of the site-diverse
cancers produced by exposure to VC, renders exposure
to these and structurally similar emissions dangerous
and inherently more difficult to access in a retrospective epidemiological study. Prior to the establishment of the 1 ppm plant emission limit set
by OSHA, worker exposure to VC ranged from 300 to
1000 ppm. Plastics workers have been well exposed
to quantities of VC, PVC and VDC capable of producing
site-diverse cancers before the enactment of current
standards. The up to twenty year period of latency
following exposure to VC indicates there is a substantial cohort in New Jersey which may yet manifest
the various site-diverse cancers cited earlier. The
current exposure limit to VC and VDC is 1 and 10 ppm
respectively. Time will tell if these levels are, in
fact, below that which may induce the cancers described earlier. Table 10 lists the location of VC,
PVC and VDC polymer and related product manufacturers
in New Jersey.

TABLE 10
POLYVINYL CHLORIDE AND VINYLIDENE CHLORIDE MANUFACTUR-
ING PLANTS IN NEW JERSEY [101, 102]

PVC Plants

Producing Company	Plant Location	Area Popula- tion Density Persons/Km
Occidental Petroleum	Burlington	152.9
Hooker Chemical Company	Burlington	152.9
Tenneco Chemicals, Inc.	Burlington	152.9
Tenneco Chemicals, Inc.	Flemington	61.8
Givaudan Corporation	Clifton	---
Pantasote Company	Passaic	1,646.7
Janna Corporation	Franklin Township	---
B.F. Goodrich Company	Pedricktown	63.7

VDC Plants

BASF-Wyandotte	South Kearny	---

Community Risk to Cancers

The EPA estimates that some 4.6 million and 3.5 million persons reside within a five mile radius of plants that synthesize, polymerize or fabricate materials based on VC and VDC, respectively.[103] The implication here is that if you live in one of the high population density counties, you have been or are exposed to these vapors. However, the five mile radius exposure well applies to residents of remote and sparsely populated Pedricktown in south Jersey (see Table 10). It is pure speculation about what levels of VC, PVC and VDC communities were exposed to prior to the 1970's.

More recent studies conducted by DEP under the Office of Cancer and Toxic Substances Research program indicate VC emissions are present only in trace (ppb) quantities in areas of northern New Jersey. These atmospheric levels are below the levels seen to cause cancers in laboratory animals. However, and with a necessary redundancy, the health effects of long-term, low-level exposures have not been determined.

The Petroleum Industry

Background

There are few naturally occurring substances as critical to world-wide economics and simultaneously presenting a great cancer risk as crude petroleum oil. Petroleum is an extremely complex mixture of organic compounds; mainly liquids of the paraffin series, some gases (e.g., methane), and solids and traces of inorganic compounds (e.g., metals). Petroleum may be refined into some 6,000 products and petrochemicals.[104] Crude petroleum oil derivatives have been demonstrated to cause several forms of human cancer. Many of the derivatives, e.g., polycyclic aromatic hydrocarbons, metals (e.g., cadmium and uranium) and coal tar dyes have been discussed already in this work. Practically all phases of refinery processes release hydrocarbons.[105] Catalyst recovery releases particulates and odors, heat exchangers release water vapor, waste sludge releases sulfur dioxide and all phases of storage of hydrocarbons release their more volatile moiety. Wastestream processes such as drying, sweetening, water washing and asphalt blowing generate large quantities of toxic wastewaters. More properly, the adverse environmental contribution is due to water pollution; however, there is an initial refinery ambient air impact. Known and suspect carcinogens derived from petroleum (as a result of processes) and their corresponding target organs of the human body, are given in Table 11.

Cancer Mortality in Counties with Petroleum Industries

An epidemiological study was conducted by the National Cancer Institute (1977) on cancer mortalities over the period 1950-1969 in petroleum industry counties.[106] There was a significantly higher mortality rate for cancer of the nasal cavity, sinuses, lung, testes, stomach and skin.* Bladder and liver cancers were not found to be excessive in this study, Surprisingly, in lieu of the constant presence of benzene, there were no excess leukemias. The study is weak in that it did not establish a history on the residents, e.g., other exposures to carcinogens, and duration of residency, and the absence of these factors was cited by the authors. This study, albeit the weaknesses, enhances other data indicating that petroleum industry workers and those living in the neighboring communities run a higher than average cancer risk.[107, 108] Additional NCI epidemiological studies** conducted in Texas, a state with the heaviest concentration of petrochemical and refinery workers, indicates the workers have a higher than average chance of mortality due to brain cancer.[109]

----

*   Study group consisted predominantly of white males.

** Co-sponsored by OCAW (Oil, Chemical and Atomic Workers International Union).

TABLE 11
SITE-SPECIFIC TUMORS ATTRIBUTED TO PETROLEUM
AND ASSOCIATED REFINERY PROCESSES

Agent	Affected Organ
Coal tar (crude petroleum)	lung, larynx, skin, scrotum, urinary bladder in humans
benzene	leukemogen in humans
coal tar dyes	bladder cancers in humans
arsenic	lung, skin cancers in humans
cadmium	prostate, kidney cancers in humans, fibrosarcomas in rats
chromium (hexavalent)	lung, nasal sinuses cancers in humans
lead	cancers in laboratory animals
nickel	lung, nasal passages cancer in humans
soots, tars, oils	skin, scrotum, lung, bladder cancers in humans
vinyl/vinylidene chloride	cancers at several sites

Petroleum Refining in New Jersey and the
Cancer Risk

As many as eight petroleum refineries have
operated in New Jersey and five are described in Table
12.[110] Collectively, they have the capacity to refine
646,131 barrels of crude oil daily. Superficially it

159

appears from Table 12 that the health impact of refinery
operations began with the inception of Exxon (Standard
Oil) in 1882. However, prior to that time, crude oil
was used as a medicine in the treatment of respiratory
infections and other ailments. And that impact is
discussed in chapter 7, "New Jersey Yesteryear".

Total employment at the state's refineries is
given at 8,291 in 1977. The aforementioned NCI brain
cancer studies were conducted at two nationwide
refineries, represented in New Jersey by Texaco and
Mobil. The implication of these studies is that there
may be a parallel, higher than average incidence of
cancers at these New Jersey refineries. Studies are
in progress to assess the situation.

Suspicions of a PCB/skin cancer link at Mobil
Oil Company's plant and laboratory, on the part of
company officials, were confirmed in an epidemiological study conducted by Dr. Anita Bahn of the University of Pennsylvania in 1976.[111, 112] Of a study
group of 92 workers exposed to PCB's, three manifested malignant melanoma and two, cancer of the
pancreas, a total significantly higher than expected
of a cohort of this size. The use of PCB's at Mobil
as an experimental substance and a catalyst during
the period 1949, and 1954-1957, demonstrates the
diverse, extra-petroleum nature of exposure to
carcinogens in the refinery environment.

There is also a cancer risk as a result of exposure to petrochemicals, as derivatives of petroleum, and some examples of these manufacturers and
associative industries are listed in Table 13. A
large percentage of New Jersey petroleum industry
workers appear to be exposed to a wide variety of
substances which present a cancer risk. Extensive
evaluation of their exposure to fugitive emissions
(pollutants that escape to the air from valves, duct-
work, fires, road dust, etc.) is required.

TABLE 12
NEW JERSEY PETROLEUM REFINERIES

Name	Location	Date Established	Employment
Exxon (Standard Oil of New Jersey)	Linden (Union County)	1882 (Standard Oil)	1,200 - operations/ maintenance/shop Florham Park: 2,500 - research 500 - chemists
Chevron, U.S.A., Inc. (Standard Oil of California)	Perth Amboy (Middlesex County)	1947	640 (65% operational)
Amerada Hess Corp.	Port Reading (Middlesex County)	1958 (closed 1974)	460
Texaco, Inc.	Eagle Point Plant Westville (Gloucester County)	1948	750-800 total 180 - chemists 300 - maintenance 300 - production
Mobil Oil Corp.	Paulsboro (Gloucester County)	(offspring of Standard Oil)	1,400 - refinery/ ancillary operations 1,000 - research 1,000 - engineering (Princeton)

161

TABLE 13
PETROCHEMICAL DERIVATIVES/MANUFACTURERS

Product	Company	Location
oils, wood preservatives	Sanivan Laboratories, Inc.	Camden
cutting oils	Baker Caster Oil Co.	Bayonne
	Oakite Products, Inc.	Berkeley Hgts.
graphite	Fiske Brothers Refining Co.	Newark
rerefining	Diamond Head Oil Refining Co.	Kearny
creosote oils	Everseal Manufacturing Co., Inc.	Ridgefield

SOURCE: Thomas Register of American Manufacturers and
Thomas Register Catalogue File, 1980, vol. 5.

Diverse Activities with Cancer Risks

Glass Manufacture

There are seventeen glass container manufacturing plants in the state, principally in southern New Jersey. The contribution of these facilities to the New Jersey air pollution burden is sulfur, oxides of nitrogen, silicon and chromium. Glass plant employees have been diagnosed as suffering from several occupationally related diseases:[113] corneal scarring, pleural asbestosis, silicosis, pulmonary fibrosis, obstructive lung disorders.

Two hundred thirty employees of the Midland Glass Company in Aberdeen Township are currently involved in litigation over 700 occupational disease claims, such as those cited above. Lung cancers are

not at issue here. However, the pulmonary diseases
are cited because they may render workers' lungs
susceptible to carcinogenesis. Especially in an
environment with more than background sulfur dioxide
and silica levels. Sulfur dioxide is ciliatoxic
and silica is cytotoxic. Perhaps what has also been
overlooked in the evaluation of the glass manufacture
workplace environment is exposure to glass itself as
a fiber or a dust. Stanton, et.al., have produced
pleural (lung lining) neoplasms in rats as a result
of glass fiber implantation.*[114]

Automakers

In August of 1980 General Motors (GM) asked the
New York Sloan-Kettering Cancer Center to conduct an
epidemiological investigation of cancer deaths at
their Ewing, New Jersey, Fisher Body plant.[115, 116]
Three thousand, five hundred workers are employed at
the Ewing plant. Three prior studies indicated that
model makers showed a higher than expected incidence
of colon and rectal cancers. Studies conducted by
the United Auto Workers and the Michigan State
Department of Health indicate that the lung cancer
rate at General Motors' Flint plant was twice the
national average. General Motors' Flint representa-
tives said there were no carcinogens in use at their
plants.

General Motors has good reason to initiate epidemiological studies at other New Jersey facilities.
In 1975, Dr. Joel Kopelman interviewed a 29 year hard-
ware plant veteran of the Hyatt-Bearing plant in
Harrison and Clark, New Jersey.[117] Further question-
ing indicated that the patient, who was then hospitalized for colon cancer, had undergone a partial
laryngectomy. Further, several of his co-workers had
also developed laryngeal cancer. Drs. Kopelman,
Thind and Louria of the New Jersey Medical School
suspecting an industrially related cancer cluster,

---

*   Inhaled fibers reach human pleura by a different route.

attempted to engage General Motors in an investigation. General Motors officials were initially
responsive, later becoming *unavailable*.

Economic Poisons -- Use/Exposure

   Background

   The expression "economic poison" includes all
preparations intended to be used as insecticides,
herbicides, rodenticides, nematocides, fumigants,
defoliants and repellents. These preparations also
present health hazards of varying degrees. Their
need in an area with the acronym "Garden State" is
fairly obvious. About 36,000 people are employed
in New Jersey in the agriculturally related industries* (vegetable, poultry, fruit field crop farming and nursery and greenhouse products). The economic poisons are used to affect pest control and stop
losses in these industries as well as in the forests.
Further, they are used to combat nuisance insect
pests (e.g., mosquitoes) and those that affect
property damage (e.g., termites and wasps). The
DEP licenses users of economic poisons, i.e., certified pesticide applicators.**[118] The DEP classifies
economic poisons as prohibited, specially restricted
and restricted. License holders may purchase economic
poisons from any category.

   The Movement of Economic Poisons through the
   Environment

   The environmental transit of the economic poisons
follows several steps: the point of chemical synthesis, exposure to applicators, airborne residues,

_____

* Mining occupations are included in this value.

** The title "Certified Pest Control Operator" is also preferred.
   New Jersey was one of the first states to certify Pest
   Control Operators.

settling on plants and animals and in the soil and
ultimately elution into groundwater. The route an
economic poison will take is a function of its chemical and physical properties. Some economic poisons
such as most organic herbicides and fungicides, methyl-
carbamate and organophosphorous insecticides are water
soluble and fortunately, biodegradable or hydrolysable.
Organochlorine insecticides of low water solubility represent a class of very persistent (non-biodegradable)
pesticides.[119] Organochlorine pesticides concentrate
in food chains and are stored in fatty tissues in
humans and animals.

Problems Associated with Economic Poisons in
New Jersey

Sevin, a carbamate, cholinesterase-inhibiting
pesticide, used to control the Gypsy moth was used
in the southern New Jersey counties of Cape May,
Atlantic and Ocean. A "rash" of birth defects and
problem pregnancies linked to the spraying of Sevin
almost brought about an end to its use in the spring
of 1980.[120] The State Department of Health conducted a quick survey which concluded there was no
connection between the observed birth defects and the
Sevin spraying programs, much to the disbelief and
disappointment of the areas' pregnant mothers. Sevin
was declared safe and spraying to control the gypsy
moth continued. The State Department of Health
(DOH) continued to investigate the incidences of
reported birth defects. Dr. George Halpin, Director
of Parental and Child Health Services in the DOH,
who directed these studies, concluded there was in
fact a "cluster" of birth defects in Cape May County.[121] Instead of the normal 2 per 1,000 birth
defects, per live births, southern Cape May County
was showing 8.5 per 1,000. Although the cause remains
unidentified, Sevin (or other pesticides) were
ruled out. It was pointed out that the herbicide

2,4,5-T*, widely used in Cape May County, was not
evaluated as a cause (cf. economic poison exposure
in New Jersey).

    Other Economic Poisons in the New Jersey
    Environment

    A review of the types of economic poisons in
New Jersey with a potential long-term health impact
begins with the data being provided by the DEP's
Program on Environmental Cancer and Toxic Substances
(PECTS). The presence of certain economic poisons
in the state's groundwater was determined. However,
the initial impact of these chemicals began with
exposure to pesticide applicators, farmers and
migrant laborers. At least 20% of all dusts and
sprays are used in residential, commercial establishments, public buildings and parks. South Plainfield,
New Jersey with a population of 21,000 is a good
example. According to the EPA, "residents of these
areas could be exposed to HCB [hexachlorobenzene]
residues resulting from emissions from the plants**
even if the plants are not currently producing HCB."122
HCB has been used as a grain fungicide and as a
pentachlorophenol feed stock. It has been shown to
cause liver tumors in hamsters. Ultimately, these
economic poisons settle on the soil where they pass
through by elution and enter the groundwater. An
analysis of the state's groundwater then reflects the
history of the economic poisons in use over the past
thirty years in New Jersey and it is given in Table
14.123 A list of over-the-counter, economic poisons
in use in New Jersey is given in Table 15.

_____

* Contaminants of 2,4,5,-T (an Agent Orange component) have been
   Dioxins, which are powerful animal teratogens, and acnegenics
   and hepatotoxic. (Sebaceous gland irritants and liver poisons
   respectively).

** The Hummel Chemical Co. in South Plainfield, produced HCB
   in 1976.

TABLE 14
SECOND PRELIMINARY REPORT ON GROUNDWATER

Economic Poison	EPA Drinking Water Standard, ppb	N.J. Pesticide Control	Carcinogenicity
Benzene hexachloride, BHC	none	P	liver/capillary tumors in hamsters
Lindane (gamma BHC)	4	R (more than 25%)	animal carcinogen (liver tumors and lung metastases in mice)
Aldrin	(1)	SR	liver cancer in mice, Fetotoxic, Teratogen, growth retardant in hamsters
Dieldrin	(1)	SR	liver cancer in mice, Fetotoxic, Teratogen, growth retardant in hamsters
Heptachlor	0.1	SR	malignant tumors in mice
Heptachlor epoxide	0.1	--	currently under test

TABLE 14 - continued
SECOND PRELIMINARY REPORT ON GROUNDWATER

Economic Poison	EPA Drinking Water Standard, ppb	N.J. Pesti-cide Control	Carcinogenicity
Toxaphene	5	SR	long-term high doses causes liver cancer in mice
Methoxychlor	100	?	Animal data inconclusive
Mirex	none	Voluntary cancellation by manufacturer	malignant tumors in mice
Endrin	0.2	P	Fetotoxic, growth retardation, teratogen in hamsters
Chlordane (velsicol, octa-klor)	(3)	R	animal carcinogen
DDT, isomers	(50)	P	hepatocarcinogen - mice (oral), liver cell tumors metastasized to the lungs

SOURCES: Economic Poisons, Reference No. 123, EPA Drinking Water, Reference No. 123, standards

( ) = recommended standard
P = prohibited
R = restricted
SR = specially restricted

168

TABLE 15

COMMERCIALLY AVAILABLE ECONOMIC POISONS IN NEW JERSEY

Trade Name	Specific Component	Specific Effect
Conqueror liquid vegetation killer, Ortho Triox-weed killer, Pentasol, Dowcide, weedone	Pentachlorophenol (May be contaminated with Dioxin and Furans)	Produces chromosome breaks Fetotoxic
Ortho - Rose/Flower Jet Duster	Malathion	May react with cellular DNA
Bonide rose and flower spray or dust	Sevin	Produces mutations in barley, teratogenisis in guinea pigs and beagle dogs
Ortho Lindane borer and leaf miner spray	Lindane (20%)	Plant/animal carcinogen
F & B weed killer	Sodium arsenite	Epidemiological evidence of carcinogenicity
"Pest Strips"	Dichlorvos	Mutagenic in submammalian species

SOURCES: Epstein, S.S. and Legator, Marvin S., The Mutagenicity of Pesticides, The MIT Press, Cambridge, 1971.
Proctor, N.H., Ph.D. and Hughes, James P., M.D., Chemical Hazards of the Workplace, J.B. Lippincott Company, Philadelphia, 1978.
Am. Ind. Hyg. Assoc. J. (42), January 1981, A-16.

169

Only one well of those tested showed an economic
poison in excess of the recommended limit. That
well, showing 0.6 ppb of heptachlor epoxide was
closed. These studies continue to show the presence
of very low-level concentrations of the economic
poisons in the state's groundwater. Although most
of the economic poisons shown in Tables 14 and 15
may be demonstrated to cause animal cancers, there are
no data yet to prove or disprove their ability to
cause human cancers as a result of long-term, low-dose
exposure. Singular opinions have been expressed that
cancer of some kind will occur in some individuals who
may not have manifested it in the absence of exposure
to at least Aldrin-Dieldrin*.[124]

Could there possibly by any toxicity or cancer
risk in merely walking through your neighborhood
farm and garden supply center? Well, when the author
conducted his shelf research in a major South Jersey
farm and garden supply center in Sewell, he was most
alarmed. There were open bins of Rotenone, Sevin**
and Malathion. The threshold limit value for these
pulmonary irritants, which also affect the nervous
system, are 5, 5 and 10 ppm respectively. They also
produce a variety of other adverse symptoms. A
former employee described working conditions there as
lacking in industrial hygiene and that the handling
of chemicals there was "geared to death." Further,
they indicated that if there was ever a fire - they
wanted to be in Cape May County. Amongst their other
negative memories were the recruitment of teen-age
employees who were given no training in the handling
of toxic substances and the presence of inadequately
ventilated areas. This establishment emerges only as
a potential for what may exist in other suburban areas
of New Jersey.

---

* Opinion of Dr. Walter E. Heston, Chief of the Laboratory
  of Biology, National Cancer Institute

** cf. gypsy moth - Cape May County alarm

There is considerable cancer risk in the use and application of the heavy metal pesticides. They contain metals which have a distinct history as carcinogens in humans and animals; arsenic, lead, cadmium and selenium. The properties and levels present in selected areas, of these metals (excluding selenium) has been described already in Table 7.

Economic poisons that are animal and human carcinogens -- the prohibited, restricted and specially restricted -- continue to be used in New Jersey. The DEP has reduced environmental residues of the economic poisons through their program of testing and authorization of dealers, and natural biological control. In addition, they sponsor about twelve yearly pesticide application training courses.

New Jersey Vietnam Veterans

Throughout the period 1962-1971, the United States Army used a chemical herbicide known as "Agent Orange" to accomplish defoliation in South Vietnam.[125] Agent Orange is actually a mixture of chemicals: 2,4,5-trichlorophenoxyacetic acid [2,4,5-T containing Dioxin (TCDD)] and 2,4-dichlorophenoxy-acetic acid (2,4,-D).[126] The impurity in Agent Orange, Dioxin*, is rated as a highly toxic substance. Dioxin has been demonstrated to cause birth defects, cancers and miscarriages in laboratory animals. In humans, Dioxin has been determined to cause memory loss, loss of consciousness, chloracne, and liver dysfunction. All of the effects of Dioxin have not been completely evaluated.

The Monsanto Company completed a mortality study on a small group (121 workers) who were exposed to Dioxin as a result of an industrial accident some thirty years ago. Their retrospective study indicates

---

* Dioxin is also a contaminant in a widely used wood preservative, pentachlorophenol.

chloracne resulted from the exposures but no excess cancer or cardiovascular disease was apparent.[127]

In March 1979, the EPA placed an emergency suspension on 2,4,5-T. Both the Dow Chemical Company and Monsanto refute those studies conducted on animals, citing delinquencies, inconsistencies, and no excess cancer deaths in their own studies.[128]

Throughout the course of spraying Agent Orange in Vietnam, about 56,000 New Jersey veterans may have been exposed.[129]

Approximately 12 million gallons of herbicide sprays (of which two-thirds were Agent Orange) were sprayed over Vietnam.[130] The solvent was kerosene, a suspect carcinogen itself. The diluted strength of Agent Orange used in Vietnam was between 13-17 times more concentrated than the concentration permitted to be used in the United States. Veterans throughout the United States have filed disability claims with the Veteran's Administration, citing 2,4,5-T as the cause of a variety of disorders including nervous disorders, birth defects in their progeny and cancers. New Jersey Vietnam veterans are now collectively represented by the New Jersey Agent Orange Commission. The Commission was established by Governor Byrne's signing of Bill 3401 in February 1980. Dr. Peter C. Kahn, a Rutgers research professor, is conducting an epidemiological study on all New Jersey Vietnam veterans who enroll in the program.[131] Dr. Kahn is well aware of the many pitfalls his study will encounter. Particularly, what was the life-style of the veteran in the "Nam"; diet, smoking (including marijuana) and exposure to dapsone (an anti-malarial, now a suspect carcinogen), just to mention a few. Further, Agent Orange components* have been used right here in New Jersey.

* 2,4,5-T and 2-4-D (high volatile esters) are restricted use herbicides in New Jersey.

Miscellaneous Industrial Processes

It is not possible to give all the industrial processes to be found in New Jersey the sort of evaluation
given to those already covered. The data are simply not
available to the author or the occupational groups have
not been subject to epidemiological studies yet. Finally, adequate space would necessitate the use of several
volumes. However, in keeping with the purpose of this
chapter, to establish an environmental inventory of
cancer risks, additional processes may at least be
listed (See Table 16). Air pollution is a common
denominator in these processes listed there. Therefore, the lung and skin are target organs. However,
many specific pollutants have the ability to induce
cancers throughout the human body.

TABLE 16
MISCELLANEOUS INDUSTRIAL PROCESSES WITH
CANCER RISKS IN NEW JERSEY

Industry Process :	Pollutant Source :	Specific Pollutant :
Auto scrap processing	smoke, fumes particulates	paints, plastics, oils, metals
Brake shoe de-bonding	particulates, smoke	phenolic resins, asbestos
Heat treating	smoke, organic vapors gases	metals
Pipe coating equipment	toxic organic vapors	asphalt, coal tar, metals, asbestos, fiberglass
Wire reclamation	particulates, smoke gases	metals, sulfur dioxide, polyvinyl chloride vapors, hydrocarbons

Industry Process :	Pollutant Source :	Specific Pollutant :
Fish canneries	gases, particulates	nitrosamines, trimethylamine
Woodworkers	wood dust particulates	specific agent not yet identified; excess sinonasal cancers observed
Kraft pulping industry	gases, particulates	sulfur compounds
Baked lithograph	smoke, fumes	aldehydes
Phthalic anhydride plant	organic vapors	hexane, phthalic anhydride, naphthaline
Vegetable oil vulcanization	organic vapors	mercaptans
Synthetic detergents	volatile hydrocarbons	petroleum distillates, linear alkylated benzenes
Varnish manufacture	gases	resins, oil, solvents
Fertilizer manufacture	toxic, acidic gases	hydrofluoric, sulfuric and phosphoric acids
Insecticide manufacture	organic vapors, particulates	ethylene dichloride, economic poisons
Carbon black manufacture	gases, particulates	hydrocarbons

Industry Process:	Pollutant Source:	Specific Pollutant:
Asphaltic concrete	dust	asphalt, asbestos (?)
Asphalt roofing paper and shingles	vapors, particulates	petroleum crude oil, still bottoms
Oil and solvent re-refinishing	vapors	hydrocarbons
Rubber compounding	large particulates	amines, sulfur compounds, antioxidants (nitrosamines)
Cement manufacture	dust	asbestos, silica
Coke manufacture	gases	sulfur compounds, hydrocarbons
Coffee bean roasting	organic vapors	pyridine, fufural, phenol, formic acid, naphthalene
Iron/steel industry	gases, particulates	iron oxide, oxides of nitrogen, sulfur dioxide
Metal salvage	particulates, dusts	lead, metallic chlorides, sulfur compounds, plastics
Brass/bronze smelting	particulates	zinc, lead, tin, copper
Secondary aluminum smelting	particulates	chlorides, fluorides

175

TABLE 16 - continued
MISCELLANEOUS INDUSTRIAL PROCESSES WITH
CANCER RISKS IN NEW JERSEY

Industry Process:	Pollutant Source:	Specific Pollutant:
Electroplating	mists	chromic acid
Paint-baking ovens	vapors, particulates	inks, varnishes resins, lacquers
Wire enameling	smoke, fumes	resins, solvents, varnishes
Drum reclamation	smoke	diverse chemical residues
Bearing manufacture	gases	chromium and cadmium plating wastes, cutting oils
Feed/grain mills	dusts	aflatoxins, economic poisons
Municipal sewage treatment	gases, mists	almost anything!
Glass manufacture	particulates	silica, sulfur dioxide, oxides of nitrogen, chromium
Rubber manufacture	gases	nitrosamines
Electronic components	vapors, dusts	solvents, metals oils

SOURCES: Thomas Register, Higgins, Frederick B., Jr., Ph.D.
(Ref. 105) and DEP documents

176

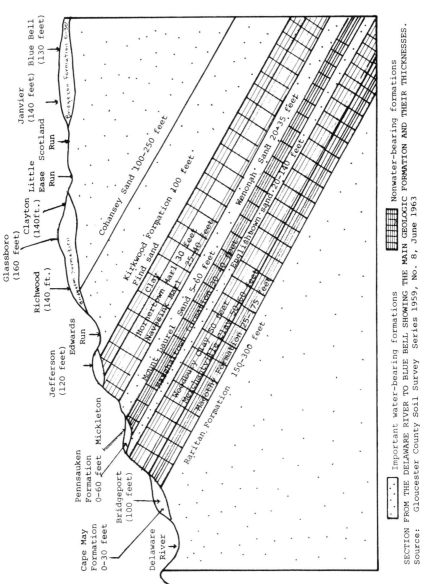

Important water-bearing formations | Nonwater-bearing formations

SECTION FROM THE DELAWARE RIVER TO BLUE BELL SHOWING THE MAIN GEOLOGIC FORMATION AND THEIR THICKNESSES.
Source: Gloucester County Soil Survey Series 1959, No. 8, June 1963

FIGURE 9

Water Pollution

Background

   Water from streams, lakes, rivers and the ocean
is evaporated by radiant solar energy, whereupon it
becomes atmospheric vapor. Subsequent precipitation
returns this vapor to the earth's surface, recharging
ground and surface waters and completing the hydrologic
cycle. Groundwater is pumped to the surface from water
bearing formations called aquifers. A cross sectional
analysis of the state from its western boundary to the
Atlantic Ocean would reveal these aquifers, i.e., the
Magothy and Raritan, Englishtown, Mt. Laurel-Wenonah,
Kirkwood Cohansey, as shown in Figure 9. In addition
to evapotranspiration, water moves underground through
these aquifers.

   A statewide Water Supply Master Plan begun in 1977
based on public purveyor supplies indicated that New
Jersey's 21 counties consumed almost 1,000 millions of
gallons daily (mgd) of which 372 mgd were derived from
groundwater sources and 581 mgd from surface waters.
That same EPA study gave a summary of the breakdown of
water diversions from purveyors by county. Collectively,
that data show a lot of ground and surface water is
used daily within the state and the northern New Jersey
communities' water sources are mainly from surface
supplies. Further, half of the water provided by purveyors in southern New Jersey is derived from groundwater. There are entire counties in south Jersey such
as Camden and Gloucester where groundwater is the main
source of potable water. The principal sources of
water pollutants with the potential to induce cancers
are from the improper disposal of hazardous wastes at
landfills, industrial accidents, illegal dumping and
industrial effluents.

Landfills

   There are approximately 400 solid waste disposal

type operations in New Jersey and over 200 entail landfilling. There are more than 80 landfills in the
counties of Burlington, Camden and Gloucester alone.[133]
The landfills were originally intended for the receipt
of municipal wastes; however, they also received
hazardous wastes. The DEP requires that liners be
placed on the bottom of landfills, that they have methane
venting systems and leachate test wells.[134] However,
none of the older sites have them. One reason is cost;
Socioenvironomics once again. Fortunately, some major
landfills are positioned over clay layers which retard
downward migration of leachate. Here the term retard
is synonymous with "time bomb" because there are many
incidents of contamination of the state's drinking
and recreational waters attributable to landfill
leachate.

A reasonable question at this point is how much
time must lapse before we know the full impact of
improper waste disposal on the state's groundwater
and surface water supplies? The answer, unfortunately,
is an equivocal one, running the gamut of a few days
to many years based on previous landfill kinetic experiences. For example, in 1972 arsenic poisoning
in a small Minnesota community was traced to contamination of groundwater supplies by an arsenic-based
pesticide applied to surface crops for grasshopper
infestation some 38 years earlier.[135] The speed and
distance of travel of a pollutant through soil will
vary with the soil type. Heavy spring rains on a
sandy soil are ideal conditions for the rapid elution
of chemical wastes as opposed to a dry summer, clay
soil condition in a landfill area. Table 17 shows
the relative distances and time of travel for some
landfill pollutants.

The DEP estimates that there are at least 500
unlicensed, illegal hazardous waste haulers in New
Jersey.[136] Their contribution to New Jersey landfills
would result in 48% of 411 wells tested by 1980
indicating the presence of chlorinated hydrocarbons.
The results of the state's water monitoring program
are discussed at the end of this section. There are

numerous instances where landfills have contaminated
groundwater in New Jersey. A few major incidents are
described here:

TABLE 17
RELATIVE DISTANCES OF CONTAMINATION FOR VARIOUS
TYPES OF INDUSTRIAL LANDFILL POLLUTANTS

Pollutant	Observed Distance of Travel	Time of Travel
Tar residues	197 feet	--
Picric acid	several miles	--
Picric acid	3 miles	4-6 years
Mn, Fe, hardness*	2000 feet	--
Miscellaneous chemicals	3-5 miles	--
Chromate	1000 feet	3 years
Phenol	1800 feet	--
Phenol	150 feet	--
Chlorides	200 feet	24 hours
Gasoline	2 miles	--
Chemical weedkiller	20 miles	6 months
Radioactivity	--	5 days

SOURCE: General Electric "Solid Waste Management Technology
Assessment." Table 17 appeared in Pollution Engineering, January 1977, Vol. 9, No. p. 51.

Price's Pit, Egg Harbor Township, Ocean County

This 20-odd acre landfill on the border of
Pleasantville and Egg Harbor Township became
characterized as "the most serious environmental
problem in the United States," in 1981.[138] The landfill was opened as a sand and gravel operation and
began to receive toxic wastes from 1968 until closure in November 1972. It is estimated that at
its peak, Price's Pit received 100,000 gallons of

---

* Mn=manganese; Fe=iron

toxic wastes weekly.[139] In 1978, strange odors were
detected in potable well water adjacent to Price's
Pit. One area resident drinking that water related
how he felt like a million pins were sticking in his
side.[140] His kidney was later removed and he died
on July 17, 1981. His survivors attributed not only
his death to the ingestion of the contaminated well
water, but their rashes, headaches and a grandson's
infirmity requiring leg braces, as well. Two area
wells have been closed due to contamination and 37
others in the area are also endangered or contaminated.

Atlantic City obtains 80% of its drinking water
from 13 wells located 3400 feet northeast of Price's
Pit. Leachate, which has been estimated to be proceeding at a rate of 10 inches daily, could reach these
wells in 1983. An EPA test well water analyses
taken 1000 feet from Price's Pit is given below:[141]

COMPOUND	CONCENTRATION, PPB PARTS PER BILLION
Dichloroethane	128,500
Cadmium	180
Lead	170
Benzene	7,900
Polychlorinated Biphenyls	170

In a landmark decision, a Federal judge concluded
that contributors to the toxic and carcinogenic wastes
in Price's Pit were in part responsible for pollution of Atlantic City's drinking water. Some of the
companies cited in a September 1981 Justice Department suit were: Union Carbide Corporation, Amaco Chemical Company, Hoffman - La Roche, Rollins Environmental
Services, Marvin Jonas Incorporated.[142]

The Kin-Buc Landfill, Edison Township, Middlesex County

This landfill occupies a total of 220 acres and 30' border along the Raritan River in Northern New Jersey. It is located in Edison Township in densely populated Middlesex County, (1,877.2/square mile) near the town of Sayreville. Waste treatment operations began there in 1968 and by 1976, Kin-Buc was receiving 500,000 gallons of chemical waste daily from fourteen states, including New Jersey.[143] It is difficult to summarize the many toxic and carcinogenic chemical wastes received during its period of operation; polyvinyl chloride, benzene, lead, pharmaceuticals, paints and plastics. There have been numerous fires at the site and a bulldozer operator died as a result of an explosion stemming from improper waste disposal techniques.[144]

On January 16, 1976, Kin-Buc literally regurgitated, spewing 20,000 gallons of a black inky chemical vomitus into the Raritan River. The site was closed in late 1976. Although Middlesex County relies on surface water, not predictably requiring the area's groundwater until the year 2000, Kin-Buc reports on the status of its cumulative abuse through leachate and gas release and eventually it will through *fires*.

Jackson Township Landfill, Jackson Township, Burlington County

This 135 acre landfill is located in the most pristine area of the state; the pinelands, more specifically in the Legler section of Jackson Township. The landfill was opened by municipal authorities in 1972 with the expressed intent to receive only municipal wastes. However, the DEP has identified at least 41 different organic chemicals believed to have been accumulated over a six year period; including benzene, chloroform, trichloroethylene, tetrachloroethane, and dichloroethylene, which have polluted the underlying Cohansey aquifer.[145] Approximately 200 families were drinking polluted water between 1972

and 1978. These residents experienced a wide range
of toxic symptoms; kidney stones and disorders, miscarriages, skin rashes and sores, which they attri-
bute to the drinking water.[146]

Bridgeport Rentals and Oil Services, Inc.
Logan Township, Gloucester County

In the fall of 1980, the DEP's Bureau of Potable
Water substantiated some Logan Township residents'
long-term suspicion. Their groundwater was polluted.
The source of the pollution is thought to be derived
from a 24 acre site, Bridgeport Rentals and Oil
Services, Inc.[147] There are about 50 storage tanks
and a fragile eleven acre lagoon at that site from
which chemical leachate is thought to be progressing
in a northerly direction. The groundwater supply of
about 90 Logan Township residents has been contaminated by the chemical leachate. DEP records indicate
their own awareness of oil leachate from the site
into an adjacent marsh and the Delaware River as early
as 1969. Groundwater samples taken 50 feet from the
lagoon have been determined to contain arsenic, benzene, mercury, vinyl chloride, 1,2 dichloroethylene,
tetrachloroethylene, 1,1 Dichloroethane and trichloroethylene.[148] An analysis of an area resident's
drinking water will be given and discussed at the end
of this section.

LiPari Landfill, Borough of Pitman, Gloucester
County

New Jersey residents living in the vicinity of
landfills not only live with the threat of groundwater pollution, but with daily air pollution. The
LiPari Landfill in Mantua, New Jersey, occupying
about ten acres, contains some 46,000 barrels of
liquid chemical wastes.[149] These wastes, parented
by the Rohm & Haas Chemical Corporation, Owens-
Illinois, Columbia Records (Pitman, N.J.), Almo, Inc.,
and the Jones Waste Removal Company have polluted
nearby Alcyon Lake with literally hundreds of
toxins and carcinogens, including:[150, 151]

phenanthrene	arsenic	naphthalene
endrin	mercury	chromium
cadmium	benzene	PCB's
lead	nickel	bis (chloro-ethyl) ether, (BCEE)

At least one leachate stream from the LiPari Landfill may be seen on the surface before it runs into Alcyon Lake. In 1979, the DEP confirmed the presence of BCEE* in the air in Pitman, 100 yards away from the major leachate stream. BCEE has produced dose related hepatomas in mice.

A summary of other south Jersey landfills posing varying degrees of threats to groundwater and surface waters is given in Table 18.[152] Fifteen abandoned dump sites regarded as top priority clean-up projects by the DEP, are listed in Table 19.

Industrial Effluents -- Into the Delaware River

Intentional Discharges Under NPDES**

More than 120 chemical companies discharge their effluents into the Delaware River and some of them are identified in Figure 10.[153] Sheldon and Hites identified about 100 compounds present in Delaware River water and were able to determine their chemical structure and their source as either municipal or industrial.[154] Further, they determined "the river can act as a carrier, sink or reactor causing trans-

---

* Trichloroethylene, Tetrachloroethylene and Benzene were also detected in the air in ppb quantities.

** National Pollutant Discharge Elimination System, 1972 Water Pollution Control Amendments prohibit point source pollutant discharge into waterways without a permit. All discharges are to cease by 1985.

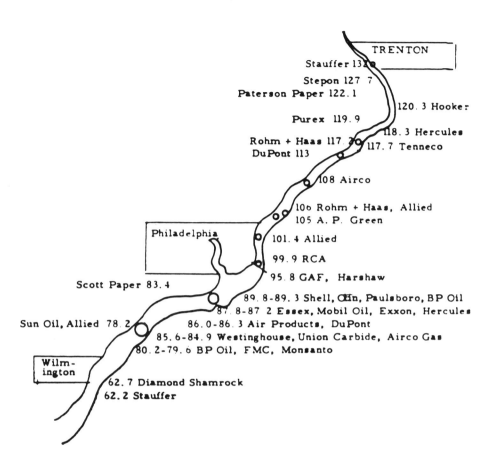

FIGURE 10
Delaware River Between River Miles 60 and 140
Showing Locations of Chemical Companies
(Side Not Significant)

TABLE 18

EPA LAND FILL SITE STUDY DATA - 1976

Name Location	Size	EPA Ground/Surface Water Threat Potential	Type Wastes Accepted	Leachate Collection System
MAC Deptford Township	40 acres 75' depth	not a serious regional threat; adjacent ground water somewhat contaminated; potential for explosive gas build-up	industrial solid wastes; evidence of acceptance of illegal liquid wastes	none
Kinsley Deptford Township	60 acres 50' depth	moderate threat to groundwater quality; large threat to shallow ground and surface water	municipal wastes animal wastes sewage sludge chemical/ industrial wastes	installed
Henry Harris Mantua Township	20 acres 40-50' depth	regional groundwater pollution potential considered high	municipal septic and non-chemical wastes; evidence of illegal liquid chemical wastes	3 monitoring wells
Fazzio Camden County	50 acres 80' deep	low	presently closed; previously accepted municipal solid wastes, industrial wastes and sewage sludge	none
Newfield Borough of Newfield	3 acres 20' deep	moderate	non-chemical and inert industrial wastes, local brush and leaf litter	none

186

TABLE 18 - continued

EPA LAND FILL SITE STUDY DATA - 1976

Name Location	Size	EPA Ground/Surface Water Threat Potential	Type Wastes Accepted	Leachate Collection System
Amadei Gloucester Township	50 acres 80' deep	high; leachate suspected of migrating deep into underlying aquifier	--	none
National Park National Park Township	45 acres 20' deep	insignificant	construction debris	none
Camden Old Camden City	90 acres 40' deep	low - moderate	closed for 25 years	EPA test wells only
King of Prussia Winslow Township	7 acres	high; local groundwater severely polluted with organic solvents and other contaminants; EPA rates area as a health hazard	abandoned; formerly liquid chemical wastes; liquid/solid chemicals still present (visibly)	none
Helen Kramer Mantua Township	50 acres 40' deep	leachate a threat to downstream surface waters. Caught afire in July '81, burned about 6 weeks, fire-hose run-off enhanced leachate	sanitary wastes; leachate indicates the presence of phenolic compounds, cadmium, lead manganese, mercury	yes

187

TABLE 19
"TOP PRIORITY" GROUND WATER POLLUTION SITES
(AS OF DECEMBER 1981)

Site	Location	Pollutant
	(NORTH JERSEY)	
Gordon Chemical Services*	Jersey City Hudson County	Methylene chloride styrene, dichloro-ethane, industrial solvents
Chemical Control Corp.*	Elizabeth Union County	PCB's sludge
Lone Pine Landfill (144 Acres)	Freehold, Monmouth County	Benzene, vinyl chloride, toluene
Intersection - Rt. 539/537	Upper Free-hold, Monmouth County	Hazardous wastes
Bog Creek Farm (4 Acres)	Howell, Monmouth County	Paint wastes
Burnt Fly Bog (15 Acres)	Marlboro, Monmouth County	PCB's, used automotive oil
Metallic Corporation	Franklin, Sussex Township	Trichloroethylene
Chem Sol Incorporated	Piscataway	Organic chemicals, PCB's
Aircraft Radio and Control	Boonton	Metal plating wastes, organic chemicals
	(SOUTH JERSEY)	
Spence Farm	Plumstead, Ocean County	Miscellaneous organic chemicals

188

TABLE 19 - continued
"TOP PRIORITY" GROUND WATER POLLUTION SITES
(AS OF DECEMBER 1981)

Site	Location (SOUTH JERSEY)	Pollutant
Goose Farm*	Plumstead, Ocean County	PCB's Laboratory wastes
Pijak Farm	Plumstead, Ocean County	Drum/Liquid wastes
Illegal Dump (6 Acres)	Hamilton, Atlantic County	40 different chemicals, including benzene, carbon tetrachloride, and lead
Chemical Leaman Tank Lines, Inc.	Logan Township, Gloucester County	Organic chemicals
Williams Porperty* (2 Acres)	Swainton, Middle Township	Organic solvents

SOURCES: New Jersey Hazardous Waste News, Volume I, No. 6, September 1981, Gloucester County Times, July 21, 1981

---

* Clean-up initiated at these sites.

formation of compounds to more or less hazardous
species." Although their prime interests were
analytical, they raised the question "it is logical
to ask if there is a correlation among cancer
incidence (in the Delaware Valley), organics in the
drinking water and organics in the Delaware River."
Their original data listed about 158 volatile organics
(of varying toxicities and at least ten suspect
carcinogens).

The approximate high level total concentration
of volatile organics at the Delaware low-level inter-
ceptor is approximately 0.01%. This implies that a
million gallons of typical Delaware River water could
contribute as much as 100 gallons of extremely toxic,
carcinogenic chemicals to New Jersey aquifiers, since
the Delaware River replenishes south Jersey aquifiers.
Some of the chemicals detected in Delaware River water
are given below:[155]

naphthalene	methylphenanthrene
substituted benzenes	ethylene glycol de-
pyrene	rivatives
phenol	plasticizers
cresol	

During times of drought in the Delaware Valley
there is concern for the movement of the salt line
(water salinity gradient) up the Delaware River. It
should be underscored that toxins and carcinogens
from industrial plant effluents will be even more concentrated during times of drought. Further, their
impact on aquifer replenishment will be enhanced.

Delaware River Oil Spills

Fuel oils are a complex mixture of hydrocarbons.
Upon being spilled into the Delaware Bay, the more
volatile fraction evaporates. The remaining less
volatile fraction is degraded by microorganisms.
There is also a complex solubilizing process, not
quite thoroughly understood.[156]

Naturally occurring and additive type organic

compounds in the fuel oil, transfer from an oily surface
film into the water. Fatty, carboxylic and naphthenic
acids, phenols, cresols, substituted hydrocarbons,
additives and process solvents are thought to be
typical components transferred. This complex mixture of toxins and carcinogens may, like industrial
effluents, eventually be transferred to south Jersey
groundwater aquifiers. Some examples of Delaware
River oil spill incidents are given below. Some oil
from spills may have been recovered or burned in fires
precipitating the accident or following it:[157]

Place/Ship/Date	Potential Quantity Spilled, Gallons
Cape May, New Jersey Tanker Olympic Dale Ran aground; refloated, 1975	small quantity out of 5,000,000
Marcus Hook, Pa. M/T Corinthos struck by M/T Edgar Queeny, 1975	13,000,000 crude
Trenton, New Jersey Pipeline break, 1975	200,000 kerosene
Marcus Hook, Pa. Olympic Games, 1976	134,000 Arabian crude

State Water Quality Monitoring

     Odor, appearance and adverse symptoms serve to
warn us about the use and ingestion of chemically
polluted water. However, somewhere at this moment,
some New Jersey resident is drinking water containing
pollutants below this level of symptomology. The
state's water quality is well defined for organic
chemicals, the metals and certain physical characteristics, and they are given in Table 20.[158]

TABLE 20
DRINKING WATER QUALITY STANDARDS FOR INORGANIC
AND ORGANIC CHEMICALS APPLICABLE TO GROUNDWATER

MANDATORY STANDARDS: EPA/NJDEP

Inorganic Chemicals	Maximum Contaminant Level--EPA* and DEP(in milligrams per liter)
Arsenic (As)	0.05
Barium (Ba)	1.00
Cadmium (Cd)	0.01
Chromium (hexavalent $Cr+^6$)	0.05
Fluoride (F)	2.00
Lead (Pb)	0.05
Selenium (Se)	0.01
Silver (Ag)	0.05
Nitrate (EPA only)	10.00 as N
Cyanide (CN) DEP only)	0.20

Organic Chemicals	Maximum Contaminant Level--EPA* only(in milligrams per liter)
Chlorinated hydrocarbons:	
Endrin	0.0002
Lindane	0.004
Methoxychlor	0.1
Toxaphene	0.005
Chlorophenoxys:	
2,4-D	0.1
2,4,5-TP	0.01

---

* Although these standards are already in effect, water
  suppliers do not have to submit chemicals anlayses
  demonstrating compliance until mid 1979.

192

TABLE 20 - continued
DRINKING WATER QUALITY STANDARDS FOR INORGANIC
AND ORGANIC CHEMICALS APPLICABLE TO GROUNDWATER

RECOMMENDED STANDARDS: (New Jersey only)

Substance	Recommended Concentration (in milligrams per liter)	
	Maximum	Minimum
A.B.S./L.A.S.*	0.5	
Chloride (Cl)	250.0	
Copper (Cu)	1.0	
Fluoride (F)	1.5	1.0
Hardness (as Ca CO_3)	150.0	50.0
Iron (Fe)**	0.3	
Manganese (Mn)**	0.05	
Nitrate (NO_3)	30.0	
Phenolic Compounds (as phenol)	0.001	
Sodium (Na)	50.0	
Sulfate (SO_4)	250.0	
Total Dissolved Solids	500.0	
Zinc (Zn)	5.0	

---

* Alkyl-Benzene-Sulfonate and Linear-Alkyl-Sulfonate, or
  similar Methylene Blue Reactive Substances contained
  in synthetic detergents.

** A public water supply, prior to distribution, shall be
   subjected to an appropriate removal process if the raw
   water contains concentrations exceeding 0.6 ppm iron
   or 0.1 ppm manganese. (Many study area supplies are
   subject to this provision.)

Regarding organic chemicals, an arbitrary 100
ppb (0.1 ppm) maximum level has been set. This interim
limit is based on the presence of trihalomethanes
(including chloroform, bromoform and other related
hydrocarbons) which may be formed in municipally
supplied water as a result of the chlorination or
bromination process. There really is no defined
limit set for the presence of organic chemicals at sub-
toxic levels because no one really knows the long-term
effect of the consumption of water of this nature.

Paralleling the state's air monitoring program
described earlier, the DEP initiated a statewide
groundwater monitoring program in 1978 (Program on
Environmental Cancer and Toxic Substances). Some of
the two hundred and fifty wells, in twelve counties
(Bergen, Cumberland Essex, Hudson, Hunterdon, Monmouth,
Morris, Passaic, Salem, Somerset, Union and Warren),
some near landfills, were tested. In their first report
of March, 1978 chloroform, carbon tetrachloride,
trichloroethylene, and trichloromethane were the most
predominant organic compounds.[159] Seven wells exceeded
the 100 ppb level proposed by EPA for organic compounds.
Those pesticides commonly present, lindane, heptachlor
and DDT were at concentrations below 0.1 ppb. Heavy
metals, normal groundwater constituents, were present
in nearly all samples. Summarily, the DEP concluded
that no well studied contained any substances at concentrations posing a threat to human health. Diametrically opposed to this complacency was the consumption
of chemically polluted water in Jackson Township, described earlier.

In December 1978, the second DEP report covering
163 wells from nine counties (Atlantic, Burlington,
Camden, Cape May, Gloucester, Mercer, Middlesex, Ocean
and Sussex) was released.[160] 1,1,1-trichloroethane,
1,1,2-trichloroethylene and 1,1,2,2-tetrachloroethy-
lene were found in most samples. Occasionally,
trichlorobenzene, chloroform, 1,1,2-trichloroethane
and meta-dichlorobenzene were also detected. For
the first time, two wells found to be contaminated
with trichloroethylene and trichloroethane, in Camden

and Middlesex respectively, were taken out of service.

Pesticide contamination, predominating in agricultural areas, was of a low level. PCB's were found in 32 wells. One Camden County well, contaminated with heptachlor epoxide at a concentration of 0.6 ppm, was closed. The DEP then concluded that the substances found in the wells studied were under certain conditions toxic and recognized carcinogens. Further, they conceded to the existence of data linking toxic drinking water pollutants and increased cancer mortality while citing the absence of data on the effects of long-term consumption of the low level pollutants. As the state's water monitoring program continued, over 500 wells would be closed as a result of testing by late 1980.

New Jersey State Drinking Water and Cancer Mortality

Just what is the cancer risk from drinking chemically polluted water as described in this section? The EPA has a set of proposed criteria, projecting the excess cancers resulting from the consumption of water containing benzene and chlorinated hydrocarbons shown in Table 21.

Earlier in this section, reference was made to the later discussion of chemically polluted water from Logan Township. The volatile organics analysis of two residents' drinking water is given below:[161]

| | Concentration, ppb | |
Chemical	Mikeleski Residence	Newton Residence
trichloroethylene	68.8	---
chlorobenzene	34.8	---
1,2 dichloroethylene	238.0	---
benzene	6.8	2.1
tetrachloroethylene	103.0	---
1,1 dichloroethylene	5.3	1.4
1,2 dichloroethane	148.0	1.6
methylene chloride	---	1.8

TABLE 21
FEDERAL WATER QUALITY CRITERIA FOR SELECTED CHEMICALS

EPA Proposed Criteria (ppb) for Drinking Water[1]
One Additional Cancer Per:

Compound	10 million People	1 million People	100,000 People	Other Criterion[2] Level	SNARL[3]
Benzene	0.15	1.5	15	---	---
Chlorobenzene	---	---	---	20	---
Chloroform	0.021	0.21	2.1	(See Note 4)	---
Dichlorobenzenes	---	---	---	230	---
1,1-Dichlorethane	(Insufficient Data for Establishing Criteria)				
1,1-Dichloroethylene	0.013	0.13	1.3	---	---
1,2-Dichloroethylene	(Insufficient Data for Establishing Criteria)				
Methylchloroform (or 1,1,1-Trichloroethane)	---	---	---	15,700	33(life-time exposure)
Phthalate esters	---	---	---	5,000 to 160,000[5]	---
Tetrachloroethylene	0.02	0.2	2.0	---	15 (one-year exposure)
Toluene	---	---	---	17,400	20 (ten-day exposure)
1,1,2-Trichloroethane	0.027	0.27	2.7	---	---

TABLE 21 - continued
FEDERAL WATER QUALITY CRITERIA FOR SELECTED CHEMICALS

EPA Proposed Criteria (ppb) for Drinking Water[1]
One Additional Cancer Per:

Compound	10 million People	1 million People	100,000 People	Other Criterion[2] Level	SNARL[3]
Trichloroethylene	0.21	2.1	21	---	225 (one-day exposure) 25 (one-day exposure) 10 (lifetime exposure)[6]
Xylenes		(Not on EPA Priority Pollutant List)			

NOTES:
1. Proposed interim risk levels, presently under review, precise target risk level not yet established. 2. Based on non-carcinogenic data; used when carcinogenic data is insufficient. 3. SNARL=Suggested no-adverse response level (non-carcinogenic effects) in ppb. 4. Interim maximum contaminant level for total trihalomethanes (including chloroform) is 100 ppb. 5. Depending on the particular phthalate ester. 6. Present accepted Massachusetts state standard.

SOURCE: Water and Wastes Engineering, February, 1981, p. 32.

Obviously, the consumption of water as described above at the Mikeleski residence results in a cancer risk greater than the EPA projection (cf. Table 21). The concentration of tetrachloroethylene alone raises the additional incidence of cancer from one to about 50 in a population of 100,000. Further, consider the synergistic effects of the consumption of such a mixture of chemicals along with the exposure to air pollutants in the same area.

Ionising Radiation

Nuclear Power Plants

There are two nuclear power plants in New Jersey currently providing electrical energy; the Oyster Creek Nuclear Power Plant and the Salem Nuclear Generating Station. Other units are under construction or proposed as indicated in Table 22. The units in operation as well as those proposed have pressurized water type reactors. New Jersey is a densely populated and highly industrialized state. It has been argued that the future residential and industrial energy needs may not be achieved economically through the use of oil, coal or natural gas.[162] And there are opposing views which cite evidence of our ability to meet our energy needs without nuclear power.[163] Nuclear fuel is reportedly capable of supplying all U.S. reactors for the next 40,000 years. Then is nuclear energy a saviour for our future electrical energy needs or a *Trojan horse*? In order to answer this question holistically, many serious issues should be reviewed:

TABLE 22
COMMERCIAL NUCLEAR POWER REACTORS IN OPERATION OR PLANNED FOR NEW JERSEY

Site	Plant Name	Capacity, Net kW(e)	Utility	Commercial Operation
Toms River	Oyster Creek Nuclear Power Plant: Unit 1	650,000	Jersey Central Power & Light Co.	1969
Forked River	Forked River Generating Station: Unit 1	1,070,000	Jersey Central Power & Light Co.	1983**
Salem	Salem Nuclear Generating Station: Unit 1	1,090,000	Public Service Electric & Gas Co.	1977
Salem	Salem Nuclear Generating Station: Unit 2	1,115,000	Public Service Electric & Gas Co.	1979
Salem	Hope Creek Generating Station: Unit 1	1,067,000	Public Service Electric & Gas Co.	1984**
Salem	Hope Creek Generating Station: Unit 2	1,067,000	Public Service Electric & Gas Co.	1936**
Little Egg Inlet	Atlantic Generating Station: Unit 1	1,150,000	Public Service Electric & Gas Co.	1986**

199

TABLE 22 - continued
COMMERCIAL NUCLEAR POWER REACTORS IN OPERATION
OR PLANNED FOR NEW JERSEY

Site	Plant Name	Capacity, Net kW(e)	Utility	Commercial Operation
Little Egg Inlet	Atlantic Generating Station: Unit 2	1,150,000	Public Service Electric & Gas Co.	1987**
*	1990 Unit	1,150,000	Public Service Electric & Gas Co.	1990**
*	1992 Unit	1,150,000	Public Service Electric & Gas Co.	1992**

SOURCE: Energy Research & Development Administration, "Nuclear Power Reactors in the United States," June 30, 1977

* Site Not Selected

** Construction at these cites was already temporarily abandoned by 1982.

mining	employment
milling	utility rates - who will
enrichment &	pay for Three Mile Island?
fuel fabrication	energy alternatives
reprocessing	waste storage
nuclear weapons	

However, health is the primary concern here. Ionisation radiation of sufficiently high doses may cause
cancers of the skin, thyroid, breast, lung, bone and
blood, as well as chromosomal damage received in
utero.[164] Specific biological effects have been
assigned to certain doses:[165] All clinical or observed
effects are found in exposures exceeding 25,000-30,000
MREM (25-30 Rads)*.

The Federal Radiation Council (FRC) has established the following exposure guidelines:[166]

1. no more than 5 rem/year whole-body expo-
    sure for radiation workers
2. no more than 0.5 rem/year whole-body
    exposure to any individual or a general
    population
3. no more than 0.17 rem/year (170mrem)
    whole body exposure average dose to
    the general population

New Jersey Resident Radiation Exposure

There are many natural and artificial sources
of radiation in the environment. Examples of sources
are cosmic radiation, soils, diagnostic x-rays and
radioactive fallout. New Jersey residents receive
an estimated 125 millirems (mrem) yearly from all
sources.[167] Residents living in close proximity to
the Salem nuclear generating station receive less
than one additional mrem yearly as a result of station

---

* The biological effect of radiation in humans is measured in
   millirems. Rem's (1000 mrem) and Rad's are used somewhat
   interchangeably.

operation.[168] There are additional releases of radiation to the air and water from nuclear generating stations.   These releases are monitored continuously and
have been determined to have no adverse health effects.

New Jersey Nuclear Power Plant Workers
Radiation Exposure

Industry-wide, less than 0.2% of all nuclear
power plant workers were determined to have received
no more than 5 rem (5,000 mrem) during the period
1947-1970.[169] Further, approximately 95% of the
workers received annual doses of one rem (1000 mrem)
or less. These exposures are within the FRC limits
stated above. Since nuclear power plants are relatively new in New Jersey, there are no similar
statistical reports. However, there have been exposure incidents. In two incidents in October of
1980 at the Salem I Nuclear Generating Station, five
workers were exposed to radiation ranging from 0.03
rems (30 mrems) to 1.6 rems (1600 mrems).[170] These
workers were reportedly not sickened by their exposures. Other incidents have occurred involving
operational or constructional factors:

          April 1979 - Oyster Creek facility cited
                       by Nuclear Regulatory
                       Commission for faulty gauges,
                       monitoring and backup equip-
                       ment, etc.[171]

          May   1979 - Inspection of reactor core
                       during refueling shutdown
                       reveals damage to numerous
                       uranium bundling belts at
                       the Salem I facility.[172]

          March 1981 - Gas release within plant of about
                       0.02 mr intensity.[173]

Radioactive Waste Storage in New Jersey

The operation of a nuclear power plant results in
the formation of low and high level wastes. There

were commercial burial sites for low-level wastes
throughout the states.   Radioactive wastes remaining
in spent reactor fuel rods were once shipped to
other reprocessing plants.   However, these facilities were suspended under the Carter administration.[174]
Since that time, high-level wastes have been stored
at each nuclear plant.   The Public Service Electric
and Gas Company (PSE&G) of New Jersey has requested
that the Atomic Safety and Licensing Board grant
them permission to expand their storage capacity.[175]
If the request is not granted, the Salem I plant
will have to *close* by the mid 1980's.   Many environmentalist organizations (e.g., The Delaware Safe
Energy Alliance and the West Jersey Sierra Club)
have protested against increased waste storage.[176]
The principal apprehension has been the failure of
the federal government to present a nationwide
permanent waste disposal plant.   Secondarily, there
is no confidence in the concept of "safe waste
storage."

        Nuclear Power in New Jersey - Short/long-term
        Effects

        The bottom line to the presence of nuclear power
plants in New Jersey is that not one single cancer
related effect is *currently* manifest.   Mind you,
nuclear energy is relatively new to the state.   The
most pronounced, yet difficult to measure effect, is
the fear that the very presence of these plants
engender.   Salem I area resident Richard Hinchman,
Jr., said, "The plant scares me in a way, but I'm not
scared to death or anything."[177]   The question must
be asked, "what is the total psychological impact
of nuclear energy near those facilities in New Jersey?"
The fear is present and may occupy an undefineable
role in the psychosomatic etiology of the cancers.
What about the potential for the most devastating
events; core meltdown or a nuclear explosion?   The
Three Mile Island accident demonstrated the potential
for a core meltdown.   Even though it did not happen,
a meltdown is still the most feared nuclear accident.[178]
The detonation of a nuclear explosion is a well-planned
event and these conditions are not present at a

nuclear plant.[179] Risk assessment studies indicate
that the chances of a citizen being killed by a nuclear incident is about 100 times less than being
killed by an earthquake.[180]

There are a lot of unknowns about the hazards
of nuclear energy. We do know how much radiation
every resident receives including extra-nuclear
plant radiation. There appears to be no increased
community risk to the development of radiation induced carcinogenesis. However, the BEIR Report and
the Gofman and Tamplin studies indicate that a 30
year exposure to 5 rems of radiation* would increase cancer mortality by between 1-5% and 10%
respectively.[181, 182] This increased cancer mortali-
ity rate burden would manifest itself initially in
a very discrete cohort -- the New Jersey nuclear
power plant worker, for whom a 5 rem/yearly (not a
30 year total) exposure was established. Dr. Ernest
Sternglass, Professor of Radiation Physics at the
University of Pittsburgh, says the increased worker
exposure will contribute to a genetic burden and
defective children in the future.**[183] A ten year
prospective epidemiological study of 197 nuclear-dock-
yard workers showed a "significant increase in chromo-
some damage with increasing exposure."[184] Excluding
an explosion and a meltdown, it is the unknown long-
term health effects of exposure to low level radiation
that may be the major cancer risk nuclear power stations pose in New Jersey. These effects will manifest themselves first in the nuclear power plant
workers and their progeny before any adverse effects
show up in the community.

----

* total exposure over a 30 year period

** A radiation worker may with approval exceed the 5 rem/yearly
   exposure rate provided his/her average exposure per year
   since age 18 will not exceed 5 rem per year.

Radioactive Residuals at Formerly Utilized Ore
Sampling Sites

Former Manhattan Engineering District (MED and
Atomic Energy Commission (AEC) sites for uranium ore
sampling during the 1940's and 1950's were decom-
missioned and returned to public and private industry for unrestricted use. These sites have been re-
evaluated to determine if the original decontamination
procedures were safe according to today's standards.
At least two of these sites are in New Jersey, Middlesex[185] and Deepwater.[186]

Middlesex Site

The site is presently the location of a Reserve
training center for the U.S. Marine Sixth Motor Transport Battalion. Several on-site buildings (thaw
house, boiler shop, garage) showed fixed alpha contamination in excess of NRC limits, which are 100
dpm*/100 cm^2 and 300 dpm/100 cm^2 respectively for
average and maximum allowable concentrations. Process room exterior surfaces showed alpha contamination by direct reading of up to 10^5 (1,000,000)
dpm/100cm^2; however, most readings ranged between 200
and 3000. Other on-site measurements indicated radon
and radon daughter measurements were in excess of
non-occupancy limits. Off-site measurements in adjacent private buildings showed radon daughter levels
to be in excess of background readings. External,
off-site gamma radiation was as high as 58 μr/hr, but
most values were near the background values. Soil
radium concentrations of 2400 pCi/g in a southerly
drainage ditch indicate radioactive run-off from the
site is occurring. The study concluded with a
recommendation for extensive radon daughter measurements in the area.

_____

* Surface radiation units - disintegrations per minute of α
  radiation

Deepwater

Portions of the Chambers Works at the E.I. DuPont
Deepwater plant were formerly used for contract operations with MED/AEC. The 700 acre complex is in close
proximity to the residential areas of Deepwater, Penns-
ville and Penns Grove. In general, the Department of
Energy (DOE) does not consider existing radiation
a hazard to employees. However, uranium has been
found on surface and underground deposit areas and
in one remaining uranium processing building, #845.
Alpha and beta-gamma contamination radiation levels
there exceed current guidelines for release of buildings to unrestricted use. DOE's greatest concern
for undue radiation exposure derives from the possible use of site-soils for crop growing or other
activities resulting in the dispersal of dusts.
Groundwater sample concentrations were determined
to be well within safe limits.

The Charlotte Mine

Between 1958 and 1968, some 95 tons of uranium
ore were removed from the Charlotte Mine in Byram
Township (Sussex County).[187, 188] The radioactivity
of the remaining tailings, which cover an area of 50
square yards, were declared a radiological hazard
to the public by the DEP (Bureau of Radiation Protection). In June 1981, this hazard was brought to
the attention of the DEP by a Byram Township Planning Board Member whose master's thesis subject was
the hazard posed by the remaining mine tailings.
Analysis of soil samples show uranium and radium
concentrations of 1500 pico Curies/gram and 1100
pico Curies/gram respectively. These values exceed
both state and Federal standards for cleanup of
contaminated sites (40 pCi/g uranium and 5 pCi/g
radium) by factors of 37 and 220 respectively. It
was determined that you would have to remain in the
mine area for 10 days to accumulate a year's permiss-
able radiation dose (500 mrem).[189] The DEP indicated
the major at risk population would be children playing in the area, who represent the most radiosensi-
tive fraction of the general population. The DEP

has recommended that the mine tailings be returned
to the shafts and the area secured with fencing.

There is at least one additional site in New
Jersey with residual radiation as a result of past
processing operations. Thorium was processed at
the Maywood Chemical Works, in Bergen County, during
the period 1915-1956.[189] Again the Nuclear Regulatory
Commission concluded, the low-level radiation in the
area is not a health threat. It may well be that
there is no present health threat from the sites
described in this section. However, we will never
know the genetic damage done to those New Jersey
residents who worked at the sites when they were
active. And what about their progeny?

Transportation of Radioactive Materials (RAM)

In recognition of the growing number of RAM
shipments in the U.S., 2.5 million in 1977 alone,
the Nuclear Regulatory Commission and Department of
Transportation conducted a state surveillance survey
in 1977.[190] New Jersey, a corridor state and one
of nine with the highest frequency of RAM transports,
was chosen for that study. The NRC/DOT concluded
there was no public health or safety problem due to
RAM transport. However, the Federal Radiation
Council (FRC) has established a general public exposure limit of not more than 500 mrem/year. And
the NRC/DOT study indicates that some freight handlers
in New Jersey were receiving annual exposures in excess of FRC recommendations. Although the NRC/DOT
survey was only maintained over a three month period,
those data were extrapolated to a yearly exposure
rate. A personal exposure badge and area monitoring
evaluation indicated that at least two employees
would receive a whole body exposure of 1730 and 2700
mrem/year, respectively. Other RAM exposures noted
in the study were to truck drivers and airline freight
terminal workers. It should be noted that many transportation incidents involving RAM result in the loss
of radioactive sources (cf. chapter 3). The unknowing
handlers of these materials are at a cancer risk.

The NRC/DOT study concluded with only a call for increased enforcement activities.

Industrial Radiation

     Certain industrial uses of ionising radiation
sources posing occupational hazards are not under
the NRC jurisdiction. In December 1976, NIOSH under-
took a survey study to determine the potential hazards
to radiation workers from such sources as electron
microscopes, particle accelerators, electron beam
welders, radiographic devices and high voltage elec-
tronic test equipment.[191] The survey encompassed
ten states determined to employ the majority of the
aforementioned ionising radiation sources, of which
New Jersey was one. The time period covered by the
study was from 1970-1974. The study concluded there
were no "extraordinary hazards from the use of industrial x-ray machines, accelerators or radium sources."
However, there were specific problems in New Jersey
and a table of inspections and violations is given
below:

Total Number of Inspections/Violations in New Jersey
                    1970-1974

X-ray Sources		Accelerators		Radium Sources	
Inspec-tions	Viola-tions	Inspec-tions	Viola-tions	Inspec-tions	Viola-tions
158	194	10	3	48	10

The major x-ray source violations in New Jersey consisted of no surveys, uncalibrated instruments, inadequate records and operator training. Detailed
accelerator and radium source violation evaluation
were not given. Of ten reported incidences, only three
involved personnel exposure to radiation of varied
and uncertain intensity.

The total population occupational exposure,*
extrapolated over a one year period, 1974, was estimated to be 2800 man-rem's and 7500 man-rem's, for
radium sources and industrial x-rays respectively.
These exposures are respectively 22 and 60 times more
than that received from natural background radiation
(and radiation effects are cumulative). The major
disturbing revelations of the study particularly pertaining to New Jersey is that approximately one-fourth
of the survey incidents involve a loss of a radium
source which compliments the incidents cited under
"transportation accidents". Further, Jenkins and
Haas estimate that on a national basis, only 30%
of the analytical x-ray accidents are reported and
verified. The incidents likely to go unreported
usually result from intoxication, fatigue, moon-
lighting, carelessness and gross negligence.

Radioactive Wastes - Atlantic Coast

During the period 1946 to 1967 approximately
33,998 barrels of radioactive wastes were dumped from
barges off the Atlantic Coast.[192] One of the sites
is approximately 111 miles southeast of Atlantic City.
Sediment samples taken at the site indicate that
more than 25% of the drums are leaking and that radioactivity is confined to an area of within ten feet.[193]
According to the director of the surveillance and
emergency preparedness division of the EPA's Office
of Radiation Programs, the wastes pose no hazard.
The Atomic Energy Commission knew of possible leak-
age of radioactive materials as early as 1961.[194]
There are two routes of return of the radioactive
wastes to New Jersey residents. Radioactive wastes
could eventually be transported by ocean currents to
our coastal zone. Further, the dumping site is in
an area of commercial fishing. The health threat
here is not necessarily from eating irradiated fish.
Rather, it is in the remote possibility of eating fish

---

*   on a statewide basis

who had ingested radioactive wastes. Fish could
accomplish this by their eating lower on the food
chain (smaller fish, benthic organisms, plankton,
etc.) and that diet having spent a good deal of its
life cycle in a radioactive environment. The drums
could provide a reef-like microcosm and attract marine
life. Just what is the possibility of a New Jersey
fisherman bringing in a catch that actually fulfills
this scenario at depths of 6000-9000 feet? It may only
be determined by further environmental monitoring.
Investigations have rightly begun not only to determine current health risks from these sites, but also
from reported air dumping as well.[195]

Non-Ionising Radiation Sources

Low Level, Low Frequency Electromagnetic Fields

The physiological and psychological effects of
low-level, low frequency electromagnetic fields
on animals has been demonstrated in the laboratory.
Decreases in growth of plant and animal tissue and
behavioral changes have been observed.[196, 197] Adverse and unusual effects (e.g., a skin-crawling sensa-
tion) have been reported by New Jersey residents living
in proximity to high voltage electric power lines.[198]
Wertheimer and Leeper established a direct relationship between residence in proximity to electrical
wiring configurations (particularly at voltage step-
down points) and childhood cancers in Colorado.[199]
Fulton, et.al. conducted a similar study in Rhode
Island and concluded no relationship existed between
Leukemia and electric power line configurations.[200]

Although New Jersey residents living in proximity
to overhead power lines have experienced unusual
physiological effects, they have been advised by
Public Service Electric and Gas Company (PSE&G)
officials that there is no danger from overhead power
lines. Steven Brogdan, South Jersey District
Engineer for PSE&G, indicates that their towermen,
performing live-line maintenance have reported no

adverse symptomology as a result of their occupation.*
Further, he reports that New Jersey power companies
do not have a unique or higher-than-other states ratio
of high voltage power lines to land area.

Radiofrequency Radiation

The adverse thermal effects of radiofrequency
radiation (greater than 10,000 μw/cm^2**), increases
in body temperature, heat stress, cataract formation,
cardiovascular effects and brainwave pattern changes,
are well documented in the literature.[201] There is
much less documentation on the effects resulting from
exposure to less than 1,000 μw/cm^2; however, changes
in respiration, appetite loss, headaches and central
nervous system disorders have been observed. Some
of the sources of radiofrequency radiation in the
state are microwave ovens, radio broadcast trans-
missions, reflected and standing radio waves and enhanced fields from antennas.

In an attempt to accomplish a thorough search
for the cause of the occurrence of clusters of
childhood leukemia and Hodgkin's disease manifesting
in the spring of 1976 in Rutherford, New Jersey, non-
ionising radiation surveys have been sponsored and
other data acquired in that area by the state's Department of Environmental Protection and Health:[202]

Ross Peterson Survey

This survey was conducted by James Ross and Ron
Peterson of the National Bureau of Standards and
Bell Laboratories, respectively. Essentially, they
reported overall roof-level values of 2.4 μw/cm^2

---

*   Per telephone conversation December 26, 1980 . However, these
    towermen wear specially insulated suits.

** Microwatts/centimeter square

for frequencies between 10,000 and 12 billion cycles
per second. Most of these frequencies were attributed to area AM radio stations.

National Bureau of Standards Survey

A second survey was conducted by Reis and Larsen
of NBS and this team used an instrument and techni-
que which provided controversial results. Nonetheless, in general, no levels exceeded 1 $\mu w/cm^2$. A
value of 10.5 $\mu w/cm^2$ was obtained at a gym score-
board jack. However, on driving out of Rutherford
on Route I-495 toward the New Jersey Turnpike, a value
of 530 $\mu w/cm^2$ was obtained.

The DEP and DOH relying heavily on the Ross/
Peterson survey results, NBS data and OSHA workplace
standard of 10,000 $\mu w/cm^2$, concluded it would be
fruitless to continue to investigate non-ionising
radiation as a cause of the Rutherford Cancer clusters.
Dr. Arthur W. Guy of the University of Washington,
Bioelectromagnetics Research Laboratory, concurred
with the DEP/DOH. However, he felt further epidemiological studies on groups exposed to excessive
electromagnetic fields should be conducted.[203] Dr.
Louis Slesin, then a Senior Research Associate with
the Natural Resources Defense Council, cited the
10.5 $\mu w/cm^2$ value as being higher than any ground level
reading reported by EPA in an eastern seaboard survey.[204] Further, he cited the I-495 reading as being
250,000 times higher than New York City median ground
level readings. Dr. Slesin's evaluation was in response
to a request for evaluation on the data by Rep. Andrew
Maguire (D-7th Dist.) who has been an advocate of
further evaluation of electromagnetic radiation in
Rutherford and the Meadowlands.[205]

* * * *

It may be observed from Figure 11, that the
national position of New Jersey in manufacturing has
declined (cf. Figure 11 to Figure 7).

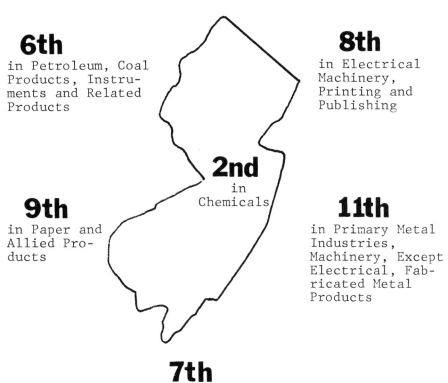

5th
in Rubber and Plastics

6th
in Petroleum, Coal
Products, Instru-
ments and Related
Products

8th
in Electrical
Machinery,
Printing and
Publishing

2nd
in
Chemicals

9th
in Paper and
Allied Pro-
ducts

11th
in Primary Metal
Industries,
Machinery, Except
Electrical, Fab-
ricated Metal
Products

7th
in Leather and Leather Products,
Food and Kindred Products, Textile
Mill Products, Apparel and Related
Products, Stone, clay and glass
Products, miscellaneous manufacturing

FIGURE 11
New Jersey Position in National
Manufacturing status (1979)

Chapter 4 / REFERENCES

1.   The Story of the Great Seal of the State of
        New Jersey, Educational Services,
        Archives and History Bureau, New
        Jersey State Library, July 1973.

2.   Wilson, Harold F., et.al., Outline History of
        New Jersey, Rutgers University Press,
        New Brunswick, 1950, p. 77.

3.   Ibid., p. 76.

4.   Cunningham, John, Made in New Jersey, the
        Industrial Story of a State, Rutgers,
        the State University, New Brunswick,
        c. 1954.

5.   Ibid.

6.   Krawiec, Stella, Ph.D., The Chemical Industry
        in New Jersey, Office of Economic
        Research, Division of Planning and
        Research, New Jersey Department of
        Labor and Industry, July 1978.

7.   Laccetti, Silvio R., Ph.D., Ed., The Outlook
        on New Jersey, Wm. H. Wise & Co., Inc.,
        Union City, New Jersey, 1979, p. 481

8.   Cunningham, John T., I'm From New Jersey,
        The National Geographic, vol. 117,
        no. 1, January 1960, pp. 1-45.

9.   Ibid.

10. Gould, Harry, Speak Now or Behold Offshore
        Drilling Plans, The Philadelphia
        Inquirer, January 25, 1976.

11. Grass Roots: An Agricultural Retention and
        Development Program for New Jersey.
        New Jersey Department of Agriculture,
        New Jersey Department of Environmental
        Protection. October 31, 1980.

12. Formaldehyde Foam Fight Fashioned, Industrial
        Chemical News, March 1981, p. 8.

13. Leary, Warren E., Nitrosamines in Animal Feed
        May Effect Tests for Cancer, Washington
        Post, September 13, 1978, p. A17.

14. Eisler, Barbara, Air Pollution in New Jersey:
        Problems, Programs and Progress,
        American Lung Association of New Jersey
        and the Department of Environmental
        Protection, 1979, p. 19.

15. Hill, T.A., Siedle, A.R., Perry, Roger, Chemical
        Hazards of a Fire-Fighting Training
        Environment, American Industrial Hygiene
        Association Journal, Vol. 33, No. 6, June
        1972, pp. 423-430.

16. Aoki, Kunio, M.D., and Shimizu, Hiroyuki, M.D.,
        Lung Cancer and Air Pollution, National
        Cancer Institute, Monograph 47, 1977,
        p. 17-20.

17. Fraumeni, Joseph F., Respiratory Carcinogenesis:
        An Epidemiologic Appraisal, Journal of
        the National Cancer Institute, Vol. 55,
        No. 5, November 1975, pp. 1039-1045.

18. Katz, Ronald M., B.S., and Jowett, Dand, Ph.D.,
        Female Laundry and Dry Cleaning Works
        in Wisconsin: A Mortaility Analysis,
        American Journal of Public Health, Vol.
        71, No. 3, 1981, pp. 305-307.

19.   Keith, Larry H., and Telliard, William A.,
          Priority Pollutants II-A Perspective
          View, Environmental Science & Tech-
          nology, Vol. 13, No. 4, April 1979,
          pp. 416-422.

20.   Runion, Howard E., Benzene in Gasoline,
          American Industrial Hygiene Associa-
          tion Journal, Vol. 36, No. 5, May 1975,
          pp. 338-349.

21.   Irving, W.S., Jr., Ph.D., and Grumbles, Thomas
          G., M.S., Benzene Exposures During
          Gasoline Loading at Bulk Marketing
          Terminals, American Industrial Hygiene
          Association Journal, (40), June 1979,
          pp. 468-473.

22.   Brief, Richard S., Lynch, Jeramiah, Bernath,
          Tibor; and Scala, Robert A., Benzene
          in the Workplace, American Industrial
          Hygiene Association Journal, (41)
          September 1980, pp. 616-623.

23.   Pitts, James N., Jr., Chemical and Biological
          Implications of Organic Compounds
          Formed in Simulated and Real Urban
          Atmospheres, Ecotoxicology and
          Environmental Safety, 2., 1978,
          pp. 199-217.

24.   Proctor, Nick H., Ph.D. and Hughes, James
          P., M.D., Chemical Hazards of the
          Workplace, J.B. Lippincott Company,
          Philadelphia, p. 388, 1978.

25. Battista, S.P., Ciliatoxic Components of
        Cigarette Smoke. In: Wynder, E.L.,
        Hoffman, D., and Gori, G.B., (Eds).
        Proceedings of the Third World Con-
        ference on Smoking and Health, New York,
        June 2-5, 1975., Vol. 1, Modifying the
        Risk for the Smoker, U.S. Department of
        Health, Education and Welfare, Public
        Health Service, National Institutes of
        Health, National Cancer Institute, DHEW
        Publication MO. (NIK) 76-1221, 1976,
        pp. 517-534.

26. Report of Governor Brendan Byrne's Hazardous
        Waste Advisory Commission, Trenton,
        New Jersey. (Draft Copy)

27. Ibid.

28. Ibid.

29. Ibid.

30. Ibid.

31. Protection Needed from PCB Hazards, The Gloucester
        County Times, Editorial, June 3, 1979, p. A6.

32. Rollins Environmental Assessment, Draft copy,
        New Jersey Department of Environmental
        Protection, 1980.

33. Higuchi, Kentaro (Ed.), PCB Poisoning and
        Pollution, Kodansha Ltd., Tokyo/Acade-
        mic Press, New York, 1976.

34. Proctor, Nick, H., Ph.D. and Hughes, James
        P., M.D., Op. Cit.

35. Reid, T.R., Paulsboro Cancer Rate Stirs Nation-
        wide PCB Probe, The Evening Times,
        Trenton, N.J., August 26, 1976.

36. Jerome, Lawrence E., Defusing the PCB "Time
         Bomb," Oceans, May 1979, pp. 60-63.

37. Budiansky, Stephen and Josephson, Julian,
         Waste Disposal Chemistry, Environ-
         mental Science & Technology, Vol. 14,
         No. 5, May 1980, pp. 508-510.

38. Proctor, Nick H., Ph.D., and Hughes, James
         P., M.D., Op. Cit.

39. North, Barry E., The Impact of PCB Incinera-
         tion on Atmospheric PCB Concentrations.
         An Assessment of the Atmospheric Dis-
         persion of PCB's. School of Public
         Health, Columbia University, December
         27, 1979, pp. 1-30.

40. Ibid.

41. Hazardous Waste Advisory Commission, Op. Cit.

42. Report of the Office of Hazardous Substances
         Control (OHSC) of the Department of
         Environmental Protection Toxic Substances
         Program, Trenton, N.J., April 3, 1979.

43. Baum, Bernard, Ph.D., Parker, Charles H.,
         and DeBell & Richardson, Inc., Solid
         Waste Disposal, Vol. I, Incineration
         and Landfill, Ann Arbor Science Pub-
         lishers, Inc., Ann Arbor, 1974.

44. Waldbott, George L., Health Effects of Environ-
         mental Pollutants, The C.V. Mosby
         Company, Saint Louis, 1973, Chapter 23.

45. Ibid.

46. Personal Correspondence from G.W. Collyer Insu-
         lated Wire Company, January 25, 1977.

47. Hill, T.A., Siedle, A.R.; and Perry, Roger,
          Chemical Hazards of a Fire-Fighting
          Training Environment, American Industrial
          Hygiene Association Journal, Vol. 33,
          No. 6, June 1972, pp. 423-430.

48. Pier Burns, (AP), The Gloucester County Times,
          March 4, 1980, p. A4.

49. Perth Amboy Residents Take Chances During Blaze,
          (AP), The Gloucester County Times, July
          8, 1980, p. A4.

50. "Time Bomb," 20,000 Chemical Drums Burn (AP),
          The Goucester County Times, April 23,
          1980.

51. Bozzelli, Joseph W., Ph.D., Kebbekus, Barbara
          B., Ph.D., and Greenberg, Arthur, Ph.D.,
          Analysis of Selected Toxic and Carcino-
          genic Substances in Ambient Air in New
          Jersey, New Jersey Department of
          Environmental Protection, Office of
          Cancer and Toxic Substances Research,
          May 1980.

52. Treitman, Robert D.; Burgess, William A., and
          Gold, Avram, Air Contaminants
          Encountered by Fire-fighters, American
          Industrial Hygiene Association Journal,
          Vol. 41, No. 11, November 1980, pp.
          796-802.

53. Ibid.

54. Archer, S.R., and Blackwood, T.R., Status Assess-
          ment of Toxic Chemicals: Asbestos,
          EPA-600/2-79-210C, U.S. Environmental Pro-
          tection Agency, Cincinnati, Ohio, December
          1979, p. 5.

55. Millette, J.R., Pansing, M.F. and Boone, R.L.,
    Asbestos-Cement Materials Used in Water
    Supply, Water/Engineering & Management,
    March 1981, p. 48-51, 60, 97.

56. Harrington, Malcolm J., et.al., An Investigation
    of the Use of Asbestos Cement Pipe for
    Public Water Supply and the Incidence of
    Gastrointestinal Cancer in Connecticut,
    1935-1973, American Journal of Epidem-
    iology, Vol. 107, No. 1, 1978, pp. 96-103.

57. Kanarek, Marty S., et.al., Asbestos in Drinking
    Water and cancer Incidence in the San
    Francisco Bay Area, American Journal of
    Epidemiology, Vol. 112, No. 1, 1980,
    pp. 54-72.

58. Langer, Arthur M. and Wolff, Mary S., Asbestos
    Carcinogenesis, Chapter 3, Inorganic
    and Nutritional Aspects of Cancer,
    Schrauzer, G.N., (Ed.) Plenum Publish-
    ing Corporation, New York, 1978.

59. Blejer, Hector P., M.D., D.H. and Arlon, Robert,
    Pharm. D., Talc: A Possible Occupational
    and Environmental Carcinogen, Journal
    of Occupational Medicine, Vol. 15,
    No. 2, February 1973, p. 96.

60. Langer, A.M., Wolff, M.S., Rohl, A.N., and
    Selikoff, I.J., Variation of Properties
    of Chrysotile Asbestos Subjected to Mill-
    ing, Journal of Toxicology and Environment-
    al Health, 4, 1978, pp. 173-188.

61. Selikoff, I.J., M.D., Hammond, E.C., Sc.D.,
    Churg, J., M.D., Mortality Experience
    of Amosite Asbestos Factory Workers,
    Mount Sinai School of Medicine of the
    City University of New York and the Ameri-
    can Cancer Society, New York, N.Y., Pre-
    sented at the IVth International Pneumocon-
    iosis Conference, Bucharest, Sept. 29, 1971.

62. Selikoff, I.J., M.D., Seldman, Herbert, M.B.A.,
         and Hammond, E. Cuyler, Sc.D., Mortality
         Effects of Cigarette Smoking Among Amosite
         Asbestos Factory Workers, Journal of the
         National Cancer Institute, Vol. 65, No. 3,
         September, 1980, pp. 507-513.

63. New Asbestos Threat Reported, Chemical Week,
         Vol. 122, No. 11, March 15, 1978, p. 25.

64. Wilk, Tom, DuPont Repaupo Plant Fined $63,000
         by OSHA, The Gloucester County Times,
         April 18, 1979.

65. DuPont Plant Cited for Health Violations (AP),
         The Gloucester County Times, July 31,
         1980.

66. Anderson, Henry A., Lilis, Ruth, Daum, Susan
         M., Fischbein, Alfred S., and Selikoff,
         Irving J., Household-Contact Asbestos
         Neoplastic Risk, Annals of the New York
         Academy of Sciences, Vol. 271, May 28,
         1976, pp. 311-323.

67. Stollman, Rita, 144 Join Class-Action Asbestos
         Suit, The Record, June 17, 1975, p. A-9.

68. Winans, Foster R., Courts Flooded with Asbestos
         Litigation, The New York Times, August
         3, 1980.

69. Gould, Harry, The Silent Threat Overhead, The
         Philadelphia Inquirer (New Jersey Metro
         Section), January 10, 1977. Section B.

70. Asbestos Issue: A Matter of Principle, The Johns
         Manville Company, April 1979.

71. McQueeny, James, Cancer Peril: DEP Wants to Halt
         Sales at Condominium Complex, The
         Sunday Star-Ledger, September 1976, p. 18.

72. Archer, S.R. and Blackwood, T.R., Op. Cit.

73. Jenkins, Catherine L., Ph.D., Scientific Basis
         for the Proposed Regulation of Dyes De-
         rived from the Chemical Substances Benzi-
         dine, 3,3'-Dimethylbenzidine, and 3,3,'
         -Dimethoxybenzidine, National Science
         Foundation Public Service Resident Center
         for Occupational Hazards, Inc., New York,
         N.Y.

74. Archer, S.R. and Blackwood, T.R., Status Assess-
         ment of Toxic Chemicals: Benzidene, EPA.
         600/2-79-210e, U.S. Environmental Pro
         tection Agency, Cincinnati, Ohio,
         December 1979.

75. Ibid.

76. Ibid.

77. Jenkins, Catherine L., Ph.D., Op. Cit.

78. Ibid.

79. Shottenfeld, David, M.D., and Haas, Joanna,
         F., M.D., Carcinogens in the Workplace,
         CA-A Cancer Journal for Clinicians, Vol.
         29, No. 3, May/June 1979.

80. Ibid.

81. Blot, William J., Ph.D. and Fraumeni, Joseph
         F., M.D., Geographic Patterns of Bladder
         Cancer in the United States, Journal of
         the National Cancer Institute, Vol. 61,
         No. 4, October 1978, pp. 1017-1023.

82. Mason, T.J., McKay, F.W., Hoover, R., et.al.
         Atlas of Cancer Mortality in U.S.
         Counties, 1950-1969. DHEW Publication
         No. (NIH) 75-780, Washington, D.C.,
         Government Printing Office, 1975.

83.   Blot, William J., Ph.D., and Fraumeni, Joseph
         F., M.D., Op. Cit., p. 1013.

84.   Mason, T.J., McKay, F.W., and Hoover, R. et.al.,
         Op. Cit.

85.   Occupational Safety and Health: A DuPont Company
         View, E.I. DuPont de Nemours & Co., Inc.,
         Wilmington, Del., Rev. 9/1/77, pp. 1-58.

86.   Ibid.

87.   Steyer, Robert, Jersey Rated High in Cancer of
         the Bladder, Newark Star Ledger, October
         28, 1979.

88.   Blot, William J., Ph.D. and Fraumeni, Joseph F.,
         M.D., Op. Cit.

89.   Jenkins, Catherine L., Ph.D., Op. Cit.

90.   Letter from Watler R. Payne, CSP, Director of
         Safety and Industrial Hygiene, Toms
         River Chemical Company, Toms River, N.J.,
         February 8, 1980.

91.   Archer, S.R., and Blackwood, T.R., Op. Cit.

92.   Friedman, Mendel, Diamond, Martin J., MacGregor,
         James T., Mutagenicity of Textiles Dyes,
         Environmental Science & Technology, Vol.
         14, No. 9, September 1980, pp. 1145-1146.

93.   Archer, S.R., and Blackwood, T.R., Op. Cit.

94.   Khan, Z.S., and Hughes, T.W., Source Assessment:
         Polyvinyl Chloride, EPA-600/2-68-004i,
         U.S. Environmental Protection Agency,
         Cincinnati, Ohio, May 1978.

95. Tierney, D.R., and Blackwood, T.R., Status
        Assessment of Toxic Chemicals: Vinylidene
        Chloride, EPA-600/2-79-210o, U.S.
        Environmental Protection Agency,
        Cincinnati, Ohio, December 1979.

96. Tabershaw, Irving R., M.D., and Gaffey, William
        R., Ph.D., Mortality Study of Workers
        in the Manufacture of Vinyl Chloride and
        its Polymers, Journal of Occupational
        Medicine, Vol. 16, No. 8, August 1974.

97. Ibid.

98. Rawls, Rebecca, Studies Update Vinyl Chloride
        Hazards, Chemical & Engineering News,
        April 7, 1980, p. 27.

99. Dorigan, J., Scoring of Organic Air Pollutants:
        Chemistry, Production, and Toxicity of
        Selected Synthetic Organic Chemicals,
        Mitre Corporation, September 1976.

100. Tierney, D.R., and Blackwood, T.R., Op. Cit.

101. Khan, Z.S., and Hughes, T.W., Op. Cit.

102. Tierney, D.R., and Blackwood, T.R., Op. Cit.

103. Ibid.

104. Brady, George S., and Clauser, Henry R.,
        Materials Handbook, McGraw-Hill Company,
        New York, 1977.

105. Higgins, Frederick B., Jr., Ph.D., et.al.,
        Air Pollution Potential of Industrial
        Processes, Landtect Corporation,
        Philadelphia, May 1970.

106. Blott, William J., Brinton, Louise A., Fraumeni,
       Joseph F., Jr., and Stone, B.J., Cancer
       Mortality in U.S. Counties with Petro-
       leum Industries, Science, Vol. 198,
       October 7, 1977, pp. 51-53.

107. Brain Tumor/Petrochemical Link Probed, Chemical
       and Engineering News, Vol. 58, No. 44,
       November 3, 1980, p. 6.

108. Fox, Jeffrey L., Brain Tumor Risk in Petro-
       chemical Workers, Chemical and Engineer-
       ing News, Vol. 58, No. 45, November 10,
       1980.

109. Oil Refineries Refute Brain Cancer Study, The
       Gloucester County Times, October 29, 1980.

110. Minde, Theodore A., New Jersey's Petroleum
       Industry, Office of Planning and Research,
       N.J. Department of Labor and Industry,
       May 1979.

111. Walcot, John, Cancer Link Studies, The Burling-
       ton Record, August 20, 1976.

112. Reid, T.R., Paulsboro Cancer Rate Stirs Nation-
       wide PCB Probe, The Evening Times,
       August 26, 1976.

113. Calendar, Jody, and Bacon, Barbara, Lawyer
       for Midland Workers Says They Suffer
       Eye, Lung Diseases, Asbury Park Press,
       July 12, 1980, Section C.

114. Stanton, Mearl F., et.al., Carcinogenicity of
       Fibrous Glass: Pleural Response in
       the Rat in Relation to Fiber Dimension,
       Journal of The National Cancer Institute,
       Vol. 58, No. 3, March 1977, pp. 587-597.

115. Scholl, Jaye, GM Eyes Cancer Study for Ewing
       Plant, Trenton Times, August 28, 1980.

116. _____, Deaths Probed at GM, Trenton Times,
          August 29, 1980.

117. Kopelman, Joel, M.D., Thind, Inderjit, M.D.,
          and Louria, Donald B., M.D., Investigat-
          ing Industrially Related Diseases (Letter
          to the Editor), American Journal of
          Public Health, Vol. 70, No. 4, April
          1980, p. 436.

118. A Decade of Progress, 10th Annual Report, New
          Jersey Department of Environmental
          Protection, 1980.

119. Cleaning Our Environment, A Chemical Perspective,
          American Chemical Society, Washington,
          D.C., 1978, Chapter 7.

120. Birth Defects, Shore Area Probed for Source of
          Problems, The Gloucester County Times,
          April 9, 1980, D-1.

121. Birth Defects Found in Cape May County, New
          Jersey Hazardous Waste News, Vol. 1,
          No. 2, February 1981, p. 1.

122. Blackwood, T.R. and Sipes, T.G., Status
          Assessment of Toxic Chemicals: Hexachloro-
          benzene, EPA-600/2-79-210g, U.S. Environ-
          mental Protection Agency, Cincinnati,
          Ohio, December 1979, p. 12.

123. Tucker, Robert K., Ph.D., and Burke, Thomas,
          A., M.P.H., A Second Preliminary Report
          on the Findings of the State Groundwater
          Monitoring Project, Program on Environ-
          mental Cancer and Toxic Substances, New
          Jersey Department of Environmental Pro-
          tection, December, 1978.

124. Highland, Joseph H., et.al., Malignant Neglect,
          Alfred A. Knopf, New York, 1979, p. 129.

125. New Jersey Agent Orange Commission, "The Vietnam
        Veterans Self-Help Guide on Agent Orange."

126. Ibid.

127. "Study Shows Few Health Effects from Dioxin,"
        Chemical & Engineering News, Vol. 57,
        No. 44, October 29, 1979, p. 7.

128. "Judge Lets EPA Ban on 2,4,5,-T Stand," Chemical
        Week, Vol. 124, No. 11, March 14, 1979.

129. New Jersey Agent Orange Commission, Agent Orange
        Seminar, Gloucester County College,
        February 28, 1981.

130. Sanders, Howard J., Herbicides, Chemical &
        Engineering News, Vol. 59, No. 31,
        August 21, 1981, pp. 20-35.

131. New Jersey Agent Orange Commission, Op. Cit.

132. The Statewide Water Supply Master Plan, New
        Jersey State Department of Environmental
        Protection, Division of Water Resources,
        November 3, 1977.

133. 208 Water Quality Management Plan, Burlington,
        Camden and Gloucester Counties, New
        Jersey, Delaware Valley Regional Plann-
        ing Commission, December 1977.

134. Rules of The Bureau of Solid Waste Management,
        N.J.A.C. 7:26-1 et. Seq. New Jersey
        Department of Environmental Protection,
        July 1, 1974.

135. "Quality Assurance for Groundwater," Environmental
        Science & Technology, Vol. 10, No. 3,
        March 1976, Part C, pp. 226-227.

136. Nordland, Rod, and Friedman, Josh, Poison at Our
        Doorsteps, The Philadelphia Inquirer,
        September 24, 1979.

137. McDonnell, Patrick, N.J. Water Among 'Most
        Contaminated' in U.S., The Gloucester
        County Times, January 18, 1971, p. B-7.

138. Mattiace, Peter, Judge Cites Owners in Price's
        Pit Controversy, Gloucester County Times,
        September 25, 1981.

139. Landfill Threatens Atlantic City Water, New
        Jersey Hazardous Waste News, Volume I,
        No. 3, March 1981.

140. Ibid.

141. Ibid.

142. U.S. Sues Firms in Poisoning of Price Pit Water,
        (AP), Gloucester County Times, September
        22, 1981.

143. Tully, Shawn, The King of Toxic Waste, New Jersey
        Monthly, Vol. 4, No. 1, November 1979.

144. Hazardous Waste Disposal Damage Report, Fatality
        at a New Jersey Industrial Landfill,
        EPA/530/SW-151, U.S. Environmental Pro-
        tection Agency Report, June 1975.

145. State of New Jersey Groundwater Pollution Index,
        1975-June 1980, Department of Environ-
        mental Protection, Division of Water Re-
        sources, Bureau of Groundwater Management.

146. Janson, Donald, Toxic Waste: A Nightmare for
        Jersey, The New York Times, February 7,
        1980.

147. State of New Jersey Groundwater Pollution Index,
        1975-June 1980, op. Cit.

148. Goldberg, Elliot, Is Area Groundwater in Peril?, The Gloucester County Times, October 30, 1980.

149. Roux, Paul H., Availability, Utilization and Contamination of Water Resources in Gloucester and Camden Counties, New Jersey. Order No. W.A. 6-00-2104-A U.S. Environmental Protection Agency, Washington, D.C., December 1976.

150. Superior Court of New Jersey, Chancery Division, Gloucester County, Docket No. C-2670-72. Department of Environmental Protection (Plaintiff) vs. Nick LiPari (Defendant) and Third Party Plaintiff, vs. Rohm and Haas Company, a Delaware Corporation, C. September 1974.

151. Letter from Richard Katz, New Jersey Department of Environmental Protection, October 22, 1979 to Dr. Lipsky (Subject: Air Samples From LiPari Landfill).

152. Roux, Paul H., Op. Cit.

153. Sheldon, Linda S., and Hites, Ronald A., Organic Compounds in the Delaware River, Environmental Science & Technology, Vol. 12, No. 10, October 1978, pp. 118-1194.

154. Ibid.

155. Ibid.

156. Lysyj, I., and Russell, E.D., Transfer of Organics from an Oil Film into Water, In: Fate of Pollutants in the Air and Water Environment, Part I. Mechanisms of Interaction Between Environment and Mathematical Modeling and the Physical Fate of Pollutants, Suffet, I.H., (Ed.), Wiley-Interscience Publication, John Wiley & Sons, Inc., New York, 1977, pp. 135-144.

157. Oil Spills and Spills of Hazardous Substances,
        Oil and Special Materials Control Division,
        Office of Water Program Operations, U.S.
        Environmental Protection Agency, Washing-
        ton D.C. , March 1977.

158. 208 Water Quality Management Plan, Op. Cit.

159. Burke, Thomas A., M.P.H., and Tucker, Robert
        K., Ph.D., A Preliminary Report on the
        Findings of the State Groundwater Monitor-
        ing Project, Program on Environmental
        Cancer and Toxic Substances, Department
        of Environmental Protection, March 1978.

160. Tucker, Robert K., Ph.D., and Burke, Thomas A.,
        M.P.H., Op. Cit., December 1978.

161. New Jersey State Department of Environmental
        Protection, Tabulation of Analytical
        Data from Public Water Supply, Memos.
        No. 80-295 and 80-323, August 26, 1980
        and September 16, 1980, respectively.

162. Nuclear Energy, Questions and Answers, Public
        Service Electric & Gas Co., The Energy
        People.

163. Shut Down, Nuclear Power on Trial, The Book
        Publishing Co., Summertown, 1979, pp.
        176-178.

164. Cairns, John, Cancer: Science and Society, W.H.
        W.H. Freeman and Co., San Francisco, 1978,
        Chapter 7.

165. Nuclear Power Information Fact Sheets, Atomic
        Industrial Forum Inc., Public Affairs
        and Information Program, Washington,
        D.C., May 1979, p. 1-11.

166. FRC, Federal Radiation Council, Report #1,
        May 1960.

167. The Salem Generating Station, Public Service
        Electric & Gas Co.

168. Ibid.

169. Eisenbud, Merril, Sc.D., Health Hazards from
        Radioactive Emissions, American Medical
        Association Congress on Environmental
        Health, April 20-30, 1973, Chicago, Ill.

170. NRC Fines PSE&G $90,000 for Radiation Exposure
        Incidents, The Gloucester County Times,
        February 22, 1981, p. A-10.

171. Salem A Plant Control Room 'A Disaster?', (AP),
        The Gloucester County Times, April 12,
        1979, p. D-1.

172. More Nuke Damage Found at Salem, The Gloucester
        County Times, May 17, 1979, p. A-1.

173. Radiation Leak Reported at Salem Nuclear Plant
        (AP), The Gloucester County Times, March
        11, 1981.

174. Collings, Amy, Atomic Waste Storage Protested,
        The Gloucester County Times, March 16,
        1979, p. D-1

175. Ibid.

176. Ibid.

177. Goldberg, Elliot, Farming in Shadow of the
        Nukes, The Gloucester County Times,
        July 15, 1979, p. A-8.

178. "The Nuclear Power Controversy," Union of
        Concerned Scientists, Cambridge, Mass.

179. Nuclear Energy, Questions and Answers, Public
        Service Electric & Gas Co., The Energy
        People.

180. The Comparative Risks of Different Methods of
         Generating Electricity, American Nuclear
         Society, Document PPS-3, October 1979.

181. Advisory Committee on the Biological Effects
         of Ionizing Radiations, The Effects on
         Populations of Exposure to Low Levels
         of Ionizing Radiation, Washington, D.C.,
         National Academy of Sciences, 1972.

182. Tamplin, Arthur R., and Gofman, John W., Popula-
         tion Control through Nuclear Pollution,
         Nelson-Hall, Chicago, 1970.

183. Shut Down, Nuclear Power on Trial, Op. Cit.

184. Evans, H.J., Buckton, K.E., Hamilton, G.E., and
         Carothers, A., Ratiation - Induced
         Chromosome Aberrations in Nuclear Dock-
         yard Workers, Nature, Vol. 277, February
         15, 1979, pp. 531-534.

185. Formerly Utilized MED/AEC Sites, Remedial Action
         Program, Radiological Survey of the Middle-
         sex, New Jersey, U.S. Department of Energy,
         November 1977.

186. Formerly Utilized MED/AEC Sites, Remedial Action
         Program, Radiological Survey of the E.I.
         DuPont de Nemours and Co., Deepwater
         New Jersey, U.S. Department of Energy,
         December 1978.

187. Tosch, Kent, Eng, Jeanette and Rauch, Frederick,
         Investigation of the Charlotte Uranium
         Mine, New Jersey State Department of
         Environmental Protection, Division of
         Environmental Quality, Bureau of Radia-
         tion Protection, June 1981.

188. Uranium Mine Hazard found in Byram Township
         Hazardous Waste News, Volume I, No. 6,
         September 1981.

189. Parisi, Albert, Radiation Report Fails to Ease
        Fears, New York Times, August 23, 1981.

190. Summary Report of the State Surveillance Pro-
        gram on the Transportation of Radioactive
        Materials, U.S. Nuclear Regulatory
        Commission, December 1977.

191. Cohen, Sandord C., Kinsman, Simon and MacCabee,
        Howard D., Evaluation of Occupational
        Hazards from Industrial Radiation: A Sur-
        vey of Selected States, U.S. Department
        of Health, Education and Welfare, Public
        Health Service, Cincinnati, Ohio, December
        1976.

192. Smith, David D., and Brown, Robert P., Ocean Dis-
        posal of Barge-Delivered Liquid and Solid
        Wastes from U.S. Coastal Cities, U.S.
        Environmental Protection Agency, Solid
        Waste Management Office, 1971.

193. Radioactive Waste Posed 'No Hazard', (AP), The
        Gloucester County Times, January 8, 1981,
        p. A-4.

194. Smith, David D. and Brown, Robert P., Op. Cit.

195. Lucas, Charlotte-Anne, N.J. Fisherman Fears a
        Radioactive Catch, The Philadelphia In-
        quirer, January 5, 1981, Section G.

196. Coate, W.B., Seed Germination and Early Growth
        Study. In: Project Sanguine, Biological
        Effects Test Program Pilot Studies, Naval
        Electronics Systems Command, Final Report,
        November 1970, pp. H-1 - H-10. Available
        from National Technical Information Ser-
        vice as ADA 717409.

197. Krueger, W.F., Giarola, A.J., Bradley, J.W.,
        et.al., Influence of Low-level Elec-
        tric and Magnetic Fields on the Growth
        of Young Chicks, Biomed Science Instrum,
        9, 1972, pp. 183-186.

198. Farm Family Claims Power Lines Hurtful (AP),
        The Gloucester County Times, April 16,
        1980, p. D-1.

199. Wertheimer, Nancy and Leeper, Ed, Electrical
        Wiring Configurations and Childhood
        Cancer, American Journal of Epidemiology,
        Vol. 109, No. 3, 1979, pp. 273-284.

200. Fulton, John P., et.al., Electrical Wiring Con-
        figurations and Childhood Leukemia in
        Rhode Island, American Journal of Epi-
        demiology, Vol. III, No. 3, 1980,
        pp. 292-296.

201. Memorandum from Richard Katz, DEP Environmental
        Scientist to Acting Director Dr. Sydney
        Gray, Summary Report on Non-Ionizing
        Radiation in Rutherford, New Jersey,
        August 6, 1979.

202. Ibid.

203. Letter from Guy, Arthur W., Ph.D. to Steven
        d'Arazien, Legislative Assistant for
        Environmental Health, Rep. Andrew
        Maguire's Office, Washington, D.C.,
        November 5, 1979.

204. Letter from Slesin, Louis, Ph.D., Senior
        Research Associate, Natural Resources
        Defense Council, Inc., N.Y. to Con-
        gressman Andrew Maguire, Washington,
        D.C., December 4, 1979.

205. Cohen, Robert, Maguire Points Up Radiation
        Findings in Meadowlands, The Star Ledger
        December 19, 1979.

CHAPTER 5

VOLUNTARY USE/EXPOSURE TO
CARCINOGENS, MUTAGENS
AND TERATOGENS

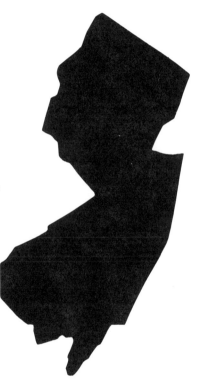

"Individuals tend to
 ignore their own
 responsibilities and
 blame harmful occur-
 rences, including
 carcinogenic exposure,
 on outside forces."

Ernst L. Wynder,
M.D., and
Gio B. Gori,
Ph.D.*

*   Guest Editorial in Journal of the National Cancer Institute,
    Vol. 58. No. 4., April 1977.

CHAPTER 5

LIFE-STYLE: A non-occupational manner of expression
characterizing human activity.

BACKGROUND

On a quantitative basis, the factors with a cancer
risk that represent the New Jersey residents' life-
style, are fewer in number than those characterizing
occupational factors. The life-style factors are however more insidious. Some of these factors trans-
verse socioeconomic groups, e.g., the use of the
"accepted drugs." Others, such as exposure to wood-
stove-derived indoor pollutants, predominate in the
suburbs. There is little data to support the concept
of a single state personality. However, an Eagleton
Poll (telephone survey) indicated that state residents under 30 years of age tend to regard the pursuit of pleasure as being of paramount importance in
life.[1] That same survey indicated that residents
over the age of 45 years tend to regard hard work as
dominating over the pursuit of pleasure. These data
are limited and shall not be extrapolated to represent the life-style of all state residents. Further
indication of a "state life-style" or factors indicative of one, shall be left to the sociologists.

In this chapter many of the life-style factors
presenting health risks to New Jersey residents are
identified. Although they are not entirely unique
to New Jersey, one common theme prevails - the element of election.

235

ACCEPTED DRUGS

TOBACCO - Background

It is the author's opinion that there is a substantial parallel between the operation of a hazardous waste disposal facility and the personal use of
tobacco:

Hazardous waste disposal technique	Smoking
Incineration	Cigarette tobacco combustion, tempera-ture profile 40-880 C.
Landfilling	Storage in body of chemicals - "trans-location"
Biological Treatment	Metabolism

Similarly, air pollution episodes occur at hazard-
our waste facilities and the parallel activity with
tobacco use is involuntary smoking.[2] It has now been
demonstrated that non-smokers who share tobacco-smoke
contaminated air with smokers, show reduced pulmonary
functioning. Tobacco smoke is known to contain over
2,000 chemicals, some of which are carcinogenic,
mutagenic or teratogenic.*[3] The principal categories
of components formed during the combustion of the
tobacco leaf are summarized below:

> • *The Gas Phase* - comprising more than 90%
> of the mainstream smoke, consisting of carbon
> dioxide, carbon monoxide, oxides of nitrogen,
> nitrosamines[c], hydrogen cyanide, volatile

---

*   indicated by a C, M or T.

aldehydes, ketones, hydrocarbons[c], sulfur
and nitrogen containing compounds, vinyl
chloride[c], formaldehyde[c] and hydrazine[c].

- *The Particulate Phase* - The "Tars", containing nicotine, nitrosamines[c], benzenes[c].
phenol, polycyclic aromatic hydrocarbons[c]
(discussed under air pollutants), and
b-naphthylamine[c].

- *Metals* - containing every metal in the
periodic table (excluding the post uranium
metals) including - nickel[c], cadmium[c] and
chromium[c]. Radioactive elements[c] - con-
tains α and β emitters (^{226}Ra, ^{210}Po,
^{210}Pb and ^{40}K). α emitters are weak sources
of x-rays, not passing through a thin
sheet of paper. However, the intimate contact of the species with soft tissue as occurs
during the chewing of tobacco, inhalation
and ingestion, insures direct bombardment
of cell nuclei and the potential initiation
of neoplasms.

- *Agricultural chemicals*[m]- Insecticide residues-
DDT (2,2 - bis p-chlorophenyl - 1,1,1 - trichloroethane), DDD, endrin, endosulfan and
other pesticides.

- *Tobacco Additives* - contain chemicals known
to be ciliatoxic (acrolein, volatile aldehydes and ketones) and diethylene glycol
regarded as enhancing smokers risk to bladder
cancers.

On the basis of epidemiological studies conducted by
the American Cancer Society, U.S. Government, other
national and European agencies, it has been concluded
that:[4]

- cigarette smoking is the major cause of
lung cancer in men and women.

- there is a *causal* relationship between
  tobacco smoking and the development of
  disease (cancer of the lung, larynx, oral
  cavity, esophagus, chronic obstructive lung
  disease, bronchitis and emphysema and coro-
  nary heart disease).

- cigarette smoking is related to cancer of
  the bladder, kidney and pancreas.

It is the author's opinion that based on the presence of virtually all of the chemicals already described in this work, in tobacco smoke - that the risk
of cancers from tobacco use be regarded as totitumoric,
i.e., capable of inducing one or more of the many forms
of cancer throughout the body. Obviously, the first
line of contact from smoking and inhalation is pre-
dominately to the lungs. However, the carcinogens,
mutagens and teratogens present in tobacco in whatever
form (cigarette, pipe, cigar or chewing tobacco) are
absorbed by the circulatory system and ingested during
use, ultimately visiting much of the human anatomy.

Tobacco Use in New Jersey and Risks to Cancers

On a national basis more than 100,000 Americans
currently have lung cancer and in 1981, 112,000 new
cases and 105,000 cancer deaths, due to lung cancer,
were predicted.[5] In New Jersey, out of an estimated
1981 all-site cancer mortality of 15,900, there will be
approximately 4,400 new lung cancer cases and 3,800
deaths. The American Cancer Society estimates that
75% of lung cancer deaths are due to smoking.*
Based on their statistics, a major source of voluntary exposure to carcinogens is clearly identified.
Since tobacco exposes the user to a totitumoric
cancer risk, it is also responsible for some portion
of the other 11,800 cancer deaths in New Jersey. How-

---

* An average of 83% in men, 43% in women

ever, bear in mind strongly, and with a generous share
of empathy for the plight of the epidemiologist, there
are other environmental pollutants with the potential
to induce cancers of the lungs and other sites, (e.g.,
asbestos).

There is little very recent epidemiological data
on tobacco use specific for New Jersey. However,
in 1968, J.F. Fraumeni conducted a study on the geo-
graphic variation in the United States of cigarette
smoking and bladder cancer mortality.[6] It should be
noted before proceeding that there are several tobacco
smoke components that are rather bladder cancer-site
specific (e.g., B-naphthylamine, 4-aminobiphenyl and diethylene glycol). Fraumeni's study, with its weaknesses, concluded that there was a strong correlation
between bladder cancer mortality and per capita
cigarette sales estimated from states tax revenues.
The deaths/100,000 population, ranged from 2.86
(Kentucky) to 6.4 for Nevada. The New Jersey index
was relatively high, 5.98, as shown in Table 23.
Although not the express purpose of his study,
Fraumeni also determined the lung cancer mortality
to have an equally strong correlation with per capita
cigarette sales.

TABLE 23
Cigarette consumption, urbanization, and mortality from
bladder cancers in selected states

State	Cigar-rettes sold per capita	Percent Urban	Deaths 1956-61	Bladder Cancer Deaths 100,000	95% Confidence interval
Delaware	3360	65.5	111	4.78	3.95-6.33
New Jersey	2864	88.6	2127	5.98	5.73-6.24
New York	2914	85.4	5720	5.30	5.16-5.44
Pennsyl-vania	2378	71.6	2526	4.89	4.73-5.06
Louisiana	2158	63.3	729	4.65	4.32-5.00

Spirometric Studies

        The American Lung Association is conducting some
important occupational health testing studies. The
respiratory ability of smokers versus non-smokers is
being evaluated at several companies of less than 150
employees. What is most valuable about their work is
that employee health is more typically neglected at
the small business establishment. Their respiratory
studies indicate that the smoker usually has reduced
respiratory ability compared to non-smokers. Some of
the establishments visited are given in Table 24.
These studies do not serve to indict environmental agents
peculiar to the institution, for example, the exposure
of firefighters to toxic and carcinogenic agents as
described in chapter 4. Rather, it is tobacco use
which separates the cohort under study and is principally responsible for the reduced respiratory capacity.
The damage done to smokers' lungs will then render them
more susceptible to being affected by any environmental
agents peculiar to the workplace and other life-style
factors. The American Lung Association usually follows-
up their health testing program with smoking cessation
clinics.

TABLE 24
OCCUPATIONAL HEALTH TESTING

SITE	NUMBER TESTED	DATE	
Teledyne	147	August,	1978
Milmay Fire Company	39	June,	1979
Atlantic City Fire Department	232	June	1979
Egg Harbor Fire Company	38	July,	1979
Atlantic City Police Department	275	September,	1979
Dover Township Fire Company	40	December,	1979
Dover Township Fire Company	41	March,	1980
Courier Post	175	May,	1980
Delaware River Port Authority	359	May,	1980
Deer Park Baking Company	83	June,	1980
Seidleman Yacht Company	36	July,	1980
Milville Tool Company	14	September,	1980
Lily Industrial Coating	27	September,	1980

Individualized stop smoking counselling was given at all occupational sites.

SOURCE: American Lung Association Records (Hammonton, N.J.
          Office).

Alcohol/Tobacco/Coffee - Background

Almost inseparable from an evaluation of tobacco use is the adjunctive use of alcohol and coffee. The associative use of alcohol and tobacco has been determined to cause cancers of the mouth, pharynx, esophagus, and liver.[7] One possible explanation for the cancers of livers could be the presence in some alcoholic beverages of nitrosamines, proven animal carcinogens with a liver specificity. Nitrosamines are thought to form during the barley malt drying phase of beer production. A Food and Drug Administration report indicated that 28 out of 30 beers evaluated showed the presence of nitrosamines, however, most were below the 5ppb acceptable level they established in January of 1980.[8] Apparently, beers contain more nitrosamines than the whiskies (e.g., Tuborg and Schlitz - 6.2 and 7.7 ppb versus Cutty Sark - 0.5, Teachers - 2 and White Label - none). There is at least one other chemical present in some alcoholic beverages with a cancer risk. More than 1.1 million lbs. of tannic acid is added yearly to foods and beverages in the U.S.[9] Half of this amount is added to beers and wines as a clarifying agent. Tannins and tannic acid are both animal carcinogens.[10] Alcohol (pure ethyl alcohol) has *not* proven itself to be an animal carcinogen, so the observations of increased cancer, accompanying tobacco use is considered an expression of synergism.

The liver may not be able to detoxify other environmental agents in the presence of alcohol, placing the
alcoholic at a *higher* risk to cancer.[11] In fact, there
is a potentiation effect with certain toxins (e.g.,
mushroom toxin and galactosamine) and the presence of
alcohol.[12] Alcohol is under study as a teratogen, producing specific defects in children.[13] Breslow and
Enstrom conducted an epidemiological study correlating
cancer mortality and alcohol/tobacco consumption in the
U.S.[14] The study was based on cancer mortality rates
for 1950 - 1967 and the authors concluded:

- Respiratory cancers were related to cigarette
  consumption

- Cancers of the upper alimentary tract, were
  related to the consumption of distilled
  spirits

- Cancers of the stomach, large bowel, kidney
  and bladder were related to beer consumption for men and breast cancers for women

- A single strong association between rectal
  cancer and beer consumption was observed

Alcohol Use in New Jersey

That same study by Breslow and Enstrom provided
an interesting and important, however singular statistic about New Jersey per-capita beer consumption, as
shown in Figure 12. Of the cohort states evaluated,
only two show a higher per-capita beer consumption
than New Jersey. The New Jersey rectal cancer mortality rate is higher than most other states as may be
observed from Figure 12. Unfortunately, the Breslow
and Enstrom study did not evaluate the state consumption of the stronger alcoholic beverages. Wine consumption it was noted was related "only marginally,
if at all, to cancer at a few sites".

However, French epidemiologists suggest that
cigarette smoking and red wine consumption may be
important risk factors for adenocarcinoma of the

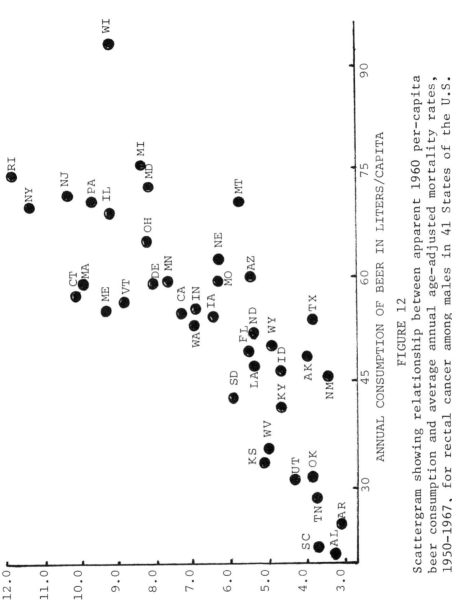

FIGURE 12

Scattergram showing relationship between apparent 1960 per-capita beer consumption and average annual age-adjusted mortality rates, 1950–1967, for rectal cancer among males in 41 States of the U.S.

stomach, in a small study group in France.[15] Breslow
and Enstrom concluded their study by citing their
sources of errors (diagnostic problems, presence of
multiple etiologic agents and reporting completeness)
and the necessity of further "direct observation of
individual human beings".

However informative the study by Breslow and
Enstrom, any evaluation based on per-capita consumption does have limitations. Some portion of the cohort
will be consuming far more or less than the average.
Supportive of the findings of Breslow and Enstrom of
a high per-capita consumption index in New Jersey really
being indicative of alcohol abuse are our more contemporary alcoholism statistics. Surveys indicate
that there are between 0.4 and 0.5 million alcoholics
in New Jersey.[16], [17] This number, approximately 7%
on a percentage basis, becomes frighteningly vivid
when applied to the ever typical county: Gloucester.*
Based on a 1980 population of approximately 199,000,**
there would be some 13,930 alcoholics in Gloucester
County alone! A review of 1978-1979 per-capita distilled spirit consumption, nation-wide (see Table 25),
does not reveal any alcoholism problem in New Jersey.
And the consumption of distilled spirits is probably
a better index of alcoholism than that of beer consumption.

Coffee - Background

A brief review of coffee bean processing is quite
revealing, and could cause a loss of an appetite for the
beverage.[18] It is the roasting of the green bean that
converts the chemicals naturally present into an inex-
plicably delicious aroma yielding bean. Ironically,
that self same delicious odor, bears the vapors of some
toxic and carcinogenic substances; formic acid,

---

* Described by pollster George Gallop as the nation's 'heart-
land'.

** U.S. Census Bureau Statistics

TABLE 25

APPARENT CONSUMPTION* OF DISTILLED SPIRITS BY STATE - 1979

State	Estimated Population (000)	Percentage of Total Population	Percentage of U.S. Total Consumption	Consumption by States
California**	22,696	10.31	12.65	1
Delaware**	582	0.26	0.33	44
Dist. of Columbia**	656	0.30	0.87	34
Nevada**	702	0.32	0.98	31
New Jersey**	7,332	3.33	3.51	8
New York**	17,649	8.02	9.01	2
Texas**	13,385	6.08	4.87	5
Pennsylvania***	11,731	5.33	3.79	7

Source: Distilled Spirits Council of the U.S., Inc.
Bureau of the Census
Department of Commerce

---

* Apparent Consumption – estimate of the gallons of distilled spirits (or any quantity of a commodity) sold at retail – based on state excise tax receipts, sales by state stores, shipments by producers to wholesalers or shipments by wholesalers to retailers.

** License state
*** Control state

naphthalene, phenol, pyridine and mercaptans. Prior to
1943, caffeine was extracted by organic solvents now
known to be carcinogenic; trichloroethylene, chloroform and benzene. Since 1943, water extraction has
replaced organic solvent extraction. Caffeine is removed from the water extracts with organic solvents
such as trichloroethylene and used in the drug and soft
drink industry.

Epidemiological Studies

One of the first studies to command the attention
of the coffee drinking public, was announced in March
of 1981. Dr. Brian MacMahon and other Harvard University researchers reported that coffee drinking could be
correlated with pancreatic cancer.[19] Dr. MacMahon and
his co-workers also concluded that the drinking of two
cups-a-day tripled the risk. The major confounding
factor in all of the research is the difficulty in
isolating singular risks of alcohol, tobacco or coffee
abuse.

Coffee drinking may be viewed as the parallel day-
time adjunct to tobacco use that alcohol is to evening
smoking activities. In addition to coffee drinking
being considered a cancer risk, it has been cited as
well as a potential fetotoxin, possibly causing birth
defects (cleft-palate and missing bones). Michael
Jacobson, co-director of the Center for Science in
the Public Interest, has sought to have the Food and
Drug Administration place warning labels on coffee
for pregnant women.[20] Accepted drug use-abusers clearly
represent a group with a very high risk of developing
cancers at diverse sites.

Controlled Dangerous Substances

The chemical substance producing the major drug
effect in marijuana is delta-9-tetra-hydro-cannabinol
(THC). Marijuana may be taken orally or by injection,
however the more typical form of use is by inhalation in
the form of cigarette smoke. "Marijuana has become a
popular and accepted form of recreation for a large

segment of the national population, including residents
of New Jersey".[21]   The use risks pertinent to the theme
of this book are currently controversial:[22]

> abnormal offspring from regular users
> development of forms of cancer
> chromosomal damage

Not subject to controversy are the cancer risks stemming
from the users exposure to the tobacco smoke constituents
alone.   The THC moiety in the "joint" burns along with
the tobacco also providing additional carcinogenic
polynuclear hydrocarbons.

In 1973, there were 420,700 national drug arrests
based on marijuana use charges.[23]   During that same
year there were 25,500 arrests based on marijuana use
charges in New Jersey.   It is noteworthy that a state
with only 3.3% of the national population garnered
about 6% of the national marijuana drug-arrest total.
The drug problem and inherent cancer risks are not
exactly peculiar to the entire state, but rather to
the northeastern sector.   In 1973 there were 47,000
addicts on probation in New Jersey.   A full 20,000
of this total lived in Newark.[24]   In any event, a cancer
risk is inherent in marijuana use - abuse and this may
be a unique problem in New Jersey.

Volatile Chemical Inhalation

Although this heading generally refers to the
practice of "glue-sniffing" or "snorting", a variety
of compounds provide such inhalable vapors.   The major
sources are:[25]

> varnish   paint-thinners
> lacquer   kerosene
> gasoline   lighter fluid
> glue   marking-pencil fluid

The volatile solvents in these compounds produce the
symptoms of intoxication (i.e., incoordination, dizzi-
ness, delirium and unsteadiness).   However, many of

these fractions contain benzene (see Table 6). Those
who practise volatile chemical inhalation deliberately
expose themselves to toxic levels of solvents which
they would normally flee from if encountered in the
ambient air. If drug-abuse is indeed disproportionately
high in New Jersey, volatile chemical inhalers should
be a high cancer risk group.

Diet and Nutrition - Background

    Basic dietary requirements to sustain life and
growth has been well documented and described as one
including carbohydrates, fats, proteins, vitamins,
minerals and water. The American diet meets these
basic needs however it is disproportionality that has
resulted in it being described as a "bad diet", or one
that is:[26]

- low in fruits and vegetables and whole grains

- high in refined sugars and other processed
  sugars

- high in total animal and vegetable fat,
  (especially saturated)

- low in fish, chicken and legumes

- high in salt

    The converse then is that a "good diet" is to be
obtained by reversing these trends according to the
observations of the U.S. Senate Select Committee and
many epidemiologists. It should be understood that
these recommendations address themselves to post-digestive dietary biochemistry, wherein natural foods induce
or inhibit tumorigenesis. There is yet another category, the preformed substances that induce tumorigenesis
on ingestion; e.g., nitrosamines, polycyclic aromatic
hydrocarbons, metals (essentially what has been already
described in chapter 4. The next cumulative and logical
question is - is there such a thing as a "New Jersey
Diet", and what is the role of post-digestive biochemistry

and preformed dietary substances, capable of inducing tumorigenesis?

The New Jersey Diet

     Very little of this discussion will be devoted to
the post digestive dietary factors because there simply
is no body of data to substantiate that on a *state-wide
basis* we New Jerseyans eat a diet that is remarkably
distinctive in the proportions of the dietary essentials
described earlier. However, The Greenberg Spatial Distribution cancer mortality study covering New Jersey,
New York and Philadelphia metropolitan regions has provided the best statistical insight into correlations
between some specific ethnic groups and certain prevalent site specific cancers.*[27] A high rate of stomach
cancers was observed in a high proportion of white
males and females from eastern Europe, especially Poland.
This cohort lived in Hudson, Mercer, Middlesex, Passaic
and Union Counties. A low correlation or risk was
identified in Germans and Italians in those same areas.
Dr. Greenberg noted that the state would have no preventive authority in the area of dietary habits and that
the rate of stomach cancer, incidence would decline as
dietary habits shift.

     White males of Italian descent were observed to be
at a high risk to mortality from cancers of the large
intestine in the counties of Hudson, Essex and Camden.
A low risk was observed in those groups originating
from the U.S.S.R., Poland and Germany. Mortality due to
cancers of the pancreas were found to be moderately
correlated with male U.S.S.R. and Polish ethnic groups.
The correlation was highest in Cape May and Passaic
Counties. Some slight correlation was noted between
cancers of the lung and Polish and Italian ethnic

---

* The study covered the period 1950 - 1961.

groups.* The study has identified several ethnic groups,
which of course suggests diet. It would provide a very
interesting theses to attempt to qualify the ethnic diets
on the basis of "stereotyping". However, that would be
foolhardy, since those "diets" are undergoing the evolution that accompanies immigration and such an evaluation
would entail a complex biochemical schema. Hence, this
author is not proceeding in that direction.

The most serious caveats and limitations that the
author(s) of the Greenberg study offer are methodologi-
cal, and the absence of confounding tobacco, alcohol and
drug use data. Further studies are in progress, and in
following their past trend, they will undoubtedly offer
some of the most significant statistical data on the
cancers in New Jersey. The significance of the Greenberg
report should be recalled from chapter 1, where some
of the evolution of the role of diet and nutrition in
the etiology of the cancers was discussed. Several
epidemiologists rate diet and nutrition highly in this
regard; e.g., Weisburger - 45% and Wynder - 50% in women
and 30% in men. [28], [29]

Deductive observations about Dietary and Nutritional
Practises in New Jersey

Although the statement was made earlier - there
is no distinct New Jersey diet, several peculiar observations and requisite recommendations for further study
may be made. The impact of the consumption of water
containing carcinogens was described in chapter 4.
That contaminated water, ingested with the "bad diet"
may place the user at an even higher risk of cancers
of the digestive system, through synergism, than when
consumed alone.

Contamination of foodstuffs may also originate
out of state. In November 1979, the state Department
of Agriculture impounded PCB-contaminated boned chicken

---

* Diet has not been cited in the etiology of lung cancer.

products entering New Jersey.[30] The contamination began
in Montana where leaking transformer oil came in contact
with poultry feed.

"Cooking out" is very definitely a statewide
spring to fall activity. Although there are no statistics to show we engage in this practise more than it
is done in other states, our many suburban and rural
areas enhance the practise of the art. Two obvious
meat food additives and their risks to cancers are suspect here, diethylstilbesterol (DES) and sodium nitrite.
DES, a synthetic female sex hormone, is used to enhance
weight gain in beef cattle and it also has teratogenic
and carcinogenic properties.[31] Although the Food and
Drug Administration has established a 7-day DES free
diet for beef cattle prior to slaughter, DES continues
to show up in beef livers after that period. DES was
banned for use in animals raised for human consumption
November 1, 1979, however, in 1980, feedlots containing
DES were still uncovered. This estrogen was once used
by women to prevent miscarriage, until rare vaginal
cancers were observed in their daughters and urogenital
lesions in their sons.

The other "cook-out" accompanyist is the frank-
furter containing the controversial sodium nitrite
which preserves, adds color to and flavors the meat.
To be added to the possibility of nitrites being converted to nitrosamines in the stomach and inducing
cancers,[32] is new evidence that the nitrite itself can
cause cancer and other toxic effects in animals.[33] There
is at least one other group of chemicals well described
earlier in chapter 4, polycyclic aromatic hydrocarbons.
These are formed during broiling and grilling processes
and will be present on the food and in the smoke about
the "pit". Again, their ingestion is accompanied by
a stomach cancer risk.

The fast food business is an established industry
in New Jersey as elsewhere. The diet offered there of
pizzas, burgers, french fries, pastries and sweet drinks
probably meets basic dietary needs. Essentially, eating
at these establishments is an adjunctive and not a sustaining activity. However, eating at these places poses

two problems for a population already at risk to cancers
of the digestive systems; the diet sponsored there is
severely opposed to that recommended by the U.S. Senate
Select Committee and eating there ingrains in children
poor dietary models. Changes are being made in these
places; fish and salad bars have been added. However,
salad vegetable fiber is not to be confused with essential dietary bulk as provided in the form of whole grain
wheat, rye, oats or sweet potatoes. Dr. Dennis Burkitt
has suggested that the minimal 4 gram crude fiber daily
intake of Americans is responsible for the high incidence of colon cancers and other diseases in the United
States.[34] According to Dr. Burkitt, dietary fiber
increases fecal bulk, feces transit time, and the
elimination of intestinal carcinogens.

Colorectal cancer mortality is second to lung cancer
mortality in New Jersey, with the estimated 1981 total
being 2400 statewide.[35] The incidence of and mortality
rate due to these cancers has not changed much in recent
years.

Cider

With our many rolling acres of terrain and apple
orchards, apple cider manufacture is a natural New
Jersey industry. Nitrosamines, previously discussed,
are known to be present in alcoholic beverages and this
includes apple cider. In one study where the average
nitrosamine level was 0.22 µg/liter, a maximum of 18 µg/l
was obtained.*[36] Recall from the tobacco/alcohol/coffee
discussion that 5.0 µg/liter has been set as a maximum
safe level. Herein lies the problem because we are
talking about a product over which there is essentially
no quality control in New Jersey. There is a substantial population drinking apple ciders who may be at
the same risk to esophageal cancer as has been observed
for consumers of other alcoholic beverages.[37] Synergism would also be manifest with tobacco usage and

---

* These ciders were of a European origin

nitrosamine intake from other alcoholic beverages. The
evaluation of cider for nitrosamine content in New Jersey
should be a high priority project for the New Jersey
Department of Agriculture.

Automotive Emissions - Background

It is stunning to uncover the statistic that with
approximately 4 million motor vehicles on the road in
New Jersey, we have more vehicles per square mile than
any other state.[38] The principal vehicle fuel source
is of course gasoline with diesel running second. Some
of the carcinogenic emissions from the combustion of
gasoline and diesel, both hydrocarbon fuels, have been
cited in chapter 4, along with total emissions resulting from fuel combustion.

Although a small portion of the vehicles contributing emissions are from what may be termed industrial
sources; i.e., commercial vehicles, approximately 90%
of vehicles on New Jersey roads are privately-owned
and thereby constitute emissions under individual control. It may be debated that all automotive emissions
should be adjudged an industrial source - since the
automobile is a means of getting to the work place.
However, the individual has some control over the means
of getting to work and could in fact elect to go by
horse, thereby contributing only biodegradeable, non-
carcinogenic pollutants to the environment. The principal pollutant emissions from transportation sources are:
sulfur oxides, nitrogen oxides, carbon monoxide, hydrocarbons and particulates, and their environmental impact has been described previously.

It may be observed from Table 4, (in chapter 4)
that transportation sources, specifically our very own
automobiles are the greatest single quantifiable source
of pollutant emissions with a potential to cause cancers. Specifically those emissions are particulates,
oxides of nitrogen and hydrocarbons. Of course the
argument becomes weaker when we talk about the quality
of the emissions. Or stated differently, which would
you rather breathe -- a lung full of auto exhaust or

industrial stack gas? In this instance the quantities
are the same but the state of the art of assessing
carcinogens does not yet enable us to make extensive
judgements on quality.

With the increased efficiency of diesel-powered
vehicles versus gasoline (33-60% greater efficiency)
increased use of diesel engines was predicted in the
early 70's. General Motors, in fact, reportedly hoped
to sell 100,000 diesel powered vehicles nationally
(including Chevrolet and GMC light-trucks and Cadillac
Sevilles) in 1978.[39] Although they fell short of their
goal, there are many private diesel-powered vehicles
on the roads; the Mercedes 240/300D, Peugot 504D and
the VW Diesel Rabbit.* In the spring of 1979, a
Newark Volkswagen dealership reported having a standing order for 50 diesel fueled automobiles and eight
additional monthly orders.[40] However, more crude oil
is required to produce diesel fuel than gasoline.
Another rapidly disappearing advantage has been the
narrowing gap between the cost of diesel fuel and gasoline. Yet the number of diesel engines in the state
increased. What then is and will be the environmental
impact of this shift, if it indeed occurs? The
principal difference between diesel and gasoline engines
emissions is the increased oxides of nitrogen and
particulate matter on the part of the diesel.[41] The
oxides of nitrogen are reduced by exhaust recycling,
however this serves to increase particulate matter
emissions. In fact, present diesel particulate emissions
are about 50-80 times more than gasoline. EPA standards
will by 1982, limit particulate emissions per mile
driven, to 0.6 grams, and 0.2 by 1985. Currently typical
emissions levels from the Volkswagen Rabbit and Oldsmo-
bile are 0.23 and 0.84 grams respectively. The cost
of the abatement technology required to meet these
standards will be passed on to the automobile buyer.

There are many data showing that inhalation of
particulate matter may lead to emphysema and cancer

---

* 12,800 diesel powered Rabbits were sold in 1977

development.   The small-sized diesel particulate
(0.1 - 0.3 μm) eludes nose and lung cilia and becomes
lodged deep in the lung.   What about hard laboratory
and epidemiological data on the biological effects
of gasoline and diesel smoke particulates; here's an
overview:[42, 43]

- Diesel Engine Particulate Extracts - mutagenic
  in Ames Test

- Diesel/Gasoline Engine particulate extracts -
  produces tumors on the skin of mice

- Diesel emissions* produces no tumors when inhaled by rats and hamsters - however, does
  produce - damage to respiratory tract,
  vesicular emphysema, interstitial fibrosis
  and cuboidal metaplasia

- Gasoline combustion emissions - produces no
  tumors, however does produce emphysematous
  lesions and renal sclerosis

There is disagreement about the impact of these
data in the scientific community.   First with the Ames
Test results, is mutagenesis synonymous with carcino-
gencity and is not the impact of particulate matter
extract on a cell more effective than on the more com-
plicated human respiratory system?   Further, most occupational morality and morbidity studies of large groups
show no excess deaths due to the inhalation of diesel
exhaust.   The single study that shows any significant
excess of cancer deaths due to the inhalation of diesel
exhaust emissions was done in our own state and the
cohort was a group of 1600 motor vehicle inspectors![44]
However, our state already has a high incidence of cancer
and the study did not specify the tumor site?   Human
studies do conclusively demonstrate what any one who
has stood behind a bus knows; diesel engine emissions

---

* Diesel smoke also contains more selenium, chromium and arsenic
  than gasoline.

produce eye irritation, objectionable odors and smoke.

The nature of the suspect and known carcinogens present on the particulate matter have been described generally as polycyclic aromatic hydrocarbons (PAH's). More specifically, examples of those PAH's considered strongly carcinogenic and occurring frequently in diesel exhausts are: chrysene, benzo (c)phenanthrene, benzo(a)anthracene and benzo(b)fluoranthene.[45] Furthermore, several other organics considered suspect carcinogens have also been detected: formaldehyde, crotonaldehyde, B-propiolactone, and styrene.[46] These data on the environmental impact of both diesel and gasoline emissions are impressive. Together they represent the major contributors of hydrocarbon pollutants to New Jersey air. There is adequate potential for both types of emissions to induce cancers of the skin and respiratory system. Several health - effects studies are being conducted by the EPA and industry (General Motors, Daimler-Benz AG, Volkswagen AG).[47] The decision to permit unlimited or to curtail diesel production rests with the EPA and is forthcoming.

A twenty member, National Academy of Sciences panel has advised the EPA not to impose stricter particulate emission standards for light-weight diesel cars.[48] Their reasons are primarily the *costs* and availability of control technology. That same panel however concedes to the need for more study on the health effects of diesel exhaust. Considering the 33,000 miles of highway* and numerous urban canyons in New Jersey, the data from all past and present studies should be evaluated thoroughly before the diesel power plant is allowed to become popular. In full recognition of the power of advertising and the economics involved, the individual still makes the final choice on his or her mode of transportation.

---

* New Jersey also has the highest ratio of multi-lane highways to other roads among the states. Conducive of a higher index of exposure to pollutants in transit.

Indoor Pollution

      Most of the air pollution data collected to date
has been acquired outdoors. The fact that the majority
of people spend 80% of their time indoors has caused
questions to be raised about the significance of outdoor ambient pollutant levels and their epidemiological
extrapolations. My evaluation of the studies conducted
indoors in the last few years indicate:

   ·   If the pollutant is generated (predominantly)
       indoors, the levels attained may equal or
       exceed outdoor levels

   ·   If the pollutant is generated (predominantly)
       in the outdoors (e.g., lead particulate) --
       indoor infiltration may result in levels up
       to 75% of outdoor levels

The following table lists some pollutants in the former
category:

TABLE 26
Indoor Air Pollutants[49]

Source	Environment	Pollutant/measured level	Ambient standard
Gas range	kitchens	oxides of nitrogen/* 500 μg/M^3	100 μg/M^3
tobacco	restaurants, church bingo, hospital waiting room	particulates/70-900 μg/M^3	260 μg/M^3
tobacco	office building conference room	2000	" "

---

*   converted to nitrate in the lungs - may contribute to nitro-
    samine formation.

TABLE 26 - continued
Indoor Air Pollutants

Source	Environment	Pollutant/measured level	Ambient standard
woodburning	homes	Benzo[a]pyrene/ 11.4 ng/M^3	none yet!
brick, stone, soil	homes	radon, radon daughters	4nCi/M^3

In the latter case with lead particulate originating predominantly outdoors, some levels are given below:

Lead Levels,[50] µg/M^3

Location	Outdoor Range	Indoor Range	Ambient standard
Site A	0.379 - 1.047	0.45 - 0.981	1.5
Site B	0.169 - 0.644	0.141 - 0.515	"

The implications of these indoor/outdoor pollution relationships are global in their impact in addition to being of concern for residents of heavily industrialized areas such as New Jersey. The data on lead shown above clearly indicate that pollutants of an extra-residential nature may concentrate in the home. This is another confounding parameter in epidemiological studies.

Earlier in this section, the statement was made that we spend 80% of our time indoors. Clearly a portion of that 80% is spent inside automobiles. In addition to being captive in an automobile with tobacco combustion emissions, there is at least one additional recently recognized pollutant in that environment. Synthetic rubber additives, specifically, nitrosamines may degas from spare tires, into the automobile interior.[51] Sources of N-nitrosamines and elimination of potential hazards are currently being investigated.

Several sources of indoor pollutants posing a cancer

risk have been identified in this section. They originate from both personal and industrial sources. Although
the responsibility rhetoric overviewed herein will
become important societal issues, the impact of indoor
pollutants on New Jersey residents should be a top
priority for the Department of Health. Further, new
threshold limit values will be required. The existing
Occupational Safety and Health Administration standards
which are the current guidelines used for exposure to
toxins in the industrial setting, will not be applicable.
Those exposures are based on an eight hour day versus
exposure in the home to indoor pollution for as long as
a 24 hour day. Clearly the role of indoor pollution in
the etiology of cancer has been much overlooked and
requires extensive evaluation.

Game and Wildlife

Every hunting season, New Jersey residents and
visitors to the state take to the woods to hunt a
variety of game; e.g., rabbits, deer and waterfowl.
The 1980 deer hunting season closed with a reported
kill of 9,941 bucks alone.[52] Table 27 is a more definitive listing of game taken by hunters during the 1970's.

TABLE 27
Average Hunter Catch of Select New Jersey Wildlife

Type Animal	Catch per hunter	Total Number of Hunters
Rabbit	5.5	124,984
Grouse	1.0	"
Quail	2.8	"
Squirrel	2.8	"
Pheasants	3.9	114,082
Ducks	6.5	27,021
Brant	2.2	"
Rail	0.3	"

SOURCE: What is hunting worth in New Jersey? Department of
Conservation and Economic Development. Bureau of
Wildlife, Trenton, N.J. circa 1970's.

None of these animal meats are subject to evaluation for the presence of carcinogens, teratogens or
mutagens (which is the function of the Department of
Agriculture regarding *wholesale* and *retail* sale of
commercial foodstuffs).* The main potable water supply
for New Jersey wildlife is surface waters, possibly
contaminated by the industrial effluents, spills and
other episodes as discussed in chapter 4. Several
studies indicate that the residues of economic poisons
used in an environment are commonly present in the
wildlife. Examples are DDT, Toxaphene, and Dieldrin.[53]
Of less importance would be the impact of air pollution
on wildlife. Collectively the water and air pollutants
which are carcinogenic, mutagenic or teratogenic would
be passed on to the hunter's table. Most experienced
hunters can probably evaluate the physical condition of
their catch. However, they have no way to determine
the animal's body burden of carcinogens resulting from
any possibly adverse environmental encounters. Secondarily, Table 27, demonstrates the hunter's participation in the not yet completely evaluated zoonotic cycle
(cf. chapter 3).

Recreational Fishing

U.S. Marine Recreational Fisheries Statistics show
that New Jersey is the most popular east coast recreational fishing area. Of 14 major Atlantic coastal
areas from Maine to Virginia, 2,725,000 anglers tried
their luck on the New Jersey coast during the period
1973-74. Half of these anglers resided in New Jersey.[54]
Point Pleasant, Atlantic City and the Cape May-Wildwood
areas are some of the most popular bank and boat sport-
fishing sites. Large quantities of fish are also taken
by boat and from bridges, piers and jetties, around
estuaries. Note well the emphasis here is on non-
commercial fishing - there is no quality control. In
1976, the DEP began a sampling program to determine the

---

* This is accomplished at best by spot checking - the
  "Basket Analysis".

levels of two specific animal carcinogens, PCB's and
Kepone, an insecticide.[55] Interest centered on PCB's
because of Hudson River pollution with that substance
in the Hudson Falls - Fort Edwards area. Similarly,
Kepones were introduced to the James River in Hopewell,
Virginia, which flows into the Chesapeake Bay and subsequently on to the Atlantic Ocean off the New Jersey
coast. Fish sampled near Fort Edward on the Hudson
showed PCB levels in excess of the FDA 5ppm limit
(Rockbass - 350ppm, Shiner Minnows - 78ppm). The PCB
levels diminished moving southward, becoming less than
the 5.0ppm limit along the New Jersey coast. Similarly,
the Food and Drug Administration ran tests on 9 fish
caught off the New Jersey coast and found Kepone levels
to be 0.03ppm (FDA limit 0.1ppm).

It should be noted that the PCB concentration in
the Hudson River is increasing, so it is plausible that
maximum PCB or Kepone concentration in fish taken off
the New Jersey coast line, has not yet reached its maximum. PCB and Kepone pollution were described here not
only because of their cancer potential, but to demonstrate the ability of carcinogens to move through the
marine environment. A much greater source of contamination is derived from sources originating in and about
New Jersey, as described in chapter 4. There are
actually more documented inland spill incidents, rendering fresh water fish unfit for consumption, than those
occurring on the Delaware River or off the New Jersey
coast; examples are given below:

> Strawbridge Lake/Pennsauken Creek
> (Pennsauken)[56] - chlordane and other
> pesticides
>
> Maurice River/Union Lake (Millville)[57] -
> arsenic
>
> Stewart Lake (Woodbury)[58] - chlordane
>
> Dillon's Pond (Monmouth)[59] - benzene

The cancer risk involved in recreational fishing

is greater than that for the ingestion of game and
wildlife in New Jersey. Economic poisons are encountered
in both activities. However, the fishing season is
much longer and there are more participants.

Ocean Dumping

 The disposal of industrial wastes in the Delaware
River and Atlantic Ocean and impact on New Jersey was
discussed in chapter 4. The subject is repeated here
with the emphasis on that moiety of the waste which
is a personal priority pollutant; our own sewage.

 During the period 1973 - 1977, the City of
Philadelphia dumped a reported 447 million lbs. of
sludge at an EPA designated dump site off the New Jersey
coast, shown in Figure 13.[60] The city of Camden (in
New Jersey) and New York also disposed of 15 million
gallons and 4 million tons of sewage sludge respectively
in waters off the New Jersey coast. Sewage sludge has
been dumped at the New York site (called the New York
Bight) since 1924. A 1976 study of proposed alternate
New York City dumping sites concluded, that the adverse
human effects would be the same as observed at the
current dump site.[61] The area is the site of intense
fishing (fin fish, scallops and clams). The buildup of
heavy metals and hydrocarbons in the sediment and water
column was determined to be minimal, but is expected to
increase. There have been reports of sediments from
disposal sites having a petrochemical odor and significant levels of pesticides.

 A considerable amount of heavy metals, which must
represent a fortune, is being dumped by the city of
Philadelphia. According to their records, 500 tons of
mercury and 1200 tons of cadmium. As described earlier,
cadmium is known to accumulate in the human liver and
is a suspect carcinogen, mutagen and teratogen.[62] By
1982, all at sea disposal of sewage sludges was *supposed*
to cease, however, the sediments at these dump sites
will continue to release toxic and carcinogenic substances for some time. As this book goes to press, ocean
dumping *continues*.

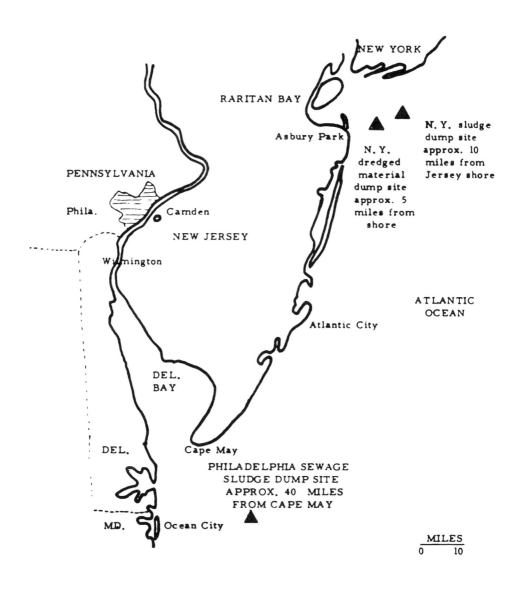

FIGURE 13
Atlantic Ocean Sewage/Sludge Dump Sites

In spite of the extensive at-sea disposal into waters about New Jersey, analysis of samples taken have not shown *mean* values of metals in excess of what is considered harmful for human consumption. The presence of the following metals in fin fish and shellfish were determined:[63]

cadmium	chromium
copper	arsenic
lead	silver
mercury	nickel
zinc	molybdenum

Toxicity, unfortunately, is not synonymous with the ability of a substance to induce cancers. An increased cancer risk at diverse sites may accompany a diet with a high proportion of fish and fin fish taken from dump site areas. Some demersal species of fish (dogfish, marlin) did show mercury levels exceeding recognized action levels. Mercury, although not a carcinogen, may on ingestion, absorption or inhalation cause severe neurological and kidney distrubances and other symptoms described in chapter 4.

Sunlight (Ultraviolet - UV)

Scotto, Fears and Gori (1975) demonstrated that there is a good correlation between exposure to the sun's rays, the degree of intensity and the incidence of skin cancer.[64] It is only the living cells deep within the skin in which cancers may arise and how deep UV will penetrate is a function of the pigment granule content in the surface skin cells. The lighter the skin complexion (or greater the absence of pigment), the greater is the hazard to a sunburn or skin cancer. Hence, the incidence of skin cancer is more common among fair-skinned people than those fortunate ones of darker hues. In addition, the thicker the skin and inherent greater shielding from UV on those cells in which cancer may originate, the lower the predisposition to skin cancer. So collectively, the person with lighter and thinner skin is much more likely to develop skin cancer than the darker-complexioned thicker-skinned individual.

It has been estimated that as many as 50% of those attaining age 65 will develop a skin cancer and, incidence does increase with age.[65]   Skin cancers originate in the epithelium or in the pigment cells (melanocytes). Those cancers arising in the melanocytes - melanomas* are rare and usually spread (metastasize), and this type is responsible for two-thirds of the deaths resulting from skin cancers.[66]   There are other causes of skin cancers beside sunlight (e.g., arsenicals, radiation, coal tars)** discussed earlier.   However, it is the elective exposure to sunlight that is being addressed here: style of dress, sunbathing, gardening, tennis, boating, fishing, etc. All of these activities are encouraged by New Jersey's many suburban and coastal areas.

The 1981 "Descriptive Epidemiology of Cancer Mortality in New Jersey: 1949-1976" report, shows: a statistically significant increase in malignant melanoma mortality rates in both males and females, over a 28-year period.

Standardized mortality ratios were greater than 1 in Ocean and Sussex Counties for men and women respectively. Better comparisons could be made with incidence data, rather than mortalities, if however the former data were available. Stein, Thind, and Louria (1978) examined malignant melanomas in Newark, Morris and Hunterdon

---

* malignant melanoma is not necessarily sun-related

** other etiological factors are: fumes and burns from molten metals and genetic DNA defects, pregnancy, oral contraceptives/other therapeutic hormone use.

Counties.*[68] They concluded that there was no pattern
to the incidence of melanoma in New Jersey, and that
data from the state-wide tumor registry might reveal
trends that lend themselves to prevention.

There are some aspects of life-style for which
there are identifiable associative risks of cancers but
essentially no epidemiological data yet to indicate a
high risk group in New Jersey. Further, it is possible
that these life-style parameters may be common to other
states. They are given here mainly to substantiate the
need for further study.

Breast Feeding

The breast milk of nursing mothers has been determined to be contaminated with many of the carcinogen,
mutagens and teratogens already discussed (e.g., insecticides, dioxin, polyhalogenated biphenyls and nicotine).[69, 70, 71] Then mothers may pass on their body
burden of environmental pollutants to their children
through breast feeding, (as well as through placental
exchange before birth). According to Gair Helfrich of
the South Jersey La Leche League, (nursing mothers
advocates), the postpartum (after-delivery) nursing
period could last as long as 18 months.[72] The natural
questions that follow are: what is the toxicity and
cancer risk to nursing infants and how many women are
nursing in New Jersey? First, there are reported instances of infant toxicity, induced by the ingestion of
contaminated breast milk.[73] In these cases, tetrachloroethane, PCB's, mercurials and hexachlorobenzene,
were cited as the pollutants. Secondarily, the cancer
risk question is answered by the standard lack of knowledge of the effects of long term, low level exposure
to carcinogens. In response to the last question,
there are approximately 142 La Leche groups of 12-15
nursing mother members each, in New Jersey.[74] There are
of course many more nursing mothers who do not belong
to any organized groups. From a risk-benefit perspec-

---

* study covered the period 1970 - 1974.

tive, human breast milk is considered superior to cows
milk, which also contains environmental pollutants but
does not confer acquired immunity on infants. Nursing
mothers should assess their own exposure to hazardous
substances (e.g., contaminated well water, drug use
and smoking), before making the decision to breast feed.
Further, they may have already passed on their body
burden of pollutants to the fetus through placental
exchange and nursing could add an additional postpartum
exposure, which could have a synergistic effect on
the new born infant. The American Academy of Pediatrics
has already recommended that prospective nursing mothers
with a history of high level - PCB exposure, have their
breast milk analysed prior to initiating breast feeding.[75]

Consumer Products

    Other than the peculiar use of alcohol, tobacco and
items discussed under diet and nutrition, the author
has been hard pressed to identify very many consumer
products posing a *special* cancer risk in New Jersey.
There is no problem in finding consumer products containing or forming carcinogens in their usage.* The
criteria for citation here must be a remarkable per-
capita consumption for New Jersey residents. Some consumer products, candidates for this criteria are now
discussed.

    Urea-Formaldehyde Foam Insulation

    Formaldehyde, a toxic and irritating chemical, and
demonstrated animal carcinogen,[76] is widely used in consumer products:

foam insulation	linoleum
particle board	vinyl car interiors
paneling	phenolic lavatory fixtures

---

*   e.g., saccharin, permanent hair dyes, and hexachloro-
    phene

cosmetics   carpet pads
permanent-press   furniture upholstery
clothing

Free formaldehyde may degas from these products causing
eye and upper respiratory system irritation, rashes and
allergic effects. There have been numerous complaints
from New Jersey residents who have urea-formaldehyde
foam (UFF) resin sprayed in place to insulate wall
cavities of existing buildings. The New Jersey Department of Health, Special Epidemiological Unit investigated
more than 100 complaints between December 1977 and
January 1980.[77] Their investigation encompassed 15
counties and indicates that between 2,000 - 3,500 New
Jersey homes are insulated annually with UFF. The
Chemical Industry Institute of Toxicology was the first
to report on a study that indicated laboratory rats
would develop nasal carcinomas when exposed to formaldehyde.[78] The Consumer Products Safety Commission,* regarding formaldehyde as a potential human carcinogen and
mutagen, proposed a ban on UFF in January 1981.[79] The
Formaldehyde Institute, (representing the UFF industry)
has cited four epidemiological studies showing no excess
human risk of cancer due to exposure to formaldehyde.[80]
The additional cancer risk due to seven years exposure
to UFF degassing has been estimated at 85 in 1 million.[81]
Since formaldehyde is a respiratory irritant, it is cited
as possibly contributing to Sudden Infant Death
Syndrome.[82] The odor detection threshold for formaldehyde has been determined to be 0.01 to 0.03ppm.
Although there is no exposure limit to this toxic substance (or any others) in the home environment, NIOSH
has established a 1ppm workplace limit. Further,
NIOSH has established that where workplace values exceed
0.5 ppm, the air should be sampled twice annually. The
New Jersey Department of Health (DOH) considers any home
environment exposure in excess of 0.1 ppm (100 ppb)
potentially harmful. Consider the following selected
results of the DOH, UFF investigation, in New Jersey:[83]

---

* The commission voted to ban all further installation of UFF
  insulation, February 1983, (effective in 130 days). Ref.
  March 1, 1982, Chemical and Engineering News.

Months since installation	Formaldehyde concentration,ppb	Symptoms Reported
1	580	mucous membrane irritation, odor
5	280	acute respiratory irritation
11	1	respiratory irritation
19	negative	odor, malaise
33	90	odor, respiratory irritation
40	negative	odor, respiratory irritation

It is easily noted from above, that occasionally adverse symptomatic complaints were lodged unaccompanied by any formaldehyde detection. This may represent "overreporting" prompted by publicity about the adverse health effects resulting from UFF in the media. The predominant remedial action following complaints are; no action, ventilation, removal or the application of a vapor barrier paint. The DOH concluded that residents of homes experiencing persistent formaldehyde odors "may represent a sub-population at special risk". Although most complaints in New Jersey have come from homeowners, the diminutive and tight living spaces, presented by the states' boats and trailers also require evaluation. Formaldehyde values as high as 4.18ppm were reported for mobile homes in a Wisconsin study.[84] Rossnagel & Associates, a prominent South Jersey Environmental Consulting Agency, has recommended the development of Public Health agency monitored allergy or sensitisation programs, in conjunction with formaldehyde complaints.[85]

Fiberglassing

Many New Jersey residents who own boats have either

repaired them with or constructed them of fiberglass.
Glass wool is usually applied to a wooden surface or
an area to be patched and a styrene polyester resin
brushed on or rolled over the glass fiber. On curing
(a process which is accompanied by the release of
toxic, irritating vapors, possibly carcinogenic) the
surface may be sanded to reduce any irregularities.
Both in the handling and sanding process, glass fibers
are proliferated into the handy person's breathing
space, along with particulates of the cured polyester
resin.

Stanton et.al., (1977) concluded on the basis of
an animal glass fiber implantation study, that glass
fibers of specific dimensions could induce pleural*
tumors.[86] Although the existing data on the carcinogenicity of glass fibers are controversial, there is
now cause for concern over *all respirable fibers*. Many
small boat supply stores in New Jersey package their
own polyesters. The plain labels may recommend that
the vapors not be inhaled, but lack information on the
hazards associated with sanding or curing. Styrene,
the fiberglass copolymer component, known as polyester
resin, is a toxic eye and mucous membrane irritant.[87]
Studies conducted to determine ambient levels in the
boating industry indicate overexposure.[88] The National
Institute for Occupational Health and Safety is considering the establishment of an 8-hour time-weighted
average of 25ppm. Styrene has been determined to be
mutagenic in the Ames Test[89] and the precautions on
use have not been passed on to the consumer.

Cesspool Cleaners

Many private homes in suburban New Jersey are
equipped with septic systems for the discharge of
sewage wastes. An integral part of this system is a
500 - 1500 gallon water-proof concrete or metal container. Wastes settle and decompose anerobically in
these containers with the effluent being discharged to

---

* space between lungs and ribs

a distribution box and ultimately through tile pipes into
a disposal field. The forerunner of the septic system,
the cesspool, consisting only of a buried concrete tank
is still extant in New Jersey. Occasionally, the blocks
of cesspools and the disposal field pipes of the septic
system become clogged with grease and oil. Commercial
degreasing agents contain "Petroleum distillates" and
"Hydrocarbons". If the home owner's well water aquifer
is in proximity to a septic system effluent, it may
become contaminated with such degreasing agents as
trichloroethylene. Owner-administered toxic septic
system contamination has already occurred in Long
Island.[90]

Chapter 5 / REFERENCES

1. (AP) Pursuit of Pleasure: N.J. hedonists more
        than match for California, Gloucester
        County Times, February 11, 1979.

2. White, James R., Ph.D., and Froeb, Herman F., M.D.,
        Small-Airways Dysfunction in Nonsmokers
        chronically exposed to Tobacco Smoke, The
        New England Journal of Medicine, Vol. 302,
        No. 13, March 27, 1980, pp. 720-723.

3. Smoking and Health, a report of the Surgeon General,
        U.S. Department of Health, Education and
        Welfare, January 11, 1979, pp. 14-35 to
        14-72.

4. Ibid. part I.

5. American Cancer Society, Cancer Facts & Figures,
        1981.

6. Fraumeni, J.F., M.D., Cigarette Smoking and Cancers
        of the Urinary Tract: Geographic Variation
        in the United States, Journal of the National
        Cancer Institute, Vol. 41, No. 5, November
        1968, pp. 1205 - 1211.

7. Schottenfeld, David, M.D., Alcohol as a co-factor
        in the Etiology of Cancer, Cancer, 43:
        1979, pp. 1962 - 1966.

8. FDA orders Carcinogens out of Beers, (AP), The
        Philadelphia Inquirer, October 26, 1979,
        p. 5-A.

9. IARC Monographs on the Evaluation of Carcinogenic
        Risk of Chemicals To Man, Some Naturally
        Occurring Substances, Vol. 10, Interna-
        tional Agency For Research on Cancer,
        Lyon,   1976.

10. Ibid.

11. Rubin, Emanuel, M.D., The Effects of Drugs and
        Chemicals on the Liver, New Jersey Society
        of Pathologists, Annual Spring Meeting
        CMDNJ - Rutgers Medical School, Piscataway,
        New Jersey, June 6, 1981.

12. Ibid.

13. Norwood, Christopher, At Highest Risk, Penguin
        Books Ltd., New York, 1980, pp. 44-46.

14. Breslow, Norman E., and Enstrom, James E., Geo-
        graphic Correlations Between Cancer Mortal-
        ity Rates and Alcohol-Tobacco Consumption
        in the United States, Journal of the National
        Cancer Institute, Vol. 53, No. 3, September
        1974,   pp. 631 - 639.

15. Hoey, John, Montvernay, Corine and Lambert, Rene,
        Wine and Tobacco: Risk Factors For Gastric
        Cancer in France, The American Journal of
        Epidemiology, Volume 113, No. 6, June 1981.

16. Alcohol Leading Killer in Nation, The Spirit, March
        10, 1976, p. 13.

17. "New Jersey And the Challenge of Alcoholism,"
        Shopportunity, September 1, 1976.

18. Kirk-Othmer, Encyclopedia of Chemical Technology,
        Vol 5, John Wiley & Sons, Inc., 1964.

19. Coffee drinking linked to pancreatic cancer, Chemi-
        cal & Engineering News, March 16, 1981, p.
        15.

20. Solomon, Goody L., Warning Label Urged for
         Caffeine Products, The Philadelphia
         Inquirer, December 27, 1978,   Section B.

21. State of New Jersey, The Commission to Study and
         Review the Penalties Imposed upon Indivi-
         duals Convicted of using Certain Substances
         Subject to the Provisions of the "New
         Jersey Controlled Dangerous Substances Act",
         P.L. 1970, C. 226 (c. 24:21 - 1 et seq.)
         and to Study the Nature and Scope of Drug
         Treatment Programs, October 1974, p. 61.

22. Drug Abuse Council, Furor Created by Recent Mari-
         juana Studies Questioned, Washington, D.C.,
         July 17, 1974.

23. State of New Jersey. Op. Cit.

24. Ibid.

25. Conte, Anthony E., Dr., and Mason, Eugene R.,
         Drug Abuse: A Challenge for Education,
         New Jersey Urban Schools Development Coun-
         cil, Trenton, New Jersey, August 1970.

26. Select Committee on Nutrition and Human Needs,
         U.S. Senate, "Dietary Goals for the United
         States", December 1977.

27. Greenberg, Michael R. et.al., The Spatial Distri-
         bution of Cancer Mortality And of High
         and Low Risk Factors in the New Jersey-
         New York-Philadelphia Metropolitan Region,
         1950 - 1969, Part I, State of New Jersey
         Department of Environmental Protection,
         Program on Environmental Cancer and Toxic
         Substances, January 1979.

28. Cancer. Op. Cit. p. 1955.

29. Cancer. Op. Cit. p. 1987.

30. Testing Detects PCB's in Feeds, Fertilizers, The
     Gloucester County Times, November 20, 1979.

31. Hodges, Laurent, Environmental Pollution, Holt,
     Rinehart and Winston, New York, 1977,
     p. 404.

32. Tannenbaum, Steven R., Moran, Dennis, Rand,
     William, Cuello, Carlos, and Correa, Pelayo,
     Gastric Cancer in Columbia. IV. Nitrate
     and Other Ions in Gastric Contents from
     Residents from a High-Risk Region, Journal
     of the National Cancer Institute, Vol. 62,
     No. 1, January 1979, pp. 9-12.

33. Nitrites and Nitrosamines: Is the hot dog an en-
     dangered species:, Consumer Reports, Vol. 45
     No. 5, May 1980, p. 311.

34. Burkitt, D.P., Epidemiology of Cancer of the Colon
     and Rectum. Cancer 28, 1971. pp. 3-13.

35. American Cancer Society, Cancer Facts & Figures
     1981.

36. Walker, E.A., Castegnaro, M., Garren, L., Toussaint,
     G., and Kowalski, B., Intake of Volatile
     Nitrosamines from Consumption of Alcohols,
     Journal of the National Cancer Institute,
     Vol. 63. No. 4., October 1979, pp. 947-951.

37. Ibid.

38. Eisler, Barbara, Air Pollution in New Jersey, Prob-
     lems, Programs and Progress, American Lung
     Association of New Jersey with support from
     the New Jersey Department of Environmental
     Protection, 1979.

39. Ketcham, Brian and Pinkwas, Stan, Diesels And Man,
     New Engineer, April 1978, pp. 23-32.

40. Diesel Popularity Eyed, (AP), The Gloucester County
     Times, March 27, 1979.

41. Ember, Lois, The Diesel Dilema, Environment, Vol.
        21, No. 2., March 1979.

42. Review of the Research Status on Diesel Exhaust
        Emissions, Their Health Effects, and
        Emission Control Technologies, Prepared
        by the Aerospace Corporation, Maryland for
        the U.S. Department of Energy,   June 1978.

43. Santodonato, Joseph, Basu, Dipak, and Howard,
        Philip (of the Syracuse Research Corporation)
        Health Effects Associated with Diesel Exhaust
        Emissions, Literature Review and Evaluation,
        Contract No. 68-02-2800, prepared for the
        U.S. Environmental Protection Agency, Office
        of Research and Development Health Effects
        Research Laboratory Research Triangle Park,
        N.C., November 1978.

44. Stern, F.B., and Lemen, R.A., Exploratory Mortality
        Study Among Workers Exposed to Carbon
        Monoxide From Automotive Exhaust, U.S.
        Dept. of Health, Education and Welfare,
        Public Health Service., 1978.

45. Santodonato, Joseph, Basu, Dipak, and Howard,
        Philip, Op. Cit.

46. Ibid.

47. Embers, Louis, Op. Cit.

48. Delay Urged In Tough Diesel Emission Rules,
        Chemical & Engineering News, Vol. 60,
        No. 1., January 4, 1982, p. 7.

49. Budiansky, Stephen, Indoor Pollution, Environ-
        mental Science & Technology, Vol. 14,
        No. 9, September 1980, pp. 1023-1027.

50. Halpern, Marc, Indoor/Outdoor Air Pollution Exposure
        Continuity Relationships, Journal of the
        Air Pollution Control Association, Vol. 28,
        No. 7, July 1978, pp. 689-691.

51. Ireland, Carol B., Hytrek, Frederick P., and
          Lasoski, Bernard A., Aqueous Extraction
          of N-nitrosamines from elastomers, American
          Industrial Hygiene Association Journal
          (41) December 1980, pp. 895-900.

52. Kinsell, Ralph, Whitetail Harvest Takes a 14 Per-
          cent increase, The Gloucester County Times,
          December 17, 1980, p. D-4.

53. "Cleaning Our Environment, A Chemical Experience",
          A Report by the Committee on Environmental
          Improvement, American Chemical Society,
          Washington, D.C., 1978, Chap. 7, Pesti-
          cides in the Environment.

54. Fisheries of the United States, 1975, U.S. Depart-
          ment of Commerce, National Oceanic and
          Atmospheric Administration, National Marine
          Fisheries Service, Washington, D.C., March
          1976, p. 27.

55. "PCB's And Kepone in New Jersey", An Interim
          Report , Cancer and Toxic Substances Pro-
          gram, New Jersey Department of Environmental
          Protection, May 1977.

56. First Annual Report of the Office of Hazardous
          Substances Control (OHSC) of the New Jersey
          Department of Environmental Protection
          Toxic Substances Program, April 3, 1978.

57. Pawling, Patrick G., State to Fine Vineland
          Chemical, The Atlantic City Press, August
          23, 1980.

58. Goldberg, Elliot, Dangerous if Eaten, The Gloucester
          County Times, June 20, 1980.

59. Pollution Confined in Monmouth Pond, Newark Star
          Ledger, May 2, 1980

60. Anastasia, George, The Assault on the Seas, Part II,
          The Philadelphia Inquirer, August 8, 1977.

61. Evaluation of Proposed Sewage Sludge Dumpsite
        Areas in the New York Bight, Marine Eco
        Systems Analysis Program Office, Boulder,
        CO. - Coordinator, United States Depart-
        ment of Commerce, National Oceanic And
        Atmospheric Administration, Environmental
        Research Laboratories, NOAA Technical
        Memorandum ERL MESA - 11. February 1976.

62. Anastasia, George, Op. Cit.

63. Pearce, John B., Report to the Working Group on
        Pollution Baseline And Monitoring Studies
        In the OSLO Commission And ICNAF Areas On
        Heavy Metals In Selected Finfish and Shell-
        fish from the Northwest Atlantic, U.S.
        Department of Commerce, National Oceanic
        And Atmospheric Administration, National
        Marine Fisheries Service, Northeast Fisheries
        Center, Sandy Hook Laboratory, Highland,
        New Jersey, 1977, pp. 1-97.

64. Scotto, Joseph, Fears, Thomas R., and Gori, Gio B.,
        Measurements of Ultraviolet Radiation in
        the United States and Comparisons with
        Skin Cancer Data, U.S. Department of Health,
        Education and Welfare, DHEW No. (NIH)
        76-1029, November 1975.

65. Clinical Oncology for Medical Students and Physi-
        cians, a multidisciplinary approach, Rubin,
        Philip, M.D., (ED) and Bakemeir, Richard
        F., M.D., (Associate Editor), American
        Cancer Society, New York, 1978, Chap. 14.

66. Cairns, John, Cancer: Science and Society, W.H.
        Freeman and Company, San Francisco, 1978.
        Chapter 3.

67. Stemhagen, Annette, M.P.H., et.al., Descriptive
        Epidemiology of Cancer Mortality in New
        Jersey: 1949-1976, N.J. Dept. of Health/
        NCI, 1981, (Vol. 1, Discussion & Analysis,
        New Jersey State Dept. of Health/The
        National Cancer Institute, June 1981).

68. Stein, David, M.D., Thind, Inderjit, S., M.D.,
        D.P.H., and Louria, Donald B., M.D.,
        Melanoma of the Skin in New Jersey, The
        Journal of the Medical Society of New
        Jersey, Vol. 75, No. 5, May 1978, pp. 391-
        394.

69. Barr, Mason, Jr., M.D., Environmental Contamination
        of Human Breast Milk, American Journal of
        Public Health, Volume 17, No. 2, February
        1981, pp. 124-126.

70. Smoking and Health, A Report of the Surgeon General,
        U.S. Department of Health, Education, and
        Welfare, Public Health Service, DHEW Publica-
        tion No. (PHS) 79-50066, January 11, 1979,
        Chapter 8.

71. Norwood, Christopher, At Highest Risk, Penguin
        Books Ltd., New York, 1980, p. 200.

72. Personal Communication, October 12, 1981.

73. Barr, Mason, Jr., M.D., Op. Cit.

74. Personal communication, October 12, 1981.

75. Cetrulo, Curtis, L., and Kurzel, Richard B., The
        Effect of Environmental Pollutants on Human
        Reproduction, Including Birth Defects,
        Environmental Science and Technology, Volume
        15, No. 6., June 1981, pp. 626-640.

76. Chemical Industry Institute of Toxicology, CIIT,
        Current Status Reports No. 3, Formaldehyde
        Draft Copy, September 1979.

77. Marshall, F.J., "Health Investigations of Urea-
        Formaldehyde Foam", New Jersey State Depart-
        ment of Health, Special Epidemiological Pro-
        ject, December 1977 to January 1980.

78. Chemical Industry Institute of Toxicology, Op.Cit.

79. Ban on Formaldehyde foam insulation proposed,
         Chemical & Engineering News, January 19,
         1981, p. 11.

80. Formaldehyde Foam Fight Fashioned, Industrial
         Chemical News, March 1981, p. 8.

81. Pittsburgh Conference on Analytical Chemistry and
         Applied Spectroscopy, Convention Hall,
         Atlantic City, N.J., March 9-13, 1981.

82. Ibid.

83. Marshal, F.J., Op. Cit.

84. Indoor Air Pollution, National Safety News, July
         1980, Vol. 122, No. 1.

85. Rossnagel & Associates, Inc., Medford, N.J. "The
         Formaldehyde Problem", Testimony for Con-
         sumer Product Safety Commission Public
         Hearing on Urea Formaldehyde Foam Insula-
         tion on January 10, 1980.

86. Stanton, Mearl F., et.al., Carcinogenicity of
         Fibrous Glass: Pleural Response in the
         Rat in Relation to Fiber Dimension, Journal
         of the National Cancer Institute, Vol. 58.
         No. 3, March 1977, pp. 587-597.

87. Proctor, Nick H., Ph.D., and Hughes, James P.,
         M.D., Chemical Hazards of the Workplace,
         J.B. Lippincott Company, Philadelphia, 1978.

88. Schumacher, Robert L., Breysse, Peter A., Carlyon,
         William R., Hibbard, Richard P., and
         Kleinman, Goldy D., Styrene exposure in the
         Fiberglass Fabrication Industry in Washing-
         ton State, American Industrial Hygiene
         Association Journal, (42), February 1981,
         pp. 143-149.

89. Ames, B.N., McCann, J., and Yamasake, E.: Mutation
         Research (31), 1975, pp. 347-349.

90. Weimar, Robert A., Prevent Goundwater Contamination
         before it's too late, Water & Wastes
         Engineering, February 1980.

ENVIRONMENTAL IMPACT ON
THE STATE OF NEW JERSEY

"Whoever attempts to
lead the nation to-
wards less cancer
had better be cor-
rect, because the
selection of the wrong
path is the equivalent
of leading millions of
Americans to certain
death".

Dr. Harry
Demopoulos,
October 4, 1979

*   from "Environmentally Induced Cancer......Separating Truth
    From Myth", A talk given to the Synthetic Organic Chemical
    Manufacturers Association, Inc., Hasbrouck Heights, N.J.

CHAPTER 6

Introduction

An overwhelming number of environmental factors
occupying varying roles in the New Jersey cancer incidence and mortality rate were described in chapters
4 and 5. Although these various factors were described
in the introduction to chapter 4 as having the potential to induce cancers, obviously some already were
prima facia causes (e.g., asbestos, b-naphthylamine
and tobacco smoke). Others were cited because deductive reasoning clearly indicates the area warrants
further investigation. The purpose of this chapter is
to summarize and evaluate the principal categories of
environmental factors described in chapter 4 and conclude with what really amounts to an environmental impact statement on an entire state. The author fully
realizes the dynamic nature of the cancer problem and
that what he has determined to be important now, may
quickly fall into obscurity. Conversely, what is recognized by many as a mere risk, may in time ascend to
the position of a number 1 public health threat.

Air Pollution

There are ample laboratory and epidemiological
data to support the concept that on a qualitative basis
the air pollutants in industrialized areas could cause
most of the cancers manifest in New Jersey public health
statistics.* The data are inadequate to determine if
the air pollutants have in fact caused these cancers.
Nonetheless, due to the high population density and
heavy concentration of chemical industries and automo-

---

* Excluding male/female colorectal and cancers of the female
reproductive organs.

biles, (compare Figures 14 and 15) New Jersey residents
living in these areas are certainly at a pronounced risk
to the development of most cancers. The DEP data on air
quality and industrialized areas clearly indicate that
workers and residents alike are subjected to more carcinogens by breathing the air then drinking water in
the state. Many wells have been closed but the air has
not yet been condemned.

The impact of air pollution in the pre-emission
regulatory years may only be speculated upon now. It
is safe to say that the era of the more gross proliferation of such pollutants as asbestos, vinyl chloride,
dyes and fugitive refinery emissions has passed.* Due
to various pressures, regulations, knowledge of chemical
carcinogens and voluntary action, industry has reduced
worker exposure to carcinogens. That is not to say
there are no current air pollution cancer risks. Many
remain to be assessed, especially where a high incidence
is manifest in a well defined cohort, and yet no
specific environmental agent has been identified. The
cancers manifest in petroleum refinery workers and
General Motors plants are good examples. The determination of the ability of the sub-toxic yet qualitatively carcinogenic air pollutant mixtures, present in
New Jersey air, to induce cancers in laboratory animals,
should be given a top priority by the state's cancer
control program. Convincingly positive results from
such tests would indicate that we are not only in serious trouble in New Jersey but everywhere.

Area sources of carcinogens continue to be a problem not only for employees but to some consumers as
well (e.g., dry-cleaning establishments, printing and
auto-body repair shops). These operations, typically
consist of small groups of employees who are not likely
to file a complaint with OSHA,** in contrast to the employees of well unionized larger industries.

---

* Ground level concentrations - not stack emissions

** Occupational Safety and Health Administration.

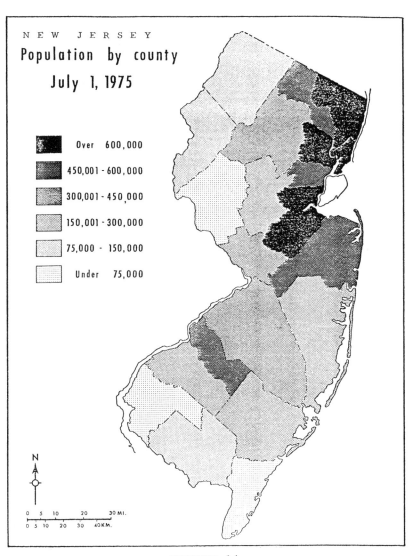

NEW JERSEY
Population by county
July 1, 1975

Over 600,000
450,001 - 600,000
300,001 - 450,000
150,001 - 300,000
75,000 - 150,000
Under 75,000

N

0 5 10   20   30 MI.
0 5 10   20   30   40 KM.

FIGURE 14

Source: Kelland, Frank S., and Marylin, C., New Jersey:
Garden or Suburb, Kendall/Hunt Publishing Co., Dubuque,
1978. (See Appendix for names of counties.)

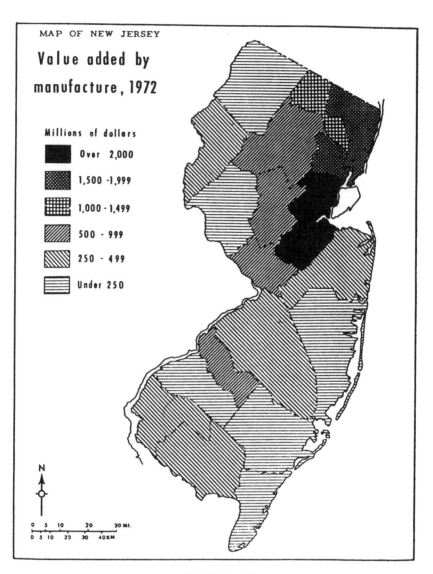

MAP OF NEW JERSEY

Value added by
manufacture, 1972

Millions of dollars

- Over 2,000
- 1,500 - 1,999
- 1,000 - 1,499
- 500 - 999
- 250 - 499
- Under 250

N

0 5 10   20   30 MI.
0 5 10   20   30   40 KM.

FIGURE 15

Source: Kelland, Frank S., and Marylin, C., New Jersey:
Garden or Suburb, Kendall/Hunt Publishing Co., Dubuque,
1978. (See Appendix for names of counties.)

It is not possible to dismiss the cancers manifest
in specific occupational groups in New Jersey in the
large and small scale chemically related industries.
The nation-wide employment in the chemical industry has
been estimated to total 1,012,500. [1] Chemical industry
employment in New Jersey is estimated to be about
120,000 by the New Jersey Department of Labor and Industry. [2] Dr. Finley, New Jersey Health Department Commissioner, indicates there are at least 167,000 chemical
industry workers in the state. This indicates that
about 11.8% of the nation's chemical industry workers
live and work in the 46th state in size. Further, on
recalling the high position New Jersey occupies in
chemical manufacture, it is easy to identify the state's
chemical industry workers as a group at a high risk for
the development of cancers.

Water Pollution

The contamination of ground and surface waters with
carcinogens is a major health problem and cancer risk
for New Jersey residents. At this very moment some New
Jersey family is drinking water containing levels of
potentially carcinogenic chemicals too low to be detected by the sense of smell or taste. By the time the sus-
picious water is tested, the process of cancer induction
may already be initiated. Although the state has been
monitoring well water for two years, the New Jersey Department of Health cannot meet the requests from residents who suspect contamination. Before the extensive
well water pollution occurred in Bridgeport, New Jersey,
the author appealed to state legislators for a more ag-
gressive and responsive monitoring program. My suggestion would have been enacted through a state-wide referendum; however, it went unanswered.*

How can it be that in an era where we sat in our
living rooms and watched men walking on the moon and

---

* Personal communication to Rep. James Florio, Assemblyman
  Martin A. Herman, and H. Donald Stewart, December 12, 1980.

read about heart-lung, kidney and liver transplants, that
New Jersey residents were forced to drink water from tank
trucks! And we wait for the next disaster area to be
heralded by some resident stricken with acute liver or
kidney toxicity!

In September 1981, Assemblyman Raymond Lesniak,
(D.-Union County), sponsored the "Hazardous Waste Discharge Act."[3] This 100 million dollar issue would help
raise money to clean up the states problem toxic waste
dumps. Ironically, the state's residents were given the
opportunity to vote on this proposal, as a referendum
in November of 1981. The state was involved in a lawsuit with the Reagan administration regarding failure to
implement the existing clean-up program, (the national
"Super Fund").[4] The Reagan Administration insisted that
it was still going over the issue for policy review.
Nevertheless, our contaminated water problems continued
in the state. The Lesniak proposal, now approved, holds
the *promise* of landfill clean-up. However, even if one
toxic waste site is cleaned-up or contained in 1982,
many residents living near the remaining sites, continue
to drink water of uncertain quality. The state has
failed dismally in promulgating an accelerated water
quality analysis program. Hopefully such an indictment
should be followed by a better idea. The author proposed a referendum permitting the state to withhold a
nominal portion of the homestead rebate, to fund state-
wide water quality analysis (for specific metals and
hydrocarbons). The analysis could be performed by
every available laboratory in the state and in neighboring states. The target areas would be determined on the
basis of pre-existing knowledge of landfill location and
resident complaints. The environmental organizations
within the state could easily provide the volunteers
for sample collection. Finally the state should have
a few vans outfitted with mini-laboratories capable of
performing on-site water analyses. Drinking water contaminated with toxic substances is now endemic in many
areas of New Jersey. Will it become epidemic? It is
not too late to deal more effectively with this the most
subtle and dangerous form of environmental pollution in
the state. Further, private wells in the state require
no tests for toxic organic chemicals, (excluding nitrate

and coliform bacteria content determinations required
for federally insured mortgages). Should the state consider making such testing mandatory? Well, anyone who
can muster the 'gelt' to buy a house these days and go
through settlement, certainly should not recoil over an
additional fee for well water quality "insurance." New
Jersey residents have already drunk, cooked with and
bathed in chemically contaminated water for indeterminate
periods. Dr. Donald B. Louria of the New Jersey College
of Medicine and Dentistry (in Newark), has said that the
increase in malignant colorectal cancers observed in
New Jersey during 1949-1976, may have been due to the
presence of organics in the drinking water.[5] Numerous
abandoned dump sites have been located in New Jersey.
Slowly, they are revealing their insidious nature by con-
taminating our drinking water.

Nuclear Power Plants

     The major demonstrable risk to the development of
cancers from nuclear power plants clearly falls on the
operating personnel. In 1980, Oyster Creek nuclear
power plant employees' radiation exposure increased by
a factor of four.[6] The other main problem is that of
the storage of radioactive wastes. You cannot build
any dwelling in New Jersey without an offsite septic or
sewage disposal system, and human waste is biodegradable! Why doesn't this preliminary requirement apply to
a nuclear power plant -- especially considering the
hazardous nature of the waste? Clearly, no more nuclear
power stations should be constructed until the waste
storage problem is solved. Any decision to treat radioactive material at the nuclear power plant site rather
than at a federal facility, would place risk factors on
the adjacent communities. Further, the reversal of
previous federal government decisions would be another
blow against trust and confidence on the part of the
general public.

Person Sponsored Pollution (Life-Style)

     The sovereignity of individual will in the etiology

of several environmental cancers has been described in
chapter 5. The most remonstrative being the use of
tobacco and the induction of cancers of the lung and
many other sites.[7] Tobacco use represents the most widely recognized environmentally masochistic practise whose
adverse effects are still denied by many smokers in the
general public. Tobacco use and the concomitant synergistic effects of other factors (alcohol, and/or asbes-
tos-exposure) is the singularly most identifiable cause
of the states lung (and other sites) cancer burden. We
are probably past the peak period for maximum combined
exposure to tobacco and asbestos. But we have not seen
the peak cancer mortality resulting from previous exposures to these carcinogens.

Of all the carcinogens, mutagens, and teratogens
studied on a world-wide basis, the data on tobacco
clearly call for an absolute ban on smoking in all public places, and a progressive ban on the growth of tobacco for anything but experimental purposes. The 1982
United States Surgeon General report reiterated earlier
themes, that most lung cancer deaths could be avoided if
Americans never smoked. Dr. Demopoulus once said, if
this (New Jersey) were Uganda and I were Idi Amin, I
would lessen the lung cancer burden in two years.[8] Such
language rings with legal paternalism. Well, society
does make such laws which hopefully will accomplish
the greatest good for the greatest number. And the
same government that sponsors tobacco related disease
studies and supports the tobacco industry - ought to
cease the hypocrisy and initiate the progressive ban of
tobacco. We are moving towards the ban in smoking in
public places in New Jersey, for the protection of non-
smokers, however painfully slow. And although I would
recommend an outright ban on tobacco, I must realistical-
ly add -- how effective would it be? Who from amongst
us could step forward and have the audacity to legislate
such legal paternalism. After all, man is an unfit
judge*- we are guilty of violating the very societal

----

*   Romans 2:1

guidelines we call on for help. At a Senate hearing on
the passage of bills regulating smoking in government
buildings, Senator Walter Foran selfishly complained the
law would stop him from smoking on the Senate floor.[9]
The laws were already on the books prohibiting smoking
in state government facilities;[10] the existing laws are
currently *ignored* routinely by DOH, DEP and DOE employees. Reiterating from chapter 1 - *"we have met the
enemy, he is us"*. Yet - judge we must or sink into an
absolutely anarchistic society. Sadly, if we cannot
deal with tobacco straightforwardly, then how can we ever
deal with the lesser environmental carcinogens which are
indicted by much less impressive data. And what does
the Tobacco Institute say - "the controversy must be resolved by more scientific research".[11] Tobacco and alcohol abuse, combined with the exposure to other carcinogenic environmental agents shall unfortunately continue
to be major person-sponsored sources of cancers in New
Jersey for some time. The percentage of smokers in New
Jersey (and nationally) is declining. However, the total
number of cigarettes sold, is increasing.

Diet/Nutrition

The New Jersey diet encompasses the same poor die-
tary/nutritional habits found elsewhere. Those dietary
practises thought by this author to be perhaps peculiar
to the state, do warrant evaluation, however. Excluding
the pre-existing superior dietary practises of some
groups, (e.g., Seventh-Day Adventists),* the dietary and
nutritional recommendations of the Federal Government
are trickling down to use at the primary school level.
Limited survey results and personal observations indicate most New Jersey adults consider their nutrition
inadequate and are basically unaware of the role of diet
in the etiology of cancer. It will prove to be far more
difficult to convince the general public about the role
of their diet/nutrition and the risk of cancer, than that
of tobacco use. Why? The effects of diet and nutrition

---

*   Strict Adventists do not smoke, or drink alcoholic beverages,
    shun tea, coffee, meat and spicy foods, prefer fruits, nuts
    and whole grains. Result - much less colon cancer.

are far less demonstrable. Secondarily, there is much less agreement in the literature about the relationship between diet/nutrition on colorectal cancers, than that of smoking on lung cancer.

Automotive Emissions

It has been clearly demonstrated that automotive emissions have the potential to cause cancers. However, epidemiologists are hard pressed to produce any studies where cohorts exposed *only* to automotive emissions developed cancers of the lung or at any other body site. There is no doubt that automotive emissions add to air pollution which is definitely linked to emphysema, bronchitis and *some* cancers. However, it is almost impossible to isolate the impact of automotive emissions from the rest of the spectrum of airborne pollutants such as asbestos, volatile organic matter, smoking, and metal particulates. Any move towards more diesel engines or any technology that will increase air pollution must be regarded with caution. Since we spend 80% of time indoors, is this concern disproportionate? Not unless you overlook the mail carrier, traffic officer or construction worker or others who spend an unusual amount of time outdoors.

Indoor Pollution

Continuing with the theme of how much time we spend indoors, indoor pollution evaluation in New Jersey is a high priority item. The sources are personal (e.g., tobacco smoke) and industrial in origin (e.g., trichloroethylene). Indoor pollution may account significantly for the incidence of lung cancer in non-smokers. The juxtaposition of airborne pollutants with the high density population areas (particularly in Northern New Jersey), underscore the need for investigation. The state Epidemiology department will probably have to place indoor pollutants high on the list of confounding factors in their cancer incidence and mortality studies. As residents tighten the integrity of their houses to reduce heat loss, the impact of indoor pollution will increase.

The implications of the indoor/outdoor pollution relationships cited in chapter 5, are global in their
health impact as well as being of concern for residents
of heavily industrialized areas such as New Jersey. The
first question to be raised is one of liability - who is
responsible for the quality of the ambient air in your
home? Clearly you have control over a pollutant source
such as tobacco. Fireplace and wood burning stove emissions are other examples. Increasing fuel oil prices
have encouraged a return to wood as a fuel source and
there are pollutant emissions associated with its combustion (cadmium, mercury and polycyclic aromatic hydrocarbons). In the fall of 1981, the author joined the
burgeoning ranks of the wood stove owners. In the first
six months of operation at least six burns were sustained. Thermal burns are cited in the etiology of skin
cancers. Many New Jersey residents are having their
first encounter with 'wood distillate' running down their
siding as a result of condensation occurring in metal
chimneys. Wood distillate is an extremely useful mixture but most homeowners will not realize the complex
mixture of carcinogens it contains. However, if the
pollutants are oxides of nitrogen from your gas range,
have you been advised of the hazard by your utility company? Or, who is responsible for the pollution of the
home environment by a family member's use of a radio-
pharmaceutical medicine? Further, if you live in North
Jersey and the pollutants are vinyl chloride, chloroform
or tichloroethylene, predominantly, of an industrial
origin, is the industry responsible for the health impact? Last, this question; should EPA/DEP regulate these
industrially derived indoor pollutants (an issue which
has already been raised)? Some environmentalists fear a
move in this direction would dilute the impetus for ambient outdoor air quality standards.

The DEP continues to evaluate outdoor pollution, but
what about indoor pollution?

Female Physiology

Female physiology was not described as a life-style
factor (excluding breast-feeding) in chapter 5. It is

discussed here briefly because it is an area where there
is control over the cancer risk.

The female reproductive organs, being far more complex than the male, manifest more site-specific cancers.
There are some cancer risk factors women have some control over:[12]

      obesity   - cancers of the breast and
                            body of the corpus uterus

      number of sex- - cancers of the cervix of the
      ual partners   uterus

Further, certain New Jersey counties have manifested
higher female reproductive organ cancer mortalities:

County	Rate	Site
Gloucester	10.6 vs 6.13 (USA)	corpus uteri, uterus and chorion epithelioma

The recent determination of an enhanced breast cancer
risk (1.4 to 1.9 as likely) in women who drink beer, wine
or liquor, is also provocative, considering the state's
alcoholism statistics.[13] In the minds of some New Jersey
residents, drinking water only *suspected* of chemical contamination is thought to be responsible for a cluster
of breast cancer cases.[14] There are other additional
suspect risk factors peculiar to female reproductive organs. However, dwelling on them could lead to dangerous
generalizations. The role of female physiology in the
etiology of cancer in New Jersey requires further evaluation.

Sunlight

The New Jersey life-style certainly could lend itself to over-exposure to sunlight. Not that our lati-
tude makes over-exposure easy, but there are many
activities that predispose an individual to a cumulatively dangerous exposure. We really have only about 5 good

months of outdoor weather, so it is easy to overdo the
enjoyment. Most skin cancers can be prevented by a
little individual common sense avoidance of over-exposure. Although skin cancers are highly curable, there
is no justification for a lack of concern. Further,
the rate of skin cancers is increasing in New Jersey.

Consumer Products

There appears to be a few consumer products that
might subject New Jersey residents to an increased risk
of cancer (e.g., urea-formaldehyde foam resins, hydrocarbon solvents and fiberglass components). However,
this assumption is made on the basis of deductive reasoning. Statistical consumer product research is required.

New Jersey - "Cancer Alley?"

Is New Jersey Cancer Alley or not? The cancer mortality rate is higher in the northeast than the national
average. If other east coast cities also have a higher
cancer mortality rate, can New Jersey be isolated and indicted as "Cancer Alley?" New Jersey must on occasion be
treated as an island because it has a unique anatomy as
described in chapter 4. When New Jersey is considered as
an island, we find that as of 1981, the cancer mortality
rate in other states increased to a degree where the New
Jersey rate ranked fourth nationally.[15]

Throughout the period of the debacle over NCI statistics, other states had a cancer mortality rate on a
par with New Jersey. On a statewide, all cancer site basis, New Jersey never was - "Cancer Alley". But -- we
certainly have several counties, (Camden, Ocean, Monmouth,
Middlesex, Union, Hudson and Essex), where cancer deaths
are significantly greater than the state average mortality rate. And if the rest of the nation is catching up
with the northern east coast region, then they are catching up with those New Jersey counties. I can agree with
the general concept of one study that expresses cancer in
New Jersey as an import, something brought in by city
dwellers escaping their crowded neighborhoods.[16] How-

ever, there are at least two problems with that concept.
The entire northeastern segment of the nation demonstrates a migration of its residents to other parts of
the nation. Secondarily, the study cites the acceptance
of the "standardization of American culture", that is
the acceptance of smoking and drinking for the shift in
cancer to the suburbs (New Jersey for one). The percentage of smokers actually fell more than 25% during the
period covered by the study (1950 - 1975).

Practically Speaking: Is New Jersey A Good Place to
Live without undue Cancer Risk?

     The proof of whether one considers New Jersey "Can-
cer Alley" is best manifested in the ability (or inability) to promote the state. Personally, I would never
leave the state because of the environmental situation
described in chapter 4. One cannot overlook those conditions or the risks associated with living in certain
areas or being engaged in certain occupations. Who would
knowingly or voluntarily move into an area with a chronic
air or groundwater pollution problem? There are micro-
cosms in the state that would be avoided. Of course
they also exist in other states. Our saving grace is the
knowledge of how much of the induction of cancer is under
individual control. Thomas A. Burke, Director of the
Office of Cancer and Toxic Substances Research in the
DEP has gone so far as to say that New Jersey is the only
state that can compare health data to environmental data.
Further, our ever improving environmental regulations
seek to protect us, and you may not find an equal if you
move to 'greener pastures'. Summarily, I can still promote New Jersey, but I will never minimize its environmental problems.

     However, what about the rest of the animal kingdom
in New Jersey, especially our domestic pets? Cats, dogs,
horses, etc., share our indoor and outdoor environmental
pollution and may display a proportionate share of our
cancer incidence and mortality. What about the impact
of the environment on their health? There is no statistical data and this is an area where some basic research
is required. Some pet owners do care enough about their

animals to have their cancer diagnosed and treated.[17, 18, 19, 20, 21] Correspondence with some very
loving pet owners indicate veterinarian diagnosed
cases of cancer of the buccal cavity, mammary ducts,
bone, muscle and lymphatic system. However, no attempt has been made to collate the available data into
anything approaching an epidemiological study. And
there is not a wealth of data because, pet owners do not
usually request autopsies on animals found dead, and pet
records may be destroyed after a five year period. Both
Drs. William Ottenheimer (veterinarian - Mantua) and
Sidney Nesbaum (New Jersey State Department of Agriculture) would like to see a New Jersey animal cancer study
conducted.[22] Such studies could improve human as well
as animal health.

Biologists have observed that the presence, absence
or condition of certain plants and animals is characteristic of polluted waters.[23] Many organisms have become
identified as biological evidence of environmental
abuse - or indicator organisms. Perhaps our domestic
pets could perform a similar service for the home environment. Haynes, Hoover and Tarone found a strong statistical correlation between the presence of manufacturing industries and bladder cancer in pet dogs.[24] This
study was conducted on data collected at 13 veterinary
medical teaching hospitals in the United States and
Canada.

How Does the New Jersey Resident Feel About Cancer in New Jersey?

The preliminary results of a state-wide New Jersey
Resident Cancer Opinion Survey have been evaluated.*
One out of three respondees felt the chances of developing cancer were greater living in New Jersey than elsewhere. A wide variety of causes was cited as the causes
of cancers, however tobacco use was legion. The American Cancer Society was most often cited as the organization doing the most to prevent or cure cancer in New

---

* Survey conducted throughout 1980 by the author.

Jersey, The most interesting statistic was the gross
over estimation of 1979, 1980 cancer deaths in New Jersey. The actual estimated number of deaths was 15,200,
and most New Jerseyans thought it to be as much as;
55,000, 85,000 or 118,000. The over-estimation indicates
several things. First, it reflects the fear, dread and
preoccupation with cancer. Further, this exaggerated
presumed data* base will render the New Jersey resident
hyper-reactive to "siting" or any other potential form
of environmental encroachment. But does this same hyper-
reactivity encourage the individual to live a more defen-
sive life-style? This is not necessarily so when the
parameter is tobacco. Diet and nutrition cannot yet be
examined similarly. Other survey results indicate there
is minimal awareness of the role of diet and nutrition
in the etiology of cancers on the part of most New Jersey
residents.

A highly personalized view of cancer in Gloucester
County comes from the Unit Director of the American Cancer Society, Mrs. Dorothy Price:[25] "Caring for a husband
with terminal cancer, being a cancer patient, a volunteer
in the fight against cancer with the Gloucester County
Unit of the American Cancer Society and now the Executive
Director of the Unit, I speak from the experiences that I
have had and am still having in dealing with the dreaded
disease.

The majority of persons today have become much more
aware of cancer and the fact that the diagnosis of cancer
does not mean an automatic "death" sentence. We have
progressed much in the way of education and communication.
Cancer has come out of the closet. Unfortunately, not
everyone has the willingness to accept the responsibility
of one's own health. There is still much to do in educating the public in the prevention of cancer. Much has been
done in the area of research and because of early detection our people can see a much more hopeful side to the
diagnosis of cancer than they could years ago. When the

---

*   mind you, the author is not demeaning the deaths of 15,200
    residents.

fear has been eliminated, the patient then can see his
course of treatment and hope for a remission or cure.
There was very little knowledge years ago of persons
surviving from cancer and living a full life. Today with
inspiration from our "survivors", education and open
communication amongst families we are now realizing the
quality of life is what really counts."

What Does Industry Think About Cancer In New Jersey?

33 New Jersey business establishments representing
approximately 190,000 employees responded to a survey
questionnaire presented by the author.* Virtually all
respondees agreed that:

> they were in compliance with OSHA regulations
> workers took advantage of protective clothing/
> equipment
> State agencies were doing enough to protect
> workers from carcinogens in the workplace

Eleven respondees indicated their workers handled known
or suspect carcinogens. Those substances were identified
as asbestos, vinyl chloride, PCB's and MOCA (4,4' -
methylenebis (2-chloroaniline). This appears to be an
under-representation as the reader will recall from
chapter 1 that S.3035 would have banned some 14 chemicals. Three respondees said they did not know if their
employees handled carcinogens or not. Six respondees
cited tobacco use as the cause of the high cancer incidence in New Jersey.** Thirty-one respondees did not
think that "Cancer Alley" was a fair or fitting title for
the State of New Jersey. Of course that means that two
industry spokespersons considered New Jersey *as such*,
which is a startling concession.

---

* surveys conducted January 1979 - March 1980, by the author

** Air, water pollution, life-style factors were also cited

Orphan Dumps

The Federal Government cites six orphan dump sites
in New Jersey and the DEP has acknowledged several hundred. The Governor's Hazardous Waste Commission has a
program to deal with the orphan dump sites. By the
spring of 1982, clean-up funds were available at both
the Federal and State level. But nothing has been done
at the so-called "priority" sites *yet*.

Radioactive Wastes

Low-level radioactive wastes from medical, research
and nuclear power plants in New Jersey are currently being shipped out of state. Increasing restrictions at
those disposal sites dictate that New Jersey eventually
establish its own site. The state faces a more immediate problem over what to do with 13,500 cubic yards of
World War II uranium extraction wastes from the Middlesex Sampling Plant, cited in chapter 4. Another 58,000
tons of the same radioactive material, placed in a
Middlesex landfill is currently releasing leachate. How
will the state ever convince a municipality of the safety
of siting a repository in any of our communities? Adding
insult to injury is a Federal Department of Energy
suggestion that certain granite formations in the state's
northern Appalachian range would make a good location for
a high-level radioactive waste respository.[26] This comes
from the same government that tells us how bad our air
and water pollution and cancer mortality rate are?? The
state should resist any such Federal Government plans.
Yet, within the same breath, I must admit the state has
the same problem as the Federal Government. It's called
"siting".

Clearly great wisdom, scientific expertise, public
trust and confidence and a remarkable budget will be required to protect the health of the states most important natural resource. Not just now, we needed it yes-
terday, and will need it for the state's future.

There are several unique sources of non-ionising
and ionising radiation in New Jersey. The most ubiquitous (other than the natural background from the sun)

non-ionising source is low-level/low-frequency electromagnetic radiation. There is a distinct concentration
from microwave sources in North Jersey, however high
voltage power lines producing measureable radiation also
traverse the state. When the DEP conducted an extensive
investigation of the clusters of leukemia and Hodgkin's
disease in Rutherford, both ionising and non-ionising
radiation were evaluated as potential causes.[27] However,
both radiation and chemical carcinogens, both present at
low levels, for which the health effects of long term
human exposure are not known, were exonerated. There is
enough residual radioactive material to affect a large
cohort at two locations in New Jersey. Some DuPont
Deepwater Facility workers are exposed to low-level
radiation and other chemical carcinogens (e.g., asbestos,
discussed earlier). Further, reservists spending a tour
at the Middlesex barracks are also an at risk group.
Clearly, there are identifiable groups in New Jersey
that are unaware of their exposure to an indeterminate,
non-ionising and ionising-radiation risk.

SUMMARY

     A great diversity of environmental factors with the
potential to cause cancers in New Jersey has been
identified in this book. Further, they have in fact
caused many of the cancers manifest in New Jersey. However the existence of an equally high all-site, cancer
mortality rate in other states throughout the 1970's
releases New Jersey from the unique stigma of the "Cancer Alley" image. Will those states with cancer deaths
anticipated to be higher than New Jersey in 1981,
(Rhode Island - 247/100,000, Florida - 245/100,000,
Pennsylvania - 212/100,000,* assume a "Cancer Alley"
image? None of them compares with New Jersey in their

---

* American Cancer Society projections are not age-adjusted.

concentration of chemical industries. New Jersey non-
theless is left with a high cancer mortality rate. And
what of the use of cancer mortality statistics alone in
assessing the position of a state in national cancer
rates? Incidence always precedes and is always larger
than the mortality rate for any disease. A very recent
study by Dr. Thind, et.al., of the New Jersey Medical
School in Newark, suggests that cancer mortality there
(1970 - 1974) resulted from "late diagnosis, poor compliance and/or suboptimal therapy".[28] Soon, the New
Jersey cancer registry will establish an accurate cancer
incidence data base.

When this work was conceived several years ago, the
author postulated that eventually he would arrive at
some graph describing the causes of the cancers in New
Jersey. However, this work has taken on more of a descriptive nature, rather than demographic. Further, the
author was very impressed along the way with the profound
words of Dr. Demopoulos, who said, "whoever attempts to
lead the nation towards less cancer had better be correct, because the selection of the wrong path is the
equivalent of leading millions of Americans to certain
death". Estimating cancer etiology as a dangerous and
yet necessary evil. Dr. Demopoulos' profound statement
was soon followed by his own cancer etiology score-card.
However, both sides of the environmental cancer liability
schools of thought have misused the score-cards and demo-
graphics to their advantage. The individual must decry
the cancer hazards of the workplace while conducting
an environmental inventory on him or herself to see if
his/her life-style is defensible. Similarly, industry
must never use the employee's life-style as a "scape-
goat" to cover up work-place hazards. Many books have
been written that state basic and simplistic measures
for avoiding cancer. This book was written mainly to ex-
pound on the great spectrum of environmental associations
that present a cancer risk. However, the identification
of adverse environmental agents becomes cancer prevention
and those ideas are summarized here:

>   Conduct an assessment on your life-style,
>   occupation and neighborhood. Remove or

avoid as many risks as possible.

- If you smoke, find a quit-smoking group and sign up.*

- If you drink alcoholic beverages - do so in moderation.

- Start a prophylactic vitamin program (C and E), whether you give up alcohol and tobacco or not. Such programs of prophylaxis are simultaneously held in high regard and ineffective by the research community. What do you have to lose? Consult your physician regarding dosages.

- Have your well water analyzed.

- Increase your intake of fiber-rich foods (e.g., bran, rye, whole wheat, nuts, peas, dried fruits, dark-green leafy vegetables, etc.)

- Replace non-nutritive drinks in your diet with fruit and vegetable juices.

- Call your county health department and arrange to have a Health Risk Appraisal. A sample form is given in the appendix.

- Take advantage of every free examination available, pertaining to cancer detection, (e.g., oral screening, hemoccult and pulmonary function).

---

* Snuff and chewing tobacco are also carcinogenic hazards.

Chapter 6 / REFERENCES

1.   Krawiec, Stella, Ph.D., The Chemical Industry in
        New Jersey, Office of Economic Research,
        Division of Planning and Research, N.J.
        Department of Labor and Industry, July 1973.

2.   Ibid.

3.   Editorial, The Gloucester County Times, September
        13, 1981

4.   State Files Suit to Force U.S. to Free Superfund,
        Washington (AP), The Gloucester County Times,
        September 18, 1981.

5.   Louria, Donald B., M.D., Cancer Patterns in New
        Jersey, Newer Aspects of its Epidemiology
        and Prevention, Seminar, Town and Campus,
        West Orange, New Jersey, November 10, 1981.

6.   Kraftowitz, Larry, Oyster Creek Workers' exposure
        to radiation quadrupled in 1980, Philadel-
        phia Inquirer, September 17, 1981, p. 11-
        B.p.

7.   New report reinforces cancer, smoking links,
        Washington (AP), Gloucester County Times,
        Nation & World, February 22, 1982.

8.   Public Hearing Before the Senate Commission on the
        Incidence of Cancer in New Jersey, Senate
        Chamber, State House, Trenton, N.J.,
        November 5, 1976.

9.   Smoking Bills Ready For Full Senate Vote, (AP) The
        Gloucester County Times, March 13, 1981.

10. Governor's Policy on Smoking, August 8, 1980.

11. About Tobacco Smoke, The Tobacco Institute, Washington, D.C., 1979.

12. Paulson, Glenn, Ph.D., and Preuss, Peter W., Ph.D., Cancer and the Environment, Let's Protect our Earth, New Jersey Department of Environmental Protection, May 1976.

13. Booze, higher breast cancer rate linked, New York (AP), Gloucester County Times, February 3, 1982.

14. Cancer cases no coincidence in Morris Co?, Montville (AP), Gloucester County Times, October 5, 1981.

15. McDonnell, Patrick, N.J. Drops from 1st to 4th in National Cancer Death Rate, The Gloucester County Times, December 21, 1980.

16. Sapatkin, Don, Cancer Moving to the Suburbs, The Trenton Times, March 18, 1980.

17-
21. Personal Communications with:
Friedman, Carolyn, January 20, 1981
Laskey, Donna, January 26, 1981
Kobel, Charles, January 10, 1981
Dante, Mary C., January 21, 1981
De Natale, Lorraine, February 11, 1981

22. Personal Communications - July 1980, November 1981

23. Hynes, H.B.N., The Biology of Polluted Waters, University of Toronto, 1974.

24. Haynes, Howard M., Jr., Hoover, Robert, and Tarone, Robert E., Bladder Cancer in Pet Dogs: A Sentinel for Environmental Cancer?, American Journal of Epidemiology, Volume 114., No. 2., August 1981.

25. Personal Communication from Mrs. Dorothy Price,
         January 27, 1982.

26. Sugawara, Sandra, Waste Study Names State Site,
         The Gloucester County Times, Ocotber 13,
         1980 , p. A-10.

27. Burke, Thomas A., et.al., An Environmental Investi-
         gation of Clusters of Leukemia and Hodgkin's
         Disease in Rutherford, N.J., The Journal
         of the Medical Society of New Jersey, Vol.
         77., No. 4, April 1980, pp. 259-264.

28. Thind, I.S., M.D., Carnes, R., M.D., Quartello, G.,
         B.A., Feuerman, M., B.A., and Louria, D.B.,
         M.D., Cancer Incidence and Mortality in
         Newark, N.J., 1970 - 1974: A National
         Comparison, CANCER, Vol. 47, No. 5, March
         1, 1981, pp. 1047-1053.

CHAPTER 7

NEW JERSEY YESTERYEAR

"A priori reasoning,
whether it be based
on sophisticated de-
ductive evolutionary
theory or on appeal
to antiquity, needs
to be re-examined.
Both the old and the
new should be investi-
gated."

Irving Selikoff,
M.D., and E.
Cuyler Hammond,
Sc.D.*

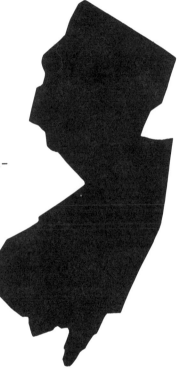

* From "Environmental Cancer in the Year 2000." From the
   Environmental Cancer Research Project of the American Cancer
   Society and the Mount Sinai School of Medicine of the City
   University of New York.

CHAPTER 7

Background

It is not difficult to find literature describing
the nature of life in New Jersey from the formative to
the pre-industrial years. Typically, most literature
describes the early inhabitants, the Lenni-Lenape
Indians, who named the territory "Scheyichbi."* The
arrival of Hendrick Hudson in 1609 and not that of the
Indians, however, serves to document inhabitancy of
New Jersey.[1] The literature may be replete with accounts
of everyday life, but not its impact on general health.

It is the intention of this chapter to apply concepts of 20th century environmental science to the life
in New Jersey during the 17th to the 19th century. The
specific goal of this chapter is to ferret out those,
at that time unrecognized chemical carcinogens. These
existed in the form of iatrogenic (physician induced),
naturally occurring remedies, or those inherent in the
daily business of eking out an existence. Further, what
was the risk of developing cancers from those exposures?
Other non-malignant diseases, prevalent at that time,
will also be discussed. The early monitoring and recognition of the cancers as a public health problem and the
paralleling evolution of requisite medical care in terms
of having an adequate corps of physicians, is also discussed briefly.

An optimistic commentary on general public health in
early 17th century New Jersey has been given to us in a
letter written by a Charles Gordon. He advised his
brother, Dr. John Gordon, still in Scotland, that he
would need to change his occupation upon arriving here.[2]
This seemingly humorous comment not only preceded the
death of its author, but of very many of the newly arriv-

---

* meaning the land of shell wampum.

307

ing Europeans. What were the early environmental factors
of this new land called a "terrestrial Canaan"?[3]

The New Jersey Environment, 17-19th Century

There are at least five essential components for the
sustenance of life: air, food, water, shelter, and medical care. The first three are old acquaintances from
chapter 3; with them we make constant contact with the
environment. There are other parameters that also render
life comfortable; they are called amenities.

General Home Environment

Shelter was the most intimate aspect of life, entailing protection from the elements and some means of
space heating. In 17th century New Jersey this usually
consisted of a fire on an earthen floor, in a hut or a
cave in a river bank. Ultimately, the living quarters
became a log, stone or brick house.[4] The log cabin
fireplace, in contrast to the much-reduced, 20th century
recreation room version, extended the breadth of the
house. The fuel was wood. Although some huts had
chimneys, the ventilation in others consisted of only
a vent in the roof, which rendered the living space a
smoky environment. Here we encounter only the first in
a series of health hazards concomitant with the "good
old days." Both coal and wood contain between 50 to
200 ppm fluoride, 0.10 to 0.25 ppm cadmium and 0.09 to
33 ppm mercury, all of which are released in the form
of either gaseous or particulate emissions during combustion.[5] These emissions were toxic lung irritants
and cadmium is carcinogenic. In addition, the carcinogenic polycyclic aromatic hydrocarbons (PAH) described
in chapter 4 would have been released into poorly ventilated living spaces.

These same fireplaces supplied light in the log
cabin environment and the Swedes on the Delaware are
credited with the introduction of "splinter sticks"
which burned vigorously giving off copious quantities
of smoke along with the light.[6] In addition, bear and
refuse grease were burned in shallow lamps hung from the

ceiling.[7] The smoky and smelly contrivances burning
hydrocarbons, undoubtedly released carcinogens (e.g.,
PAH's) into the cabin or hut environment. Continuing
with the peripheral aspects of shelter, consider the
health impact of the practise of roasting animals and
birds over the fire.[8] Animal carcasses were brought
into the home where they could readily transfer either
insects or microorganisms. Those same animals were
often smoked in a smokehouse for future use and the
hazard incurred in that practise will be commented on
later.

Communal drinking cups, the common practise of early
New Jersey life, just about insured that any communicable
disease was shared. If cancers were of a bacterial origin, they would have had every opportunity to have been
quite virulent. Although not strictly a home industry,
distilling of approximately 50 available alcoholic
beverages took place on the estate of large farms.[9] The
possible environmental impact of this practise besides
the problems stemming from the liquor production for tap-
rooms and the confinement of curfews, as early as 1668,
was the body intake of lead* from leadworm coils inside
the copper stills.[10] Almost paralleling the attitude of
water consumption in Europe, water, suspected of not being safe to drink was not a favored beverage. By 1830
there were 338 distilleries in New Jersey and an undetermined number of private copper "boilers."[11] South
Jersey (Burlington, Cape May, Cumberland, Gloucester and
Salem counties) had a population of 92,722 and could
boast of a distillery to inhabitant ratio of one to
every thousand residents.[12]

Traditionally, we spend about 25% of our lives in
bed and close evaluation of beds and bedrooms as they
existed in the settlers' lives does not reveal any latent
carcinogens. However, settlers did sleep on animal skins
which were reportedly occasionally infected with lice and
fleas which carry such diseases as relapsing and typhus
fevers and bubonic plague.[13]

---

* Lead acetate (II), trihydrate is a class I carcinogen.

Tobacco Use

The use of tobacco, introduced as early as 1686 and practised by men, women, boys and girls to cope with bordeom, added to the pollution of the home environment.[14] Tobacco underwent a usage evolution; it was initially used in pipes, later as snuff and then cigars in the 1850s. Eventually, in the 1860s, the hand-rolled cigarette was introduced, with usage being enhanced by the invention of the friction match. It was then that cigarette use became a very popular pastime. In some states, attempts were made to prohibit smoking because it was cited as the cause of the farmer's neglect of food crops. Of course, there was no Surgeon's General Office pronouncement to warn the unsuspecting settlers of the adverse health effects of smoking, but reformers campaigned not only against the evils of tobacco use but of alcohol abuse, another colonial pastime previously discussed.[16]

Much concern and intelligent analysis have been devoted to the identification of the carcinogenic constituents of tobacco smoke, as described in chapter 5. However, tobacco poses an environmental health hazard even before it is burned. Hecht and associates (1978)[17] demonstrated that nicotine, a tobacco constitutent, toxic in its own right, and used as an insecticide (black leaf 40), is converted to carcinogenic nitrosamines during the curing and processing of tobacco. The implications are obvious; there was and is exposure to these nitrosamines and other carcinogens during the curing, handling and chewing of tobacco. The surface has only been penetrated in the study of tobacco environmental carcinogenesis. The impact of tobacco use on public health is extremely well documented and is summarized in chapter 5. Needless to say, a parallel impact would have been engendered in the environments of early New Jersey settlers, correlatable with the degree of the use of both alcohol and tobacco usage.

Diet and Nutrition

Most accounts given of the flora and fauna of New

Jersey by the early settlers served to encourage more
immigration. The land was described as having a great
diversity of animals ranging from the smaller hares to
the large bear, deer, and elk. Equally diverse were
the descriptions of the wild fruits, nuts, berries,
birds and amphibians.[18] Inland and marine waterways
provided more fish than the Europeans could name from
their ichthyological nomenclature repertoire.[19] In fact,
the descriptions indicate an early decline in the environment directly proportionate to European settlement.
The settlers learned much from the Indians: how to grow
corn and the ability to recognize edible roots, tubers,
nuts and berries and many other valuable practises. In
spite of this great diversity of foodstuffs capable of
providing what could be demonstrated to be a prudent
diet by today's standards, the period 1609 to about
1800 is referred to as the "bread and meat" era. Settlers were concerned principally with the maintenance of
field crops and livestock. Cattle were raised in bog
areas and the predominant field crops were corn, rye,
beans, potatoes, pumpkin, squash, and turnips. Fruits
and berry crops were also cultivated.

     Those settlers who lived near coastal areas also
adopted some of the Indians' dietary habits. Many foods
were derived from the sea without nearly as much effort
as required for survival inland. That diet consisted
of scallops, whelks, mussels, crabs, conch, oysters, and
clams. Additional delicacies consisted of marsh hens
and gull eggs, eels and roast terrapin.[20] Throughout
all of New Jersey, hog products and venison were enjoyed.
It was not until the 1800s and the dawn of the industrial
era and railroads that farmers turned to specialty crop
raising such as asparagus, tomatoes, peas and lima
beans.[21] There is no record of cranberry farming until
after 1840. The turn of the 20th century marked the beginning of a great diversity in diet.

Impact of Diet and Nutrition

     Examination of the available foodstuffs indicate
that the essentials of a good diet were available. However, it is not possible to assess what each individual
ate of the available food supply. If the average diet of

that earlier time centered on a bread and meat staple, it
would now be described as a high carbohydrate-protein
diet.   If the carbohydrate consisted of nuts, fruits,
vegetables and whole grains (and we certainly know the
baked products were not "enriched") and the protein on
the lean side, that diet would have been closer to the
prudent diet than that of contemporary U.S.A.   Early
20th century dietary trends indicate that nutrient fats
consisted predominantly of lard and butter.[22]   Additionally, good dietary bulk fiber was avilable as rye,
corn and buckwheat.   However, it may have been the manner
of preserving both meat and fish that subjected all early
New Jersey settlers (Indians included) to the highest
risk to cancers of the stomach and other body organs.
Before the ice and refrigeration era, smoking was the
mainstay method of preserving food.   Essentially, the
meat, fish, poultry, or cheese is suspended in a chamber
where wood smoke is allowed to permeate and deposit on
the foodstuff.   Today the composition of the smoke vapors
are well known to contain carcinogens; phenols, hydrocarbons, formaldehyde and other organics.[23]   The deposit consists mainly of tars.[24]   The organic composition of the smoke chamber vapors will vary slightly with
the selection of the wood.   Hickory, oak and beech provide a smoke which contains creosote, an excellent preservative, if you wish to preserve a lumber product.[25]

Salt, (sodium chloride), has a very ancient history
as both a meat and fish preservative.   Salt effects its
preservative quality in meat and fish by tissue dehydr-
tion and subsequent bacterial growth inhibition.[26]   It
is thought that salt peter (sodium nitrate) was a salt
impurity, which was later recognized singularly for its
color preserving property.   It is not possible to determine now what were typical sodium nitrate levels in that
salt used in early New Jersey.   However, it is now known
that the correct amount of salt to use in curing was anything but a science until the latter half of the 19th
century.   This establishes the premise that many early
New Jersey inhabitants were probably exposed to more
sodium nitrate, an unrecognized carcinogen percursor,
than in more recent times.   Sodium nitrate degrades in
meat to form sodium nitrite which may react with secondary amines to form a very potent class of carcinogens,

nitrosamines.[27] Alternatively, the nitrite could react
with secondary amines in the human digestive tract,
also forming nitrosamines. Since 1925, sodium nitrite
has also been used as a color-stablizing agent. As
discussed in chapter 3 and 4, this retrospective and
controversial cancer risk still haunts us today on a
world wide basis.

It should also be noted that abdominal distress was
a common complaint of the early settlers. Obviously,
not all perishable foodstuffs were smoked; i.e., they
were eaten ostensibly, in a "fresh" condition. In the
absence of smoking, ice, or refrigeration, and a keen
sense of smell, it is likely that some of the reported
abdominal distress was food poisoning due to infections
from staphylococcus and salmonella organisms.

The Extra-Home Environment

Once outside the home environment, one encountered
the Jersey mosquito, a nuisance then as well as now. The
early settlers recognized their association with swamps
and stagnant water, an environment provided by many
areas in the state. What was not recognized and is certainly not a presumptious speculation now is that
lymphomas, attributable to the presence of the malarial
mosquito may have been present in early New Jersey. (cf.
Burkitt's Lymphoma, chapter 3).* One colonial practice
that resulted in the introduction of aromatics and PAH's
into the home environment while driving off mosquitoes
was that of generating "skeeter smoke."[28] Pineys** used
to pile pine needles and cones in a deep pan on a stove
generating a smoldering, destructive distillating smoke
which rid the home of mosquitoes, and on inattentive
occasions, burned down the house![29]

---

* Conversations with Dr. Dennis Burkitt indicate that to support
  this hypothesis, malaria would have to have been holoendemic
  and infecting 75% of children.

** A New Jersey colloquism for pine-barren dwellers.

In addition to the mosquitoes, some bearing malarial parasites, swarms of flies meandered over the settlers' food and beverages. This contributed to outbreaks of such diseases as cholera, typhoid fever, and the debilitating effects of liver and lung abcesses resulting from infection with the pathogenic protozoan, Endamoeba histolytica.[30] The common practice of walking barefoot made everyone a prime target for the hook worm larvae which enters the body through the skin, preferably that of the foot. Also to be found in the soil was the anerobic soil bacillus of tetanus, entering the circulatory system through wounds and causing a disease commonly known as lock-jaw. Tetanus would continue to be a public health problem until antitoxins were introduced between 1880 and the early 1900s.[31]

Early New Jersey Home and Farm Industries

In New Jersey colonial days, the basic needs of each family were supplied by each farm with the family members being jacks of all trades; carpenters, tanners, brewers, blacksmiths, etc. Further, they were also very often the administrators of therapeutic remedies. Consequently, their responsibility exposed them to potentially toxic and carcinogenic agents. Consider these examples:

Tanning

Records indicate that the tanning of hides as a trade began in the period 1664-1703.[32] By 1850, there were approximately 137 tanneries in the state and in 1860, Newark alone had 30 tanneries employing more than 1000 workers.[33] In the tanning process, the animal hide protein which when untreated decays, is converted with lye and tannins into a durable substance, leather, which can be moistened and dried without becoming hard. The tannins were obtained from the barks of a variety of trees (oaks, birch, beech, hemlocks, and willows). Animal hides were processed in sunken wooden vats and ascending vapors contained tannins and tannic acid. Studies conducted by the International Agency for Research and Cancer show that the subcutaneous injection of tannic acid into mice produces liver tumors.[34]

Dyeing

Prior to the construction of fulling and dyeing mills, the women of the household performed these duties almost exclusively. Occasionally, this art was practised right in the home in iron or earthen vats built into the fireplace. The dye sources and risk to cancers were the same as described under tanning.

Glassmaking

Glass may be said to be a super-cooled mixture of fused silica (sand) and other metallic and non-metallic elements.[35] The color and physical properties of the final product are a function of the metallic and non-metallic element additives. Records indicate that an early and successful glass factory was established by Caspar Wistar in 1717 along Alloway Creek in Salem County.[36] Glassmaking would become a major industry in the state because of its remarkably pure and vast sand deposits. The firing of the glass is described as follows.[37] The typical furnace in which fusing was accomplished consisted of three sections: a fire chamber, and above it the calcar and the annealing chamber where finished pieces were cooled gradually. Silica (sand) potash or lime were added to the calcar and the complete process took about forty hours. In the interim, workmen were in close proximity to maximum furnace temperatures of 2500 degrees F[o]. The furnace emissions associated with glassmaking were chlorine, silica, and boron. In addition, certain glass formulas, ruby glass for example, called for the addition of zinc oxide (known to contain fluorspar, also known as calcium fluoride, and cadmium) and red lead (a mixture of led oxides), all of which guaranteed the presence of a toxic and potentially carcinogenic environment about the furnace for the glassblower.[38]

Mining Operations -- Iron and Copper

In the early 1700s iron ore, a black stone called Sukahsin by the Lenni-Lenape Indians, was extracted from New Jersey hills.[39] The black stone, magnetite, and a

red form of ore, hematite,* are found principally in
northern New Jersey. It is difficult to comprehend
mine shafts in New Jersey; however, many abandoned shafts
may be visited in the northern part of the state today.
In addition to the deep mine shafts, bog iron, a variety
of limonite ore, was found literally on the surface
along streams in meadows and lowlands throughout the
state.

Before the rich copper deposits of Montana, Utah,
and Wyoming were discovered, New Jersey was the leading
source of that metal. A significant deposit was located
in what is now called North Arlington along the Passaic
River in northern New Jersey. Dutch settlers at the
Schuyler Mines extracted the ore as early as 1720 and
shipped it back to Holland.[40] Iron was mined in New
Jersey perhaps twenty years before copper mining began.
The counties of Sussex, Warren, Morris and Passaic were
maintained as important iron ore sources for 19th century
America until the even richer deposits of the northern
Great Lakes region were discovered.[41]

Contemporary epidemiological and animal laboratory
studies show that those engaged in mining operations
have a high risk potential for the development of cancers
of the skin, larynx, lung and liver.[42] Although copper
mining in early New Jersey consisted of the removal of
the various ores from open pits rather than deep shaft
mining, workers were still exposed to toxic and carcinogenic particulates. It may take as much as 5 tons of
ore to yield 20 pounds of copper and some of the other
metals present are a health hazard on being inhaled as
particulate matter or on being absorbed through the
skin; e.g., arsenic, lead, and nickel. Similarly, most
iron ore in New Jersey came from open pits. The principal hazardous impurities accompanying this ore are
sulfur and silica. The sulfur is not a problem until

---

*   In some parts of the world, hematite has been found associated
    with asbestiform fibers in the host rock. Personal communica-
    tion from Dr. Irving J. Selikoff, February 5, 1982.

the ore is refined; then it becomes sulfur dioxide, a
ciliatoxic agent. The silica is a hazard as a dust,
often causing silicosis.

Records show that there are 26 abandoned and inactive mines in the state of New Jersey.[43] And this
is a good indication of the extent of past mining operations. What may have been an unrecognized cause of lung
and blood cancers in early New Jersey mine workers were
the accompanying radioactive emissions due to the presence of radon daughters in the mine ores. Currently,
an excess of lung cancers, reduced pulmonary function,
and emphysema among uranium mine workers has been reported.[44] Further, that rate is higher in workers who
use tobacco. The presence of uranium in New Jersey mines
is not remote, as a 1953 U.S. Geological Survey indicates: an exceptionally high grade uranium ore (0.5%)
exists in a northwestern mountainous area of Passaic and
Bergen counties called the Ramapos.[45]

Iron Smelting

The earliest furnaces in which the ore was reduced
to metallic iron were about three feet at the base and
larger ones about ten feet in diameter and resembling
an egg.[46] A fire was kindled at the base of the furnace
and was maintained by charcoal from periods ranging from
16 weeks to 8 months. The furnace iron ore charge contained impurities which on oxidation would generate
sulfur dioxide, oxides of phosphorous in addition to
emanations of aluminate and silicate particulate matter.[47] There would also be organic compound by-pro-
ducts released as a result of the incomplete combustion
of charcoal (which itself contains incompletely decom-
posed organic matter and absorbed chemicals): e.g., benzene and naphthalene. The furnace operator and furnace
community consisted of a collection of workmen's houses,
a school, church, carpenter shop and variety store and
and these inhabitants were constantly exposed to a
variety of toxic and carcinogenic emissions. The
etiology of the resultant diseases are well established
today: respiratory distress, siderosis, metal-fever,
and cancers of the respiratory tract.[48, 49]

Woolen Cloth Manufacture

Wool manufacture began in New Jersey as a home-based industry. The first step was the shearing of sheep in the spring followed by the washing of the wool and this activity was normally performed by men. Washing was accomplished in a stream or with a weak lye solution which removed dirt and grease. A seemingly strange step was carried out at this point -- the wool was scoured with a mixture of very hot water and urine.[50] Workmen actually collected their urine in a common tub for this purpose, maintaining it until it was putrid and then using the mixture as a scouring solution.[51] This practise, entailing exposure to tub vapors, certainly provided an opportunity for the transmission of disease. Further, today we know that both human stool and urine may be mutagenic.[52, 53] The author considers that the aforementioned practise placed workmen at a slight risk to the induction of cancers.

Cedar Mining

Most New Jersey cedar swamps were discovered between 1740-1750 and they were lumbered for about 100 years.[54] Cedar was cut into shingles, fences, lumber canoes, tanks, pails, tubs, and furniture. The work hazard peculiar to this activity can be discerned from a description of a cedar swamp, where the wood was cut. The typical weather there was a micro-climate of calm, still, moist and cool air, while it was yet windy outside. There would have been a dust hazard which would also contain aromatics peculiar to that wood in addition to trace quantities of mercury and cadmium. Contemporary epidemiological studies have established the substantial risk to the development of intranasal cancers in wood workers* (sawyers) exposed to wood dusts.[55]

Pottery

The abundant clay deposits in New Jersey proved to

---

* Cedar, however, was not one of the woods to which workers were exposed to in the study cited.

be an encouragement to pottery manufacture in much the
same manner that sand deposits encouraged the early
glass-making industries. There are abundant clay deposits in the areas of Woodbrige, Perth Amboy, and
South Amboy; however, pottery was eventually manufactured all over the territory. Records show the erection
of a pottery kiln as early as 1685 for Burlington.[56] Records from the very early 17th century do not indicate
the extent of individual versus commercial "pottery"
manufacture of the necessary cooking and food storage
vessels. However, the early New Jersey colonials certainly brought the art of pottery manufacture with them
from Europe and found native Indians practising similar
arts as it was also the Indians' practise to boil ground
cornmeal to make porridge.[57] In 1863, there were ten
potteries in Trenton alone and in 1882, 16 were producing such products as drugware, sanitary ware, plumbing
fixtures, dinnerware, electrical porcelain, and tile.[58]

The principal raw materials used in the manufacture
of pottery are the plastic (the clay), the flux or solvent (feldspar in most cases, an igneous rock), and an
inert nonplastic or filler (typically flint). The total
formulation actually has undergone an evolution as well
as the glazing techniques which seal in pottery constituents. This step in the process prevents permeation
of raw materials into foodstuffs. The chief hazard to
those involved in pottery manufacture was exposure to
particulate dust in the pre-molding stage. Clays contain hydrous silicates of aluminum which are rather
innocuous in terms of ingestion. However, silicates,
when inhaled as particulates may induce silicatosis.
Glazing, which puts a shiny coat on pottery, was accomplished by the application of a mixture of silicates,
sand or oxide of lead. The absence of respiratory protection and hand cleaning hygiene would result in inhalation and ingestion of toxic lead. Nineteenth century pottery manufacturers in New Jersey were known to
suffer from lead colic, potters' asthma (silicosis),
emphysema, and consumption as a result of these exposures.[59] It is a plausible speculation that some of

the lung diseases were cancer malignancies.* One may
only further speculate on the household illnesses resulting from transport of metals from the workplace to
the home. The 1905 New Jersey Department of Labor and
Industries Report indicates that pottery workers employed in the slip or dipping rooms "rarely reached forty
years of age."[60] An interesting and early epidemiological account of the synergestic effect of life-style and
occupation is given in that same report:

> "Undoubtedly the excessive use of alcohol
> had much to do with the early breakdown
> of health and the brief average dura-
> tion of life in the case of these men
> as the unhealthy conditions necessarily
> surrounding their work."

The "unhealthy condition" the writer was referring to
was the exposure to "dusts" in the workers' ambient
air. The dust hazard persisted until the institution
of the practise of sweeping up at night and other
improvements. The hazards associated with pottery
manufacture were not limited to occupational exposures.
The virtual complete industrialization of pottery manufacture in the 19th century resulted in the dispersal
into surrounding communities of such emission products
as fluorides, silicates and ammonia.

    There were many other home-based and industrial
activities in 17th to 19th century New Jersey that resulted in exposure to toxic and carcinogenic substances;
e.g., tar-pitch mining, blacksmithing, hat-making, and
shoemaking. However, those discussed here should provide an adequate basis for the existence of a substantial
risk for the development of cancers in early New Jersey.

Women in the Workplace

    Comparing the potential exposure of women in the
late 18th century to carcinogens in the workplace en-

---

* there is no evidence that these lung diseases were lung cancer.

vironment to contemporary occupational exposures, they
fared much better then. There were only seven trades
open to women of that era: teaching, needle work, keeping boarders, domestic service, cotton mill employment,
bookbinding and typesetting.[61]   Cotton mill employment
in the 18th century meant certain exposure to fiber dust
and concomitant byssinosis.* However, it was the employment as typesetters and associative exposure to
printing inks and metals that posed the risk of developing cancers. Today, epidemiological studies show these
workers risk the development of cancers of the lung,
skin, and nasal sinuses.[62]   Type metal is known to
oxidize on exposure to air and the resultant material,
called "dross", is a combination of complex oxides of
lead, antimony and tin.[63]   Several lead salts are under
investigation to determine if they are carcinogenic
and at least one, lead acetate (ll) trihydrate, is a
positive animal carcinogen.[64]

     Employment by women in typesetting, cotton mills,
and bookbinding industries was de-emphasized in the 19th
century. Home based activities filled the void in
women's lives, in contrast to today where they have
pursued the right to take their place in industry along
with men.

Therapeutics

     The early settlers in New Jersey imported few of
the sophisticated English physicians, but they did have
a wealth of disease-producing viruses. Among those
diseases were measles and small pox which took a toll
on the defenseless Indian. The settlers themselves
suffered from small pox, malaria, mumps and yellow fever.
The absence of and ignorance concerning sanitation, resulted in contamination of water supplies, followed by
outbreaks of typhoid fever and dysentery.[65]   Although
the water contained pathogens, it was essentially void
of the gross industrial and non-industrial contaminants

---

* a chronic industrial lung disease resulting from long term
   inhalation of cotton dust or fibers

now a problem in our state. The scarcity of medical
practitioners in the scattered communities prompted
Benjamin Franklin of nearby Philadelphia to publish the
fourth edition of John Tennant's "Every Man His Own
Doctor."[66] Some of the therapeutic practices extant in
the 17th and 18th century entailed exposure to chemicals
now known to be toxic and/or carcinogenic. Several of
these therapeutic agents are listed in Table 27.

Many therapeutic agents were also used to treat
animal disorders, especially in cattle and sheep:[67]

Turpentine*	chloride of lime
powdered opium	tincture of veratrum
calomel	pulverized digitalis
carbolic acid*	powdered catechu
iron sulphate	tobacco tea*
black antimony	asafoetida
sulfur	azedarach
belladona	pulverized cinchona
tartar emetic	arsenic*

(* potential or suspect carcinogens)

Bear in mind that the formulation of these remedies by
yesteryear's self-taught veterinarians also entailed the
intimate handling of toxic and carcinogenic compounds.

A common practise used to treat an iron worker's
children suffering from the croup (laryngitis or laryngeal spasms in children) was to secure the child near
the top opening of a burning charcoal heap so as to
effect its inhalation of creosote fumes.[68] Wood creosote, a distillate product of charcoal burning, contains
mixtures of phenols, guaiacol and cresol-phenol.* One
component of the distillate, although not currently adjudged a carcinogen, is known to potentiate the carcinogenic action of another charcoal smoke component,
benzo[a]pyrene, a class I carcinogen.[69] In addition to
the inhalation therapy, a coal-tar cough syrup was

---

* Phenol was a suspect carcinogen up until late 1980 (NCI Report).

TABLE 27

THERAPEUTIC AGENTS OF THE 17th-19th CENTURY

Symptom to be Treated or Desired Effect	Active Component	Source of Active Component (s)	Contra Indications, Toxicity/Carcinogen Rating
Anesthetic	opium, morphine	papaveraceae, or poppy family	abuse leads to habituation or addiction
	aconite	aconite root, monkshod	effective doses considered toxic
	hyoscyamine, hyoscine, atropine bella-donnine and other components	belladonna plant leaf	toxicity based on alkaloid content, specifically atropine causes blurred vision, vasodilation, hyperpyrexia, delerium
	arnicin (containing 0.5-1% tannin)	arnica flowers	tannin in an animal carcinogen
	chloroforml	organic synthesis	toxic, carcinogenic
Cancer (Topical treatments)	tannins	white/red oak bark ashes	tannins are not considered toxic however, adjudged suspect animal carcinogen

TABLE 27 - continued
THERAPEUTIC AGENTS OF THE 17th-19th CENTURY

Symptom to be Treated or Desired Effect	Active Component	Source of Active Component(s)	Contra Indications, Toxicity/Carcinogen Rating
Cancer (Topical treatment) - continued	chrysophanic acid, neopodin, lapodin and tannin	yellow duck root	
	coumaric, salicylic acid, phenolic substances and others	red clover	salicyclic acid - absorption of large doses can cause increased respiration, mental disturbances
	glycerides of linolic, linolenic and isolinolenic, myristic, stearic and palmitic acids	linseed, flaxseed oil	most constituents rather innocous, having a variety industrial applications
	pinene	oil of turpentine	irritant to skin and mucous membranes, and severe kidney irritation

324

TABLE 27 - continued
THERAPEUTIC AGENTS OF THE 17th-19th CENTURY

Symptom to be Treated or Desired Effect	Active Component	Source of Active Component(s)	Contra Indications, Toxicity/Carcinogen Rating
Cancer (Topical Treatment) - continued	camphor	cinnamomum camphora (plant) or synthetic	toxic, taken orally/parentally may cause vertigo, delerium, respiratory failure and death
	antimony chloride, gold chloride, zinc chloride		skin and mucous membrane irritant
	mercurous chloride	calomel	toxic, may cause mercury poisoning
	Pb_3O_4	red lead	brain damage, neurological disturbance, changes in cellular biochemistry
	$Pb(CH_3COO)_2 \cdot 3H_2O$	sugar of lead	dust toxic

325

TABLE 27 - continued
THERAPEUTIC AGENTS OF THE 17th-19th CENTURY

Symptom to be Treated or Desired Effect	Active Component	Source of Active Component(s)	Contra Indications, Toxicity/Carcinogen Rating
Childbirth	mixture of alkaloids amino acids, sterols, gluco- sides, sugars, oil and ergotoxine, ergotamine and histamine	ergot of rye	toxic, acute poison- ing causes diarrhea, tachycardia, coma, chronic circulatory changes and gangrene
Colds, coughs, Croup		coal tar tobacco	mixture of hydro- carbons many of which are C-I carcinogens
	mercurous chloride	calomel	see above.
Diarrhea	carbolic acid (phenol)		phenol is a cocarcino- gen
Delerium	camphor	see above	see above
Fever	camphor	see above	see above

326

TABLE 27 - continued
THERAPEUTIC AGENTS OF THE 17th-19th CENTURY

Symptom to be Treated or Desired Effect	Active Component	Source of Active Component(s)	Contra Indications, Toxicity/Carcinogen Rating
Gallstones	chloroform	see above	see above
Hydrophobia (Rabies)	scutellarin○ (contains tannins)	skullcap (perennial herb)	see above
Inflammation	capsaicin T	Cayenne pepper, African chillies	contains suspect carcinogens
Laxative Relaxant	mercurous chloride protoveratrine ○ jervine pseudojervine rubijervine	calomel dried rhizome and roots of veratrum viride plant	see above
Sedative	chloral hydrate○	organic synthesis 1869	suspect carcinogen; abuse may lead to habituation or addiction

327

TABLE 27 - continued
THERAPEUTIC AGENTS OF THE 17th-19th CENTURY

Symptom to be Treated or Desired Effect	Active Component	Source of Active Component(s)	Contra Indications, Toxicity/Carcinogen Rating
Stimulant	strychnine, brucine[O] chlorogenic and other alkaloids	dried ripe seed of nux vomica plant	overdose produces respiratory arrest and death
Stomach strengthener	ipurganol, gluco-sides of con-vovulinic and ipurolic acids also B-methy-aesculetin chrysophanic acid	jalap (dried tuberous root of Exogonium jalapa rhubarb (dried rhizome and roots or rheum officinale or R. palmatum	
Toothache, neuralgia	aconite[O] morphine chloroform[I]	see above	see above

Notes: C-I Class I Carcinogen
Mode of Application: Inhalation=I
Topical=T
Oral=O
Parenteral=P

Adopted from Selections in
Pharmacognosy, Edward N.
Gathercoal, Ph.B., Ph.M. and Elmer
H. Wirth, PH.C., PH.D., Lea & Febiger
Philadelphia, 1936

328

administered orally to those manifesting respiratory
distresses as indicated in Table 27.

The investigation of the carcinogenicity of folk
medicines is very contemporary and providing some
alarming results. Kapadia et.al., (1978) evaluated the
occurrence of esophageal carcinoma in black rats given
subcutaneous injections of twelve medicinal herb extracts.[70] Those containing tannins produced tumors
in 33% of the test animals. Other common root extracts
producing tumors were sassafras and sumac. The extrapolation from subcutaneous animal injection to human
ingestion is still unproven. However, considering the
popularity of the return to nature's remedies and health
food stores in the last ten years, the importance of
the extrapolations of animal carcinogenicity to humans
is a much needed area of research.

Insect Pest Control

How did the early New Jersey farmer cope with insect
pests in the pre-chlorinated hydrocarbon, insecticide
era? They used relatively innocuous methods such as
concoctions containing black pepper and the topical
and very specific application of boiling hot water.
During the 19th century some not so innocuous chemicals
came into popular usage:[71]

carbolic acid (phenol)	oil of pennyroyal
camphor gum	(contains tannins)
turpentine	hellebore (toxic
benzine (same as	tuber extract)
benzene) and gasoline	coal tar (ben-
potassium sulfide	zene, phenol,
cuprous ammonium car-	naphthalene, etc.)
bonate	white arsenic
Paris green (an	(arsenic trioxide,
arsenic salt)	AS_2O3)
London purple	pulverized cigar
	factory residue

At this stage, the reader may begin to recognize which
chemicals are the suspect and recognized carcinogens,
based on previous readings.

The Development of the Medical Profession

Into the late 17th century, the farmer or the house-
wife continued to be the medical practitioner in each
household, with the records indicating that at least 18
professional medical men served the entire state.[72]

These early colonial medical men were called upon
to treat the complete spectrum of disorders and illnesses: tooth extraction, bonesetting, surgery, child
delivery, catheterization, administration of drugs,
dressing of wounds, and administering innoculations.

The early medical practitioners came from Europe
and quite naturally, brought with them their own
theories on the treatment of disease. Therapeutics,
the use of extracts and tinctures of herbs and plants
in the treatment of disease in America is credited to
the German physician, Samuel Christian Hahnemann (1755-
1843). Literally, he prescribed fighting fire with fire,
his motto being "Similia, similibus, curantur" (Let
likes be cured by likes").[73] In essence, Hahnemann's
prescribed treatment for a headache would be a drug
which "clinically" was found to induce a headache. Although Hahnemann is credited as the author of the
homeopathic approach, influencing emigrating Europeans,
the Indians also introduced the early settlers to
nature's medicines. Further, the use of naturally
occurring medicines also was long associated with every
culture of early mankind. In fact, the ancient Greeks
and Romans used an extract of the juniper tree as a
cancer curative. Homeopathy persists today with some
30,000 physicians promoting it and five million Americans
subscribing to it.[74]

There were also some doctors like Thomas Sydenham
in England (1624-1689) who conceived of disease as
being caused by a specific agent. He considered each
disease as a member of a peculiar species, classifiable
like plant taxonomy. Further, Dr. Sydenham is credited
with the observation of a correlation between disease
and meteorology, rendering him a founder of the science
of epidemiology.[75] Dr. Sydenham served as a consultant
to New Jersey colonials prior to the American Revolution.

On July 23, 1766, seventeen recognized professional
doctors with a common cause met at Duff's Tevern in New
Brunswick to form the Medical Society of New Jersey.
The reason is to be found in the minutes of that society
which served as an excellent record of the general
health at that time: "the low state of medicine in New
Jersey and the many differings and discouragements alike
injurious to the people and the physician..." and on it
goes to justify the need for a concurrence of legitimate
physicians to protect the public from charlatans.[76]
These efforts culminated in the establishment of a system
of examination and licensure in 1772. Although only ten
men could claim a Doctor of Medicine degree obtained in
either Philadelphia or New York, by 1800 the total number
of practising physicians increased to 300.

By 1797 the Society was able to boast 91 members and
with no medical school, apprenticeship served as a sort
of floating medical college. This practise was to last
from the colonial period through to the 19th century.

Cancers -- Early Treatment Methods

A review of the literature at the New Jersey Medical
Society Library in Trenton indicates that surgery and
homeopathy were the usual recommendations for the treatment of cancers in early New Jersey. The tendency to
recommend surgery is captured in the words of English
physician Dr. John Leake whose 1787 text was probably
used as a reference by early settlers:

> "As no certain and infallible cure is yet
> known for a confirmed ulcerated cancer,
> which inevitably destroys the constitu-
> tion by vitiating the blood; the early
> extirpation of all such scirrhous tumors
> as are moveable under the skin and unconnect-
> ed to any considerable nerve or blood vessel
> is a practice which can never be too much
> recommended, even where they may appear void
> of pain or danger; more particularly if they

> arise from external causes, and the
> constitution is otherwise good and
> found."*77

In another text, Salmon's Herbals, published in
England in 1696, and used not only in New Jersey but
throughout the colonies, homeopathy is the recommended
treatment for hard tumors and inveterate ulcers.78
There is a sad parallel between the approach to cancer
cure in the 17-19th and the 20th century. The latter
approach was through extirpation (surgery) and homeopathic remedies, which we now know contained many carcinogens. In the mid 20th century, excluding the use of
radiation therapy, surgery and chemotherapy are the
recommended approach and again, some once highly regarded
chemotherapeutics are now recognized as potent carcinogens. Another popular book of homeopathic remedies
was Dr. Chase's Recipes which recommended the topical
application of bromine and a mixture of mercurous chloride and the body of a thousand legger (the common
house centipede) for the treatment of skin and breast
cancer respectively.79 Dr. Chase and many other physicians were absolutely convinced of the efficacy of the
mercury preparation and so preparations of this nature
continued in use for many years. Dr. James B. Coleman,
Chairman of the Medical Society in the early 19th
century, was not so convinced about mercury, writing:

> "It follows from the combining affinities
> of the different preparations of mercury,
> that none but the most robust can take
> it into their circulation without ob-
> vious injury, and even in their cases
> the safety is questionable."80

However, the use of toxic chemicals such as mercury and
antimony continued along with numerous drugs.

U.S. Department of Commerce and Navigation records

---

* The citation read "found"; it may have been "sound" in the
  original.

indicate that by 1899, 13 million dollars worth of drugs were imported into this country.[81]   In 1851, a standing committee of the Medical Society suggested that a botanical review of New Jersey plants be conducted.   Their goal was to put the British Empire out of business and discover the important active ingredient in the drugs. It was not heeded.   Without entering into a great discourse on the relative merits of the use of naturally occurring drugs, it is obvious that they portend merits and deficiencies.   The active ingredients in many plants have been isolated and are in use today in natural and synthetic form.   However, inasmuch as this chapter has delved into forensic history, deductive processes indicate that physicians of yesteryear experienced difficulty in assessing the efficacy of drugs administered versus their toxicity.   To be taken into consideration also is the absence of drug quality control, individual sensitivity, and the state of the diagnostic art.   And this leads to the question: what was the incidence of cancers in early New Jersey?

Cancers in Early 17-18th Century New Jersey
Minimal or Undiagnosed?

It is easier to assess the treatment of cancers in early New Jersey than the incidence of the disease.   As discussed earlier, the New Jersey Medical Society minutes relied on voluntary reporting of individual counties and many times counties did not report because no communications were submitted.   That the society set up an approved table of fees (including the extirpation of cancers) indicates the presence of the disease early in pre-colonial life.   It is not until 1858 that such statistics as 15 cancer deaths for Essex County appear.[82]   The advent of the New Jersey State Board of Health (1877) under the leadership of Dr. Ezra Mundy Hunt proved to be an important step in the control of disease within the state.[83]

Cancers in New Jersey at the Turn of the 19th Century

Liberty has been taken in this chapter to explore the environmental causes of cancers in early New Jersey. There are no valid epidemiological statistics to corre-

late the potential causes with the actual incidence in
the years preceding 1879. After that time it is Board
of Health reports that indicate the total New Jersey
health picture as the 19th century closed and it was
marked by a decline in contagious disease. However,
with population increasing, there were greater numbers
of deaths and more non-fatal illnesses. One of the
earliest and most definitive accounts of cancers incidence and mortality comes from the 1905 Report of the
Board of Health. From that we learn the cancers rate
as indicated in Figure 16.[84] It began to show an increase from 3.70% (per 10,000) in 1879 to 5.46% in 1904.
Commentary on the increase was noted in the same Board
of Health report by the then epidemiologists:

> "No new facts have been contributed during
> the year to more fully explain the increas-
> ing prevalance of this disease (cancers)
> but observations are still being diligently
> prosecuted, and it is reasonable to believe
> that the cause of this affection and the
> mode by which it is acquired will not
> much longer elude the unremitting search
> which is being made in many laboratories."[85]

The year was 1904, the problem the same as now, the un-
remitting search.

It is interesting to note from Table 28 that the
city of Salem manifested the highest cancer mortality
rate for New Jersey in 1904.[86] Today, the county of
Salem manifests an inordinately high bladder cancer
mortality rate as discussed in chapter 4. This current
bladder cancer mortality has been attributed to employee
exposure to bladder specific carcinogens at the DuPont
Company. There is no way to determine what the site
specificity was of the 1904 cancer incidence in the
city of Salem. However, the then mortality rate is a
provocative statistic in lieu of the establishment of
DuPont in New Jersey *after* a distinctively high cancer

Years	1879	1880	1881	1882	1883	1884	1885	1886	1887	1888	1889	1890	1891
Deaths from Cancer...	378	425	451	402	461	484	498	546	574	612	579	640	642
Deaths from Cancer per 10,000 population)	3.70	3.75	3.88	3.37	3.81	3.87	3.89	4.15	4.21	4.45	4.11	4.41	4.34

Years	1892	1893	1894	1895	1896	1897	1898	1899	1900	1901	1902	1903	1904
Deaths from Cancer...	688	723	731	770	811	857	852	946	921	1,042	1,031	1,132	1,125
Deaths from Cancer per 10,000 population)	4.55	4.69	4.68	4.60	4.71	4.33	4.70	5.10	4.84	5.43	5.24	5.61	5.46

Chart Showing Deaths in New Jersey From Cancer, Per 10,000 Population, for Twenty-six Years, 1879-1904.

YEAR	Deaths from Cancer per 10,000 Pop.
1879	3.70
1880	3.75
1881	3.88
1882	3.37
1883	3.81
1884	3.87
1885	3.89
1886	4.15
1887	4.21
1888	4.45
1889	4.11
1890	4.41
1891	4.34
1892	4.51
1893	4.65
1894	4.63
1895	4.60
1896	4.71
1897	4.83
1898	4.70
1899	5.10
1900	4.84
1901	5.43
1902	5.42
1903	5.61
1904	5.46

5.60
5.40
5.20
5.00
4.80
4.60
4.40
4.20
4.00
3.80
3.60
3.40
3.20

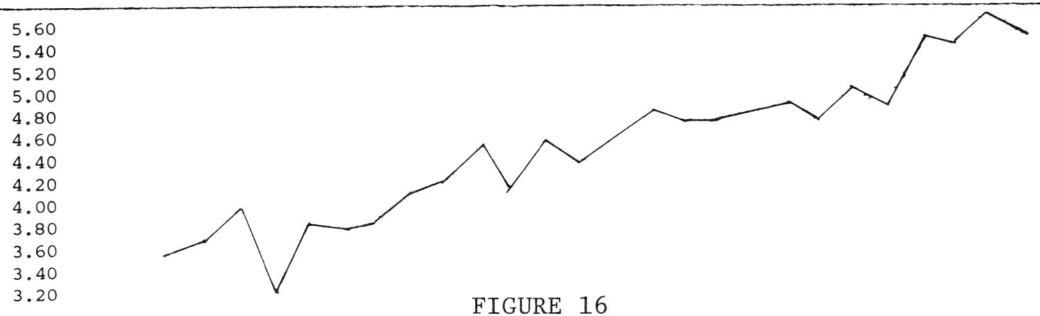

FIGURE 16

Deaths from Cancer in New Jersey for Twenty-Six Years
1879-1904

mortality rate trend was established.*87   Similar, admittedly overly generalized, conjectures may be based
on the other statistics given in Table 28.

    Here the tide of questions that challenge the mind
of today's epidemiologist surface. Was the cancer rate
always high and just unrecognizable in the gross complex community of diseases, only becoming distinct as
medical science diminished the fatalities due to non-
malignant diseases?** Was the early incidence due to
the latent carcinogens in the environment as have been
described herein, or due to the infantile types of
industries which would later earn New Jersey such titles
as "Cancer Alley"? Perhaps the New Jersey swamp miasma
and the genetic make-up and dietary habits of an even
yet shifting immigrant population were to blame.

Retrospective Environmental Toxicology

Life-Style (Excluding Home/Farm Based Activities)

    Before commencing this exposition, it must be under-
stood that the cancers' site descriptions extant at the
time of the preparation of the very early 1900s Board of
Health Reports lacked the definitive quality seen in today's literature. Examination of Table 29 indicates
that the foremost site specific cancer mortality was of
the stomach and liver.88 It is probable that certain
dietary qualities, described earlier in this chapter
(smoked fish and meat, dried and salted fish, and pickled
vegetables) were the specific etiologic factors responsible for most cancers of the stomach, and cancers in
general. Although it is not discernible from Table 29

---

* Construction began at the DuPont Company, Deepwater, New Jersey,
   Dye and Organic Chemicals Plant in 1917.

** Admittedly, the incidence of many infectious diseases subsided
   prior to the era of antibodies and immunization due to improved dietary practises and hygiene.

TABLE 28
DEATHS FROM CANCER IN NEW JERSEY FOR THE YEAR
ENDING DECEMBER 31, 1904 PER 10,000 POPULATION
BY COUNTIES AND BY CITIES OF OVER 5,000 INHABITANTS

Name of Place	Deaths from Cancer	Deaths per 10,000 Population
Atlantic County	6	2.96
Atlantic City	16	5.52
Bergen County	30	4.24
Englewood	6	8.68
Hackensack	5	4.48
Burlington County	30	6.42
Burlington City	6	8.12
Camden County	14	6.85
Camden City	54	6.29
Gloucester City	3	4.09
Cape May County	12	8.90
Cumberland County	10	3.68
Bridgeton	6	4.16
Millville	9	8.43
Essex County	21	5.88
Bloomfield	6	5.49
East Orange	8	3.28
Irvington	8	4.45
Montclair	14	8.90
Newark	171	6.11
Orange	26	10.31
West Orange	4	5.18
Gloucester County	23	7.08
Hudson County	14	4.83
Bayonne	18	4.18
Harrison	4	3.53
Hoboken	55	8.65
Jersey City	114	5.06
Kearny	8	7.13
Town of Union	7	4.20
West Hoboken	15	5.57
West New York	1	1.90
Hunterdon County	14	4.06
Mercer County	11	5.17
Trenton	39	4.76

TABLE 28 - continued
DEATHS FROM CANCER IN NEW JERSEY FOR THE YEAR
ENDING DECEMBER 31, 1904 PER 10,000 POPULATION
BY COUNTIES AND BY CITIES OF OVER 5,000 INHABITANTS

Name of Place	Deaths from Cancer	Deaths per 10,000 Population
Middlesex County	18	4.50
New Brunswick	8	3.98
Perth Amboy	11	5.38
South Amboy	1	1.43
Monmouth County	34	4.77
Long Branch	6	5.94
Red Bank	2	3.41
Morris County	22	3.70
Dover	3	4.50
Morristown	12	9.96
Ocean County	9	3.78
Passaic County	6	2.33
Passaic City	16	4.48
Paterson	71	6.37
Salem County	5	2.54
Salem City	8	13.77
Somerset County	19	6.48
North Plainfield	5	.89
Sussex County	11	4.34
Union County	8	3.80
Elizabeth	25	4.25
Plainfield	9	5.36
Rahway	5	6.30
Summit	4	6.68
Warren County	11	4.02
Phillipsburg	8	7.39

Total in Cities of Over 5,000 Inhabitants	797
Total for State	1125
Rate per 10,000 Population (State)	5.46

SOURCE: New Jersey State Board of Health Report, 1905

TABLE 29

Deaths from Cancer in New Jersey, Showing Organs Affected and Age at Death For the Year Ending December 31, 1904

Cancer	Under 1 mo.	Under 1 year	1 to 5	5 to 10	10 to 15	15 to 20	20 to 25	25 to 30	30 to 35	35 to 40	40 to 45	45 to 50	50 to 55	55 to 60	60 to 70	70 to 80	80 to 90	Over 90	Age not stated	Totals
Of the Mouth		1			1	1		1	1	1			8	11	19	14	10	1		69
Of the stomach and liver		3	3		1		6	3	11	18	25	31	58	57	131	88	13			448
Of the intestines and rectum								1	4	6	10	4	9	11	18	17	2	1		83
Of the female genital organs							2		8	13	17	25	28	21	45	20	4	1		184
Of the breast								1	1	3	12	9	11	6	17	12	3			75
Of the skin		3	1			1						1			2					8
Others			1		2	3	3	4	2	13	10	24	32	34	70	48	12			258
Totals		7	5		4	5	11	10	27	54	74	94	146	140	302	199	44	3		1125

SOURCE: New Jersey State Board of Health 29th Report, 1905

339

what portion of the stomach/liver cancers moiety is
attributable to liver cancers, malignancy there is not
typically due to dietary factors. Cancers of the liver
are associated with chronic alcohol abuse, consumption
of grain or peanuts contaminated with aflatoxin B_1, and
the ingestion of arsenical pesticides.

The second major category is cancers at various
sites (others). These sites may have been at the head,
neck, brain, eye, respiratory system (post-oral), pancreas, testes, and bone. It is noteworthy here that
cancers of the respiratory system, specifically the lung,
are absent as a single category. Considering the popular
practise of smoking, lung cancer diagnosis would now
seem to have been more prevalent. The next major category is cancers of the female genitals for which most
contemporary oncological literature cites no known
etiologic features.* The next major category is cancers of the intestine and rectum, which today would be
called colorectal. Again, for both colon and rectal
cancers, a diet high in fat, protein and carbohydrates
is cited as the specific etiological feature. An additional etiologic agent, peculiar to our portion of the
20th century, is the consumption of processed food.
Breast cancer is the next major category and again, high
fat diets have been suggested as an associative etiologic
agent. Hormonal, viral, immunological agents and the
use of post-menopausal estrogen therapy are also being
evaluated in that connection.

The last category, cancers of the mouth, may have
been engendered by the use of snuff, cigarettes, pipes,
cigars and alcohol use. However, there should have been
an associative lung or other respiratory system cancer
mortality (as mentioned above) involvement. Was it
absent or covered by the "other" category? Neither is
probable. Misdiagnosis was more likely. Dr. Isaac A.
Adler (1849-1918), an early 20th century oncologist,

---

* There is a relationship between other diseases and other risk
  factors: e.g., venereal disease and age at first intercourse--
  when the genitals are defined as the cervix uteri.

gives us some insight. He wrote, lung cancer was commonly misdiagnosed as the "ubiquitous tuberculosis, with
its multiform clinical appearances and plastic adapta-
tion to all ages and conditions."[89] Mind you, there
are no grounds here for immodesty on the part of contemporary oncologists. The misdiagnosis of pulmonary
tumors still happens.[90] So, I ask the question, "how
many of the purported 5,000 tuberculosis sufferers of
the latter 19th century actually had lung cancers?"[91]

Home and Farm Based Industry Activities

     The overall impact of most of the "home or farm
based industries" described herein (tanning, dyeing,
etc.) would have been to induce cancers mainly of the
nasal cavity, sinus, larynx, lung, urinary tract,
bladder, scrotum and skin. These sites are not speci-
fied in Table 29; however, they would fit well into the
"other" category. It would appear that home and farm
based industries may have contributed up to as much as
23% of the overall cancer mortality rate.

Remedies

     Collectively, the various organic, inorganic and
plant derivative natural remedies (see Table 27) had
the potential to cause cancers at various sites when
taken internally and topically. This statement applies
as much to remedies taken specifically for cancers as
well as other ailments.

Psychosomatic Etiologies

     In chapter 2, several causes of cancers considered
to be theories, hypotheses and speculations were reviewed. The principal perspective from which 17th-19th
century New Jersey was evaluated in this chapter was that
of chemical carcinogenesis. There is at least one other
perspective from which the potential to develop cancers
in early New Jersey could have been evaluated: the
psychosomatic etiology.[92, 93, 94] There were certainly
enough unique stress factors in 17th-19th century New
Jersey. In the 20th century we have environmental pollution in itself providing both carcinogens and a depres-

sive psychological climate, along with double digit
inflation and unemployment. In New Jersey yesteryear
for the male, stress may have been the unrelenting daily
battle against the elements, the inner depression accompanying the loss of an important life sustaining crop
due to a drought, or the loss of an entire family to a
disease epidemic. For the slave, stress may have been
indenture itself, the fear of recapture or the traumatic
termination of the family unit. For the female, stress
may have been the sheer absence of rights; in those days,
a woman couldn't vote, make a will, or start a law suit.
Her husband owned the very clothes on her back, could be-
queath their children to strangers and was legally entitled to beat her![95]

SUMMARY

The application of present day environmental science
to 17th-19th century New Jersey provides the observation
of a strange parallel to contemporary times. Numerous
sources of environmental carcinogens and associative
risks for developing cancers existed then as well as
now. And this is devastating to the "good old days" concept. The most identifiable cause of cancers affecting
most of the general population then appears to be that
due to the consumption of smoked and pickled foods and
alcohol consumption. This conclusion will probably
provoke an "aha" from those who place great emphasis on
dietary habits as a cause of today's cancers. It cannot
be over-emphasized that the speculative identification
of a predominant environmental agent causing those
cancers listed in Table 29 reflects a life's exposure
going back some 90 years or to about 1810. A gap remains of about 200 years from which there are no site-
specific data on which to make speculations. What is
available is enough life-style data to conclude that the
"terrestrial Canaan" was never carcinogen free.

Using explanations for the cause of cancers other
than chemical carcinogenicity, it would be possible to

develop other arguments for the incidence of these diseases in early New Jersey. It would have been far more
interesting and challenging to enact the purpose of this
chapter on the true first New Jersey inhabitants, the
Indians. However, there would be again no mortality data
base from which to draw conclusions.

A contrast of today's affluent life-style and health
problems with New Jersey yesteryear, reveals no affluence
at that time, and a host of environmental problems.
Then, one might ask, is the affluence of the 20th century
with a burgeoning populace and no place to dispose of the
concomitant wastes of a throw-away society where cancers
are pancresic, a better world than yesteryear's? Most
would probably prefer the 20th century, where there is
room for improvement, the methodology, but also an un-
deniable "systematic" restraint to finding cures and
effecting prevention as discussed in the summary to
chapter 1.

The brief review of the evolving medical profession
in the state and its inadequacy has been described in
this chapter. Unfortunately, with so long a history of
recognition of the problem, it is still extant as some
New Jersey cancer patients continue to journey to other
states for treatment.

If it is ever proven that the burden of the current
higher than average cancer mortality in New Jersey is
borne by industry, then the seeds were *sown* toward the
end of the period covered in this chapter. The state
population had grown to 1,883,669 with 13 cities having
populations of over 20,000. Accompanying this growth
and responsible for it was industrialization. Large
masses of people meant a corresponding amount of human
waste, and sewers, the technical answer, contaminated
water supplies. The answer was chlorination, currently
known to intorduce carcinogens as discussed in chapter
3. Industry began to make its adverse contribution to
the environment with the introduction of arsenic and
dyes into the Passaic River. Thus, yesteryear's more
local and personal pollution concluded and a century of
more sophisticated, broad scale proliferation began.

Perhaps the positioning of this chapter after the assessment and impact statement on New Jersey is more comprehensible to the reader now. For it is only through the painful acquisition of the knowledge of contemporary environmental science, in vivo and in vitro, that this post-mortem walk through New Jersey yesteryear becomes possible.

Chapter 7 / REFERENCES

1.   Kelland, Frank S. and Kelland, Marylin C., New
         Jersey: Garden or Suburb? Kendall/Hunt
         Publishing Company, Dubuque, 1978.

2.   Whitehead, William A., East Jersey Under the
         Proprietory Governments, Martin R.
         Dennis, publisher, Newark, New Jersey,
         1875, p. 466.

3.   Weiss, Harry B., and Weiss, Grace M., The Early
         Promotional Literature of New Jersey, New
         Jersey Agricultural Society, Trenton,
         N.J., 1964, pp. 12 and 25.

4.   Weiss, Harry B., Life In Early New Jersey, D. Van
         Nostrand Co., Inc., Princeton, 1964.

5.   Waldbott, George L., M.D., Health Effects of
         Environmental Pollutants, C.V. Mosby Co.,
         St. Louis, 1973.

6.   Weiss, Harry B., Life in Early New Jersey, D. Van
         Nostrand Co., Inc., Princeton, 1964.

7.   Ibid.

8.   Ibid.

9.   Ibid.

10. Ibid.

11. Ibid.

345

12. Weygandt, Cornelius, Down Jersey, D. Appleton-
        Century Company, New York, 1940.

13. Cowen, David L., Medicine and Health in New
        Jersey, A History, Princeton, D. Van
        Nostrand Co., Inc., vol. 16, 1964.

14. Ibid.

15. Ibid.

16. Ibid.

17. Hecht, Stephen S., Chen, Chi-hong B., Hirota, Norio,
        Ornaf, Raphael J., TSO, T.C., Dietrich,
        Hoffman, Tobacco-Specific Nitrosamines: For-
        mation From Nicotine In Vitro and During
        Tobacco Curing and Carcinogenicity in Strain
        A Mice, Journal of the National Cancer
        Institute, Volume 60, No. 4, April, 1978,
        pp. 819-824.

18. Wacker, Peter O., Land and People, Rutgers Univer-
        sity Press, New Brunswick, 1975.

19. Wilson, Harold F., Ph.D., The Jersey Shore, A
        Social and Economic History of the Counties
        of Atlantic, Cape May, Monmouth, and Ocean,
        Lewis Historical Publishing Co., Inc., New
        York, 1953.

20. Wacker, Op. Cit.

21 Wilson, Op. Cit.

22. Page, Louise, and Friend, Berta, The Changing
        United States Diet, Bio Science, Volume
        28, No. 3, March 1978, pp. 192-197.

23. Borgstrom, Georg, Principles of Food Science,
        Volume I, Food Technology, The Macmillan
        Company, New York, 1968.

24. Ibid.

25. Ibid.

26. Kramlich, W.E., Pearson, A.M., Tauber, F.W.,
          Processed Meats, Westport, The Avi Publishing
          Company, Inc., 1973.

27. Ibid.

28. Weygandt, Op. Cit.

29. Ibid.

30. Cowen, David L., Op. Cit.

31. Rogers, Fred B., M.D., and Sayre, A. Reasoner, The
          Healing Art, A History of the Medical Society
          of New Jersey, Trenton, 1966.

32. Weiss, Harry B., and Weiss, Grace M., Early Tanning
          and Currying in New Jersey, New Jersey Agri-
          cultural Society, Trenton, 1959.

33. Ibid.

34. IARC, Monographs on the Evaluation of the Carcino-
          genic Risk of Chemicals to Man: Some Natural-
          ly Occurring Substances, Volume 10, World
          Health Organization, New York, 1976.

35. Briscoe, Herman T., General Chemistry for Colleges,
          Houghton Mifflin Co., Boston, 1949.

36. New Jersey Bell Telephone Company Tercentenary
          Publication, Tales of New Jersey, 1963.

37. Pepper, Adeline, The Glass Gaffers of New Jersey,
          Charles Scribners Sons, 1971.

38. Ibid.

39. Cunningham, John T., Sukahsin: As Good as Gold,
          Royle Forum, March 15, 1979, pp. 3-6.

40. New Jersey Bell Telephone Company, Op. Cit.

41. Ibid.

42. Kraybill, H.F., and Mehlman, Myron M., Advances
        in Modern Toxicology, Volume 3, Environmental
        Cancer., Ed. by Myron M. Mehlman, John Wiley
        Sons, New York, 1977.

43. Inactive and Abandoned Underground Mines,
        EPA 440/9-75-007, U.S. Environmental Pro-
        tection Agency, Washington, D.C., June, 1975.

44. Archer, V.E., and Wagoner, J.K., and Lundin, J.R.,
        F.E., Uranium Mining and Cigarette Smoking
        Effects on Man. Journal of Occupational
        Medicine, 15 (3): 204-211, March 1973.

45. Fleeson, Lucinda, Seeing Red, The Philadelphia
        Inquirer, Section C., September 29, 1980.

46. Boyer, Charles S., Early Forges and Furnaces in New
        Jersey, University of Pennsylvania Press,
        Pennsylvania, 1931.

47. American Chemical Society, Chemistry in the Economy,
        National Science Foundation, Washington,
        1973, chapter 16.

48. Wynder, Ernst L., M.D., and Gori, Gio B., Ph.D.,
        Contribution of the Environment to Cancer
        Incidence: An Epidemiologic Exercise,
        Journal of the National Cancer Institute,
        vol. 58, No. 4, April 1977.

49. Waldbott, George L., M.D., Op. Cit.

50. Weiss, Harry B., and Ziegler, Grace M., The Early
        Woolen Industries in New Jersey, New Jersey
        Agricultural Society, 1958.

51. Ibid.

52. Cairns, John, Cancer: Science and Society, W.H.
        Freeman and Co., San Francisco, 1978.

53. Burkitt, Dennis, M.D., Potentials for Reducing
    Cancer's Frequency, Omega Institute,
    Cancer Dialogue 80, New York City,
    October 16, 1980.

54. Weiss, Harry B., Some Early New Jersey Industries,
    New Jersey Agricultural Society, 1965.

55. Acheson, E.D., Nasal Cancer in the Furniture and
    Boot and Shoe Manufacturing Industries,
    Preventive Medicine, Vol. 5, 1976, pp.
    295-315.

56. The Pottery and Porcelain of New Jersey Prior to
    1876, New Museum Association, 1915.

57. Wacker, Peter O., Op. Cit.

58. Op. Cit.

59. Op. Cit.

60. Op. Cit.

61. Weiss, Harry B., Life in Early New Jersey, D. Van
    Nostrand Co., Inc., Princeton, 1964.

62. Shottenfield, David, M.D., and Haas, Joanna F.,
    M.D., Carcinogens in the Workplace, CA-A
    Cancer Journal for Clinicians, Vol. 29,
    No. 3, May/June, 1979.

63. Kirk-Othmer, Encyclopedia of Chemical Technology,
    Interscience Publishers, New York, Volume
    20, Tetracyclines to Unsaturated Polyesters,
    1969.

64. Registry of Toxic Effects of Chemical Substances,
    Richard J. Lewis, Sr., Ed. Cincinnati,
    Ohio, U.S. Government Printing Office,
    Washington, D.C., January 1979.

65. Cowen, David L., Op. Cit.

66. Ibid.

67. Insects of Importance in New Jersey Nurseries, State
        of New Jersey, Department of Agriculture,
        1953.

68. Cowen, David L., Op. Cit.

69. Waldbot, George L., M.D., Health Effects of Environ-
        mental Pollution, The C.V. Mosby Company,
        St. Louis, 1973, p. 252.

70. Kapadia, Govind J., Chung, E.B., Ghosh, B., Chukla,
        Y.N., Baska, S.P., Morton, J.F., and
        Phradhan, S.N., Carcinogenicity of Some
        Folk Medicinal Herbs in Rats, Journal of
        the National Cancer Institute, Volume 60,
        No. 3, March 1978, pp. 683-686.

71   Nichols, J.L., Prof., A.Am., The Farmers Manual,
        J.L. Nichols Publishing Co., Illinois,
        1896.

72. Rogers, Fred B., M.D., and Sayre, A., Reasoner,
        Op. Cit., p. 5.

73. Garrison, Fielding H., A.B., M.D., An Introduc-
        tion to the History of Medicine, W.B.
        Saunders Company, Philadelphia, 1929.

74. How To Sell Medicine Made from Whale Vomit and
        Pokeberries, Focus, January 24, 1979,
        pp. 22-23.

75. Garrison, Fielding, H., A.B., M.D., Op. Cit.

76. The Rise, Minutes and Proceedings of the New Jersey
        Medical Society (1766-1889), Jennings &
        Hardham Printers and Bookbinders, Newark,
        1875.

77. Leake, John, M.D., Medical Instructions Toward
        the Prevention and Cure of Chronic Diseases
        Peculiar to Women, Vol. I, London, 1787.

78. Salmon, William, Herbal, published in England, 1696.

79. Chase, A.W., M.D., Dr. Chase's Recipes of Infor-
        mation for Everybody, An Invaluable Collec-
        tion of Approximately 800 Practical Recipes,
        R.A. Beal Publisher, Ann Arbor, 1871.

80. The Rise, Minutes and Proceedings of the New Jersey
        Medical Society, Op. Cit.

81   Transactions of the New Jersey Medical Society,
        1889, L.F. Hardin, Printer, 243-245 Market
        St., Newark, New Jersey.

82. The Rise, Minutes and Proceedings of the New Jersey
        Medical Society, Op. Cit.

83. Rogers, Fred B., M.D., and Sayre, A. Reasoner,
        Op. Cit.

84. Report of the Board of Health, Annual Report of the
        Bureau of Vital Statistics, John L. Murphy
        Publishing Co., Trenton, 29th Report, 1905,
        pp. 28.

85. Ibid.

86. Ibid.

87. DuPont Background, A Brief History of the DuPont
        Company, DuPont Company/Public Affairs
        Department, Wilmington, Delaware, March,
        1979.

88. Report of the Board of Health, Op. Cit.

89. Adler, Isaac A., A.M., M.D., Classics in Oncology,
        Primary Malignant Growths of the Lung,
        CA-A Cancer Journal for Clinicians, Vol. 30,
        No. 5, September/October 1980, pp. 294-301.

90. Ibid.

91. Rogers, Fred B., M.D., and Sayre, A. Reasoner,
          Op. Cit.

92. Brody, Jane E., and Holleb, Arthur I., M.D.,
          You Can Fight Cancer and Win, McGraw-Hill
          Book Co., New York, 1977.

93. Cassileth, Barrie R., and Lief, Harold, I., Cancer:
          A Biopsychosocial Model In the Cancer
          Patient, Edited by Barrie R. Cassileth,
          Ph.D., Lea and Febiger, Philadelphia, 1979.

94. McQuerter, Gregory, Cancer: Clues in the Mind,
          Science News, vol. 113, no. 3, January 21,
          1978.

95. New Jersey Bell Telephone Company, Op. Cit.

CHAPTER 8

LOGAN TOWNSHIP VERSUS ROLLINS
ENVIRONMENTAL SERVICES - A
CASE STUDY

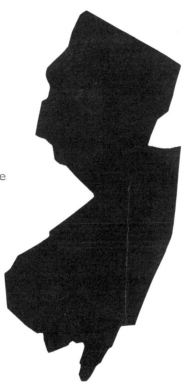

"Probably the single
most prevalent claim
advanced by the pro-
ponents of a new
paradigm is that they
can solve the prob-
lems that have led the
old one to a crisis."

Thomas S. Kuhn,
1970*

*   The Structure of Scientific Revolutions Vol. 2, No. 2 The
    University of Chicago Press, Chicago, 1970, p. 153.

CHAPTER 8

BACKGROUND

New Jersey, like many suburban areas, has many
seemingly borderless towns. When you drive through
them, one blends into another. In south Jersey, just
before reaching the Commodore Barry Bridge on Route
322, you are passing through Logan Township. As you
pass over the junction of Route 322 and 295, a pan-
oramic view of the area is enjoyed. There is nothing
remarkable on that horizon; just typically flat south
Jersey land with small farms, some new housing develop-
ments like one called "Beckett". But a singularly
incongruent 100 foot stack, belching white smoke, its
plume trailing the prevailing wind, is unusual. The
sprawling acres conceal only about 3,081 residents,*
but they, like many other New Jersey communities, are
confronted with special health hazards stemming from
imposed environmental problems that run the gamut of
complexity.

Usually, from the ranks of the silent majority,
a few people rise up who are organization-minded
activists, some with technical know-how, eager to
learn more, and all with a concern for people and
environment. One such resident is Mrs. Esther Slusarski,
who has served on the present Environmental Commission
since 1974. The commission has encountered difficul-
ties with several local industries: Monsanto, Bridgeport Rental and Oil Services, Allied Chemicals, National
Lead, American Dredge and Chemical Leaman.

However, it is the enterprise at the location of

---

* Census Report - Carl Helwig/Pureland Industrial Complex, 1980

the aforementioned solitary stack, Rollins Environmental
Services, that is the focal point of attention in this
chapter. The purpose of this chapter is to present a
case study of the conflict between that industry and
the Logan Township community. The evaluation of this
dilemma provides several lessons which should collectively present some models for dealing with contemporary, repetitive and highly predictable issues in New
Jersey. Commentary on the psychosomatic causes of cancers has been reserved for discussion in this chapter.
The sources are better than primary, as they are derived
from the author's personal involvement.*

A theme that I have stated before is that waste is
synonymous with affluence; hence, the elimination of
wastes is big business because we are a nation of affluent people. New Jersey, the 46th state in size, is a remarkably large consumer and producer state of hazardous
wastes.[1] The Logan Township branch of Rollins Environmental Serves (RES), has been in existence since 1969.
RES is a chemical waste processing facility and about 50
people are employed there, spread over three shifts. A
current RES prospectus reads "Total responsibility service for difficult industrial waste treatment and disposal."[2] Their disposal methodology was described in
chapter 4. Inherent in these processes is the emission
of noxious, toxic and carcinogenic chemicals as stack
gases. Area residents have complained about odors and
accompanying respiratory eye discomfort, thought to be
derived from RES, for several years.[3] Mrs. Slusarski,
wearing at least two hats -- Environment Commission member and Board of Health Secretary -- recalls the yearly
increase in these complaints.[4]

RES, realizing the definite inherent economic gain
in disposing of PCB's, applied for and was granted a permit to conduct a test incineration of this chemical on
August 10, 1977. Apparently satisfied with the results, the DEP permitted RES to incinerate PCB's from

---

* The author serves as DEP public participant, a technical advisor
  to Logan Township and the People for Environmental Protection.

September through December 1977, but this was not
announced to the general public.[5] After an explosion
and fire at RES on 8 December 1977, the facility was
shut down. The accident claimed six lives, injured
twelve workmen and hospitalized forty firemen for
smoke inhalation.*[6] RES was allowed to reopen in
November 1978, entering into a consent agreement with
EPA, whose regulations over PCB's then pre-empted the
state's DEP.[7] The cumulative community distrust and
fear of RES was soon to become quite evident when RES
requested permission from the DEP on June 12, 1978 to
incinerate PCB's. But much occurred before that date.

In April 1979, the DEP announced there would be
a test incineration of PCB's at RES sometime during the
month of May. Spearheaded by W.D. Wilson, a Logan Township resident and P.E.P. member,** serious picketing began outside RES on April 30, 1979. The content of the
picket signs reflected the *psychological impact* of operations at RES on local residents:

> "Jersey's Three Mile Island"
> "Not in Our Backyards"
> "Stop Cancer Death"
> "The Ovens of Germany Have Not Been
> Destroyed, Only Relocated"
> "Rollins Pollution Plant -- It Works"
> "Give Us Breath, Not Death"

By May 8, 1979, neighboring townships, Woolwich
and Swedesboro, joined in the opposition to the incineration test.[8] Rep. James J. Florio, D.-1st District,
announced a public meeting would be held with EPA and
DEP, saying "we want to find out exactly what the dangers
are, if any, and what will be done to protect residents
in the surrounding area."[9]

---

* Accounts of a reported spill vary, involving the consumption or
  containment of 66,000-200,000 gallons of liquid wastes.

** The People For Environmental Protection, a citizen's environmental interest organization

Before the meeting took place, Kenneth DiMuzio,
Logan Township Solicitor, recommended that the township be represented by an environmental consulting
firm and that they monitor the test incineration.
DiMuzio sought financial aid from the Public Advocate's
Office, Stanley C. Van Ness, Rep. Florio, D.-1st District
and Assemblyman H. Donald Stewart, D.-3, who heads the
Agriculture and Environment Committee.[10] In the long
struggle ahead to attain environmental protection in
Logan, DiMuzio would prove himself one of the most dedicated and persistent advocates of that goal. He would
put to good use his legal expertise and growing knowledge of environmental relationships.

The Logan Township-EPA/DEP Dialogue '79

The meeting between the township, concerned area
residents and the DPA, DEP and RES was held on May 15,
1979. Some 250 attendees slowly filled the local fire-
house and the public hearing began. Having taped the
opening dialogue and introductory remarks by the EPA and
DEP, I am able to summarize their introductory dialogue:

> The issue was a relatively narrow one;
> Rollins was already in existence and the
> question is should they be given the per-
> mit to incinerate PCB's. These chemicals
> are already in the environment and they
> are a major environmental problem. Their
> incineration should not be likened to the
> building of another nuclear power plant.
> EPA is committed to doing what is right,
> including weighing the risks to the commu-
> nity. PCB's have been dumped into water
> supplies because there was no appropriate
> place to dump them. PCB's must be dealt
> with. EPA does not expect you (the public)
> to come to the mass perspective.*

---

* The DEP was implying the holistic viewpoint.

The obvious overtones of socioenvironomics, risk/
benefit analysis and holism permeated these comprehensive opening remarks. Something within me said EPA
will approve the test incineration eventually. Inwardly,
I was torn between the knowledge that society must get
rid of these chemical wastes but I was not happy about
it being done in a nearby town. Besides, so much attention was being devoted here to PCB's and so little to
the health impact of a multitude of other toxic and
carcinogenic compounds formed during current disposal
methods as described in chapter 4. But cold reason,
idealism, holism and technology were not to set the tenor
of this meeting. There were some pertinent technical
questions about incineration, decomposition products,
permits, transportation accidents and enforcement by
the DEP, but the questions of adverse health effects
and residents' inability to deny PCB incineration permission, were dominant. For over four hours the EPA
and DEP took a good lambasting, attempting to answer
such comments and accusations as:

>"This is going to be the next Love Canal."
>"This is our town, we pay the taxes, why
> can't we rule it?"
>"Burn it somewhere else -- burn it in the
> desert."
>"We're fighting for our lives, I've got
> children and I want grandchildren."

These comments were delivered with emotion but
underscored some viable arguments; potential danger,
invasion of home rule, poor site location and genera-
tional health effects. One particularly vociferous
resident, Sandra Shute, taking a familiar tack, likened
the inability of the township to disapprove of the
test incineration to the lack of individual rights in
Communist Russia and Austria from which her grandparents
had fled. In June of 1979, Esther Slusarski asked for
a meeting with the then Governor, Brendan Byrne and
Commissioner Daniel J. O'Hern, DEP. This request was
handled by Senator Raymond Zane, Assemblyman Stewart and
Herman, and Congressman James J. Florio. Kenneth A.
DiMuzio, Logan Township Solicitor also attended this
meeting. Plans were set for a review of RES' PCB

proposal and an environmental assessment* of the entire
facility with citizen participation. Finally, on August
2, 1979, the EPA announced it would not only withhold
a permit to incinerate PCB's from RES, but require an
environmental impact analysis. Further EPA said it
would institute legal proceedings for previous violations
dating back to 1978.[11]

Original Community Response To RES

In 1969, when RES originally approached Logan Township municipal authorities with plans for the construction of their proposed waste disposal facility, the use
variance request stated specific binding conditions on
RES pertaining to pollution:[12]

- an adequate clay liner will prevent seepage
  of pollutants into underground waters

- no noxious smoke, odors, fumes or sounds shall
  extend beyond the boundaries. . . .

Further, the same variance indicated specific *benefits*
to the Logan community inasmuch as an industrial waste
disposal plant had contributed significantly to the
industrial development of communities elsewhere.[13] Apparently, industrial developers had even indicated they
would find Logan attractive if there were an existing
waste disposal plant. Other factors which probably
made RES attractive to municipal authorities were the
prospective tax dollars and employment.

Permission was granted! There was some dissension
however, a variance was granted to allow the RES Bridgeport facility to be built. RES officials appeared at
public hearings and vowed the facility would be pollution and odor free with only "pure steam" emanating from

---

* An evaluatory process which summarizes and predicts the anticipated impact of a proposed action.

their incinerator stack.[14] The capacity of the original
facility has been increased since its inception. The
industrial world has not followed E.F. Schumacher's
"Small is Beautiful" model.[15] New Jersey's chemical
industry and its concomitant wastes have increased com-
parably during the past ten years.

Air, water, and soil pollution with toxins and
carcinogens was no new concept in New Jersey in 1969
or elsewhere, nor was leachate an entirely foreign
word. There was no environmental commission or task
force designated to predict the adverse effects of an
industry like RES on the township and the physical
environment. Earth Day was a year away -- but the great
body of knowledge preceding it was available! The EPA
and DEP were just being established to foresee just
such problems and protect the citizens. Logan, like
many other communities, cannot be blamed for its lack
of knowledge, because the people had an overriding
quality -- trust -- now currently eroded. And there
is ample evidence of the perception of potential
economic gain. In a parallel trusting fashion, the
LiPari and Kin-Buc and Jackson Township landfill operations, Chemical Control Corporation, the Union Asbestos
and Rubber Co., American Cyanamid and scores of others
were invited into New Jersey municipalities. In yesteryear, trust was more important than the facts or the
absence of data; today, the lack of trust or the
memory of trust betrayed will inevitably outweigh the
impact of the best data.

Community Activists -- The People For Environmental Protection

Logan Township residents had banded together more
than once before to cope with environmental problems,
forming at first "COLTS," Concerned Citizens of Logan
Township and Residents Against Rollins. Mrs. Slusarski
was very sympathetic with both groups but to be an active member constituted a conflict of interest with her
other township duties. She conceived of an independent
organization which would not prohibit her environmental
commission membership from dealing collectively with RES.

Hence, the People for Environmental Protection (PEP)
was established in late May, 1979. PEP became a
spokesperson for the silent majority of the community,
attaining the attention of the state's lawmakers.

There was more than irony in the formation of a
group such as PEP, and again, Logan provided a model.
The EPA was ostensibly created to represent the public
interest in protection of the environment. However, the
DPA was not created to do for citizens what they should
do for themselves. Diane Graves, Sierra Club Conversation Chairperson, says "citizenship means taking part
in decisions and seeing that government works."[16]

So, ten years after EPA's inception, citizens'
organizations were being established all over the state.
In Bayonne, it is Bayonne Against Tanks (BAT), in
Trenton, the N.J. Public Interest Research Group (PIRG),
in Bordentown, Help Our Polluted Environment (HOPE) and
in Mantua, Citizens Help Oppose Pollution (CHOP), all
with various degress of success.[17, 18, 19, 20] The
EPA/DEP are chartered to take a more holistic viewpoint
for the greatest number. However, the EPA/DEP frequently do not act at all. In contrast, citizens in
each troubled locale tend to see their particular prob-
lem(s) as the horizon and would be quite satisfied to
see it relegated to "Timbuktu."

The Psychological and Sociological Effects of
Environmental Stress

A common denominator underlying the environmental
problems in Logan is present in many communities, nationally and internationally -- the psychological and
sociological impact. The slow wheels of government ro-
tated (imperceptibly to the community) for a few years
with the DEP engaged in the assessment process, while
RES continued to operate sans PCB's.* Logan was unique

---

* DEP permitted them to handle wastes containing less than
  50 ppm PCB's.

in that an assessment would be conducted on an existing
facility; ostensibly, the grandfather clause would not
hold. Excluding this factor, Logan shared a common problem with many other communities; festering fear, distrust,
a feeling of helplessness, and a concern for health. The
prospective environmental problem only added on to the
normal daily risks of life.

The Love Canal disaster, at the upper end of the
environmental problems scale where there were manifest
health problems, provides realistic examples of the kinds
of stress residents are subjected to.[21] Two years after
the first Love Canal residents were relocated, it is
reported that the "psychological damage from that long
running disaster may ultimately turn out to rival and
perhaps exceed the physical damage."[22] The Niagara
Falls Community Mental Health Center composed a special
pamphlet, "Coping With Stress," for residents who felt
the government did not deal with them truthfully. Of
the 237 families involved in the 1978 relocation, 40%
of the couples reportedly have either become divorced
or separated.[23] A typical problem in families was the
wife wanting to move because of health concerns and
the husband wanting to remain because of the invest-
ment in the home. New Jersey did not have a singular
"Love Canal," yet, the reaction to our many environmental problems with a cancer risk has many common elements. The landfill problems in Pitman, Mantua, Jackson and Edison Townships, and the birth defects alleged-
ly linked to Sevin use in Cape May County, have created
the same fears and possibly the same stresses present
at "Love Canal". Many New Jersey residents would like
to move away from these areas but they are caught in
the web of spiralling mortgage interest rates.

Strangely enough, in dealing with cancer as a
disease caused by specific environmental agents, an
intangible psychosomatic cause must also be considered.
Psychoanalyst Lawrence LeShan attributes cancer to a
"despair personality," manifested by those who are
unable to express anger or resentment but seemingly
emanating a benevolent aura. Included are those who
have lost a beloved parent or have experienced cumulative failures.[24, 25] Other supportive studies indicate

that severe emotional stress may act as a carcinogen.[26]

According to LeShan, you don't just develop cancers.
We are all exposed to chemical carcinogens, but those
with the predisposition are the ones who develop cancers. Further, LeShan indicates there is no single
factor in cancer etiology; genetic readiness, stress,
and other factors are all important. Dr. Barrie R.
Cassileth, Psychosocial Program Director at the University of Pennsylvania's Cancer Center, dismisses this
hypothesis as conjectural, saying "most work in this
area relies on post hoc data, such as the results of
interviews with cancer patients about recalled events or
feelings prior to diagnoses."[27] Dr. Cassileth places
more credence on immune and hormonal systems as the
possible bridge between psychosocial stress and the
development of malignancies.

However, who can argue with success? Several researchers and physicians, e.g., Stephanie Mathews-Simon-
ton, and Drs. Arthur Davis and Lawrence LeShan are reversing cancers using the psychotherapeutic approach.[28]

The cancer fear as a consequence of environmental
pollution is very real, especially in New Jersey. The
author has attended several meetings and forums and
heard the testimony of victims of cancer and other
diseases who were absolutely convinced their condition
was caused by the environmental problem being discussed.
What happens when residents in an environmentally troubled area have a long history of attempting to attain
abatement in vain? Do they become helpless, in a
psychological state where unpleasant events are uncon-
trollable? Psychologists say helplessness produces
emotional distrubance and is to be avoided.[29] The frus-
tration index and exposure to at least air pollution
will be experienced most by those living in close proximity to chemical type industries.[30]

Summarily, living in a polluted environment creates
tension because of the fear of getting sick. The resultant stress is harmful to the organism. New Jersey
residents are subjected to the stress of everyday living,
environmental pollution and perhaps an undetermined

synergistic effect of both factors.

Logan Township Community Environmental Hazards Risk Perception Survey

The author designed and tested a survey questionnaire to determine community perception of environmental
hazards and other factors in the Logan Township area.[31]
The majority of the responses indicated a feeling of
powerlessness with regard to being in on the decision-
making process about RES. Further, the majority were
afraid they would suffer from adverse health as a result of past, present, and future plant operations and
that there would be another accident. In terms of
community-received risk to cancers, the sample living
nearer to RES viewed it as a greater cancer risk than
the use of tobacco. However, the potency of this sentiment is diminished in that in New Jersey the perceived
total cancer death rate (encompassing that of deaths
due to lung cancer from tobacco use) is larger than the
actual rate. Here, a problem in risk perception by a lay
person is identified -- the lack of familiarity with
readily available mortality data. This is a major reason for the communications barrier that exists between
the lay person and the competent professional. The survey data continue to provide a cornucopia of information on parallels between the Logan community and the
rest of the state. The very first question -- "Do you
derive any benefit from the presence of RES in your
township?" -- drew in an incredibly *negative* but informative response. We each generate about 20 tons of
solid waste, directly or indirectly, annually, of which
about 1100 pounds is industrial waste.[32] Logan Township residents as well as the rest of the state enjoy
the affluence which generates wastes but refuse to see
any association between the two. As long as the "siting"
of the concomitant wastes disposal facility is "elsewhere," they would be satisfied.

Rollins Environmental Services (RES)

In the summer of 1979, pickets marched outside the

RES plant and there was a barrage of criticism from the press, PEP, state and local officials. However, company officials stood by a position from which they would never deviate -- our operations are safe![33] Jack Lurcott, Director of Corporate Development at RES, was confident that EPA would approve their permit to incinerate PCB's and this RES would accomplish with a residue of only 1 ppm in the air around the plant. Further, he contended that the plant was governmentally sanctioned because it was using environmentally sound methods of disposing of hazardous wastes. C. Edward Ashby, a former plant manager, recalled how RES already incinerated PCB's and other chemicals under a state permit, without incident, prior to the 1977 explosion. RES had provided a check for $7,000 to Mrs. Esther Slusarski to pay for the services of a consultant to review their proposed test incineration of PCB's. In a final touch of diplomacy RES opened their gates to area residents, conducting plant tours of their facility. Dr. Samuel Epstein called this an industrial strategy -- minimize the risks and propagandize the public.[34] This attempt to soothe area residents' distrust and radiate a "See how safe we are" image unfortunately came too late.

Governor Byrne toured the plant for a vis a vis education on the status of their technology and concluded facilities such as these should not be closed but improved. On into the summer of 1980, when a system overflow occurred but reportedly never reached adjacent Raccoon Creek, RES maintained its "environmentally safe" image. Maurice W. Hunt, Eastern Region Vice President of RES, took to the press to state that there was no discharge to Raccoon Creek or a request by RES for an emergency volume overflow.[35] He admitted that Rollins is not perfect ("what is?"), is not raking in huge profits due to "constant regulatory redirection" and that the undegraded, original chemicals they release to the environment pose less of a health hazard than carsuicide. Further, Hunt decried the image that RES cannot be trusted and has endangered the community for years, and concluded with the question, "Who are the better environmentalists -- those who gnash their teeth and beat their breasts without offering any practical solutions or those who invest millions of dollars to develop systems to treat wastes and prevent pollution, at the same time assuming the responsibility for all the accompanying liabilities?"

Rollins Environmental Services distributes several brochures describing their waste disposal technology. One entitled "The Proper Management of Difficult Industrial Wastes," concludes with a quotation by Dr. Barry Commoner: "Everything must go somewhere."[36] Then let us examine their records of the 'somewhere' of an environmentally safe facility. According to the N.J. DEP, Division of Water Resources, early in the career of RES, both lined and unlined waste treatment ponds were responsible for severe groundwater pollution at the facility.[37] The system of abatement wells were found to be either inoperative or inadequate. Three more wells were added to the system later. Particularly conspicuous on visiting RES is the absence of any drinking fountains supplied by wells; bottled water alone is consumed there! PCB incineration at RES prior to the 1977 accident was not as Mr. Ashby stated, "without incident." It is not known to the general public, but Raccoon Creek was polluted with PCB's. The DEP should have been thoroughly familiar with the situation, since that agency conducted the study.[38]

During the December 8, 1977 fire and explosion at RES, tanks containing 45,000 gallons of PCB's were ignited. Some PCB's may have been converted by the heat of the fires to the very toxic and carcinogenic dibenzyl furan. According to the DEP, PCB's were released into Raccoon Creek at that time.[39] Local residents have been subject to noxious odors which have resulted in DEP documented eye, nose, throat and respiratory irritation as far back as 1974.[40] The principal source of odors is from treatment ponds which have overflowed in the past. During two plant visits, the author observed that there was no toxic exposure personnel monitoring system. Such technology is readily available and widely in use. RES has also been cited for environmental abuse outside of New Jersey. Their East Baton Rouge, Louisiana, facility has been called "a serious threat to human health and the environment" because of disposal malpractice.[41] Workers of OCAW 4-367, of the Rohm and Haas

Chemical Co. in Deer Park, Texas, have described their
long standing suffering from emissions from the neighboring RES facility.[42]   They write, "steam tarnishes contacts in the instruments and other metal materials."   In
addition, it causes symptoms of nausea, eye irritation
and gastrointestinal upset.[43]   And thus everything has
gone somewhere, as we know something of the resting
places of the residuum of a "not so perfect" process. . .

According to a January 1980 Hazardous Waste Advisory
Commission Report, at least 20,000 tons of special and
hazardous wastes are generated annually in New Jersey.[44]
Approximately 20 facilities are providing off-site treatment and most have a history of accidents, mishaps and
violations.   Here RES in its relationship to Logan
emerges as a paradigm for the hazardous waste crisis in
the state.   We need these facilities but their activities
must not result in additional environmental pollution.
The technology exists to attain environmentally safe-yet-
not-perfect waste disposal.   However, the closer one of
these facilities comes to this attainment, the more costly the processes.   Mr. Hunt, plant manager at RES, said
DEP's constant regulatory redirection is preventing them
from making their due profits.   So it's *socioenvironomics*
again, and they are not in business to be environmentalists but to make money, as all waste disposal facilities managers and owners are!

The Role Of The Department of Environmental Protection

When RES opened in 1970, many of the current laws
regulating their operation did not exist.   After the 1977
fire and explosion, the EPA/DEP had the Solid Waste
Management Act, the Spill Compensation and Control Act
and more recently the Federal Resource Conservation and
Recovery Act and the Toxic Substances Control Act, and
they all have an influence on operations at RES (cf.
Mr. Hunt's constant regulatory redirection).   With regulatory and enforcement strength granted in these laws,
RES was allowed to reopen but through posting a
$200,000 performance bond and entering into a compliance
agreement with EPA in November 1978.[45]   Specifically,
incinerator operational temperatures were not at optimum

for toxic substances.

There has been considerable controversy about emissions compliance. However, as of May 1980, the EPA concluded that it had no evidence of violations of its consent order or of temperature requirements of the consent judgment since September of 1979. The EPA, in recognition of its past failure to gain public approval and acceptance in the control of toxic substances was now making an overt effort to gain citizen participation. New York and New Jersey were involved in a pilot program to attain citizen participation, involving 36 public interest groups, 11 of which were participating as volunteers. As stated earlier in this chapter, a sixteen member advisory group (REAAG)* was selected to assist in the preparation of the environmental assessment of RES.

Carl Helwig (President of Pureland Industrial Complex)** and REAGG member Ken DiMuzio, had advised the DEP of the existence of the monumental Shell Environmental Impact Statement. The Shell study was a substantial environmental inventory of a tract of land near the RES facility.[46] After months of footdragging, the DEP examined it. In addition, the DEP collected and organized all of its existing RES data and funded further studies (e.g., the Consultant Services of Battelle Columbus and the Conservation and Environmental Studies Center of Browns Mills, New Jersey).[47, 48]

It requires no seer to predict community disenchantment with the final environmental impact assessment. The DEP failed to explain publicly the significance of the assessment and to keep the community abreast of the various stages of its completion. The REAAG meetings began

---

* REAGG, Rollins Environmental Assessment Advisory Group (The author attended this group's meetings representing Logan Township and the People for Environmental Protection.)

** The Pureland Water Company, a public utility, provides two water systems in the Logan Township area.

with the involvement of the genuine "public." However,
inconvenient subsequent meeting times and locales,
eventually excluded the real public.   REAAG should have
been tasked and funded to report back to the community.
During the assessment process, the DEP aided in the ero-
sion of its own trust and confidence image in the eyes
of many REAAG members by summarily ignoring their advice
and requests on such issues as funding to complete the
assessment, whether the facility was in a flood plain,
and the hat switching conflict of interest on the part
of group's coordinator, Paul A. Giardina (who also
acted as the Director of the Hazard Management Program
for the DEP).[49] The most critical failure of the DEP was
not to institute the assessment of RES themselves. They
had to be coerced by public, private and political pressure.   Similarly, the DEP/EPA has had to be sued by
various national environmentalist organizations (e.g.,
The Environmental Defense Fund) before they would enact
critical life protecting regulations.[50]

Underscoring and undermining the entire assessment
of RES was the state's hazardous waste dilemma -- close
the facility and then what do we do with wastes?   The
Gypsy haulers and midnight dumpers would thrive as the
incidents described in chapter 4 would continue.   One
outspoken and sincere REAAG member, Kenneth DiMuzio,
wrote to the Commissioner of the DEP who will make the final decision on the future of RES: "The Hazardous waste
crisis has compromised DEP. The state needs RES because it exists and its existence alone justified per-
petuation of its operation.   The fact of ten years of
pollution at an environmentally unacceptable site is
secondary to DEP but primary to Logan Township."[51]

RES -- The Hazardous Waste Disposal Facility Model?

Currently, there is no set of regulations pertaining to the operation of an entire hazardous waste treatment, storage or disposal facility. As of now, RCRA regulations apply. The DEP will soon promulgate a long
awaited set of hazardous waste management regulations.
One of the major contributions of the RES assessment will
be the provision of a model for the rest of the state.

If the environmental assessment process does not
close RES permanently, the resultant operational guidelines will become standards for other incinerators.
This is why it behooves all those participating to make
sure the assessment methodologies are most stringent,
for the benefit of any community who may in time find
such a facility as a neighbor. Environmental pollution
has already occurred at RES, so a totally positive and
optimistic impact assessment would be a farce. Unfortunately, with the poor faith, trust and confidence image
surrounding the DEP, will the assessment statement help
them in selling a hazardous waste facility to another
community? Governor Byrne's Hazardous Waste Advisory
Commission cited the need for more hazardous waste
treatment storage and disposal facilties.[52] It also
recommended numerous improvements in the state's management and enforcement systems.[53] The state is in a very
delicate position because, the long term consumption of,
or person's living in proximity to unidentified hazardous
wastes, are some of the major undefined cancer risks
faced by New Jersey residents. Clearly, the state is
advocating the construction of more hazardous waste
treatment, storage and disposal facilities as an important means toward eliminating indiscriminate, unsafe
disposal.[54]

Accomplishing Detente Over Environmental Problems

The Role of the DEP

The EPA and, subsequently, the DEP were created to
serve as the "public advocate" for a livable environment. Outraged citizenry have said that the DEP has
sold out the public's health. Further, the DEP has
been called the Environmental Protection Agency Against
the People and the Department of Industrial Protection.
Industry cries out that the DEP regulates too much,
threatening economic sanctions. In the agency's ten
year history it has often occupied a most undesirable
position -- neither friend of the public nor of industry. And this in spite of its accomplishments.

But I argue we need to strengthen and support this

agency; it has been a most unique buffer between two
disparate entities that just have not engaged in the
fine art of listening to one another. Throughout
this work, I have stressed Galantowitz' conception of
socioenvironomics; people first, environment second and
economics last![55] It does not appear to have surfaced
adequately that the EPA's charter calling for a livable
environment is an excellent concept, but that agency
does not function in a vacuum. Many an initially
stringent, environmentally protective EPA regulation is
strangely weakened after "off the record" conversations
between that agency and the White House (at the federal
level with repercussions at the state level).

The DEP, caught in the middle, is forced to make
decisions over what is a safe level of exposure to
toxins and carcinogens. Its judgments are pronounced
in an arena where there is controversy over what is a
health hazard to begin with. The public sees any DEP
inaction as *ineptitude*. Realize from chapter 3, it has
not achieved eco-omnipotence -- hence, any decision is
a compromise -- unless it is on the side of a zero risk
society. Surveys in Logan Township and other communities confirm well that the general public is not asking for a zero risk society.[57, 58] In fact, those
living in Logan near to RES averaged a 3 on a zero to
10 elective risk of cancer scale.*

A step toward attaining detente over environmental
problems may be accomplished by rendering the EPA/DEP
more independent as Senator Edmund S. Muskie suggests --
like the Federal Trade Commission.[59] The environmental
assessment and impact statements are important tools
which accomplish detente over environmental problems.
The DEP initiates these methodologies but to do so well
requires adequate staffing. This agency needs adequate
yearly block funding to insure its existence and budget
requirements. Every letter of complaint on the DEP
should be matched by one requesting more legislative

---

* 10 represented the maximum risk of the development of cancers.

support! Where does the money come from for an increased DEP budget? Taxes -- and in an era of double
digit inflation, is this acceptable to the general
public? Public opinion polls say yes. To attain
detente over environmental problems, we also need more
positivism -- the reverence ethic -- which is an appeal
through values change and accomplished througn environmental education.

The Role of Industry

A legacy of distrust and fear is what RES, and
industry in general, has stamped, hopefully not in-
delibly, on the minds of the general public. How can
trust in industry be restored in New Jersey after pollution incidents like those in Logan, Jackson Township,
Chemical Control and Kin-Buc Landfill? Perhaps by
atonement for the ongoing era of environmental dis-
honor. Perhaps by cessation of data suppression as was
done on asbestos, bis(chloromethyl) ether and tobacco.[60, 61, 62]   Certainly, by establishing better community relationships before legal conflicts arise. Further,
by opening up the decision-making process to the pubic
and by supplying the public with new product information. Absolutely, by considering the hazardous waste
impact of technologies and products in deference to
profits. Hopefully, never by "constant regulatory
redirection." And always, by telling it like it is!

Industry lobbied hard to defeat the passage of the
"superfund."[* 63] In its original version the fund would
have been used to clean up active or inactive chemical
dump sites and spills on land or water. In addition,
there would have been provision for the reimbursement
to citizens affected by toxic wastes. In the final
version, passed in December 1980, oil spill coverage
and citizen reimbursement were deleted. 87.5% of the
fees to support the $1.6 billion "superfund" were to
come from the chemical industry.[64] They argued that

---

* PL 96-510, "Comprehensive Environmental Response, Compensation and Liability Act of 1980"

incidents such as Love Canal caused Congress to over-
react and that the "superfund" places blame and burden
of cost entirely on the chemical industry. Prior to
the passage of the "superfund," hazardous waste generators could have come forward and owned up to their contributions to New Jersey's orphan and parented dumps.
Thus, the cost of the accidental find and some of the
need for the "superfund" would have been minimized.

The Role of the Public

   The Individual

   Participation is the key to how the general public
may influence decision-making toward more acceptable
solutions. Participation requires time and that may
mean a trip to Trenton or the local municipal building
or at the very least a letter to state officials requesting more legislative support for the DEP. The individual
must ask him or herself "How much am I willing to pay for
a clean environment?" Since improper hazardous waste
disposal may disperse a cornucopia of carcinogens into
the environment, the individual must re-examine his or her
life-style, asking what is each person's role in the
affluent way of life, waste disposal equation. Is the
individual, as many Logan Township and area residents,
denying the derivation of any benefits from a facility
like RES? If that answer is yes, then they should become environmental education advocates for the sake of
the next generation who hopefully will relate better to
the environment. Lastly, in July 1980, a 90 mile
strip of land running through six south Jersey counties
was cited as at least "potentially" having the requisite underground clay layer to make it a possible
candidate location for the long term burial of certain
hazardous wastes and hazardous waste treatment and
storage facilities.[65]

   The actual site to be chosen may be in *your* area.
Some of New Jersey's near future conflicts over the
environment will be due to "this siting."

   Remember Barry Commoner's second law of ecology:
"everything must go somewhere." Detente over most of

the state's problems can be resolved by citizens being
a little reductionistic -- i.e., selfish -- by demand-
ing the best available technology and by being holistic,
trying to see the whole problem.

The Organization

Citizens should support their local and state-wide
and national environmental organizations and especially
the organizations which have achieved a high degree of
efficacy in defending the environment, e.g.:

> The Sierra Club
> The Environmental Defense Fund
> The Natural Resources Defense Council
> The National Wildlife Federation

It has been through the collective efforts of these
organizations (especially the EDF) that the EPA and
other federal agencies have been forced through legal
action and petition to enact regulations protective
of human life and the environment. All of these regulations enacted through DEP at the state level (e.g.,
pesticide bans, air emissions standards, prioritization
of pollutants, RCRA and TSCA implementation) have been
beneficial to New Jersey. No matter how sincere the
community-based environmentalist group is, it is still
basically concerned with their *own* local issue. The
group may be able to muster some technical expertise
and dedicated citizens, but it cannot compete with the
legal and technical expertise, financial support and
full time employment which is the forte of groups like
EDF or of large industries.

EPILOGUE

On May 4, 1981, an explosion occurred in the
incinerator kiln at Rollins Environmental Services.[66]
Euphemistically, RES termed the explosion - an over-
pressurization in the kiln. The ensuing community
and state reaction was a small-scale rerun of earlier
events; community outrage, temporary closure and a re-
opening on a one year permit basis. Logan Township

officials again legally sought to have RES closed. The
new political regime in office in the winter of 1982,
did not pursue the lawsuit against RES. On January 20,
1982, RES presented Logan Township with a check for
$113,880.[67] This was the first payment under New
Jersey's Hazardous Waste Facilities Siting Act, requiring that such facilities pay local communities as much
as 5% of their gross receipts earned from treatment,
storage or waste disposal. Would these payments become
a palliation for the effects of 'Siting', a legally
paternalistic enigma? RES continues to dispose of our
nemismatic wastes, which cumulatively present a far
worse environmental impact than PCB's. However, Logan
demonstrated the power of community involvement -- no
PCB's have been incinerated in that community since
December 1977! As of July 1982, the stalled and
belabored environmental assessment of RES continues....

Chapter 8 / REFERENCES

1. Report of Governor Brendan Byrne's Hazardous Waste
       Advisory Commission, Trenton, New Jersey,
       January 1980.

2. Rollins Environmental Services, Inc., Brochure 102,
       pp. 1-8.

3. Rollins Environmental Assessment, Section 2.6.2.2.4.
       Odors, Appendix 2, p. lxxxvi-lxxxix. New
       Jersey Department of Environmental Protec-
       tion, draft, 1980.

4. Personal Communication. May 22, 1979.

5. Ibid.

6. Rollins Environmental Assessment, draft, Background,
       1980.

7. Ibid.

8. Ursillo, Donna and Goldberg, Elliot, "2 Towns
       Protest Chemical Burn Plan," Gloucester
       County Times, May 8, 1979. p. A-1.

9. Wilk, Tom, "Rollins, Picketers Comply with Order
       Protest of PCB Burn Test." Gloucester
       County Times, May 3, 1979, p. A-1.

10. Goldberg, Elliot, "PCB Burning," Gloucester
       County Times, May 10, 1979, p. A-1.

11. Wilk, Tom, "EPA Plans Suit Against Rollins," Glou-
       cester County Times, August 2, 1979, p. A-1.

12. Logan Township Zoning Ordinance No. 28, 1969.

13. Ibid.

14. Ibid.

15. Schumacher, E.F., Small is Beautiful, Harper &
     Row, Publishers, New York, 1975.

16. Personal Communication

17. Bishop, Gordon, Newark Star Ledger, "Antipollution
     Group Vows to Fight Bayonne Chemical Tank
     Expansion," February 25, 1980.

18. Newark Star Ledger, January 19, 1980.

19. Carey, Art, "N.J. Chemical Waste Landfill Spurs
     Fears," Philadelphia Inquirer, October 23,
     1978, p. 1-C.

20. Hordt, Bob, "Landfill Cancer Fears Spur Anti-
     pollution Efforts," The Gloucester County
     Times, May 11, 1980, p. A-3.

21. Kolata, Gina Bari, Love Canal: False Alarm Caused
     by Botched Study, Science, Vol. 208, 13
     June 1980., pp. 1240-1242.

22. Holden, Constance, Love Canal Residents Under
     Stress, Science, Vol. 208, 13 June 1980,
     pp. 1242-1244.

23. Ibid.

24. McQuerter, Gregory, Cancer: Clues in the Mind,
     Science News, Vol. 113, No. 3, January
     21, 1978, pp. 44-45.

25. Cancer Dialogue 80, An International Symposium
     of Physicians, Scientists and Researchers,
     New York City, October 16-19, 1980.

26. McQuerter, Gregory, Op. Cit.

27. Cassileth, Barrie R., Cancer: A Biopsychosocial
         Model, The Cancer Patient, Edited by
         Barrie R. Cassileth, Ph.D., Lea & Febiger,
         Philadelphia, 1979. pp. 17-31.

28. Cancer Dialogue 80, Op. Cit.

29. Seligman, Martin E., "Helplessness, on Depression,
         Development and Death," W.H. Freeman and
         Company, San Francisco, 1975.

30. Zentner, Rene D., Shell Oil Company, Preceptions
         of the Chemical Industry by Its Neighbors,
         Paper presented for the 179th Annual Meet-
         ing of the American Chemical Society,
         Houston, Texas, March 23-28, 1980.

31. Dixon, Eustace, A., (Ph.D. Candidate), Pitman
         and Logan Township Area Environmental
         Hazards Risk Perception Survey. Pre-
         liminary Report on Procedures, Findings and
         Recommendations, August 1980 (unpublished).

32. Miller, Jr., G. Tyler, Living in the Environment:
         Concepts Problems, and Alternatives, Wads-
         worth Publishing Company, Inc. Belmont,
         1975, P. E9-1.

33. Goldberg, Elliot, "Rollins Officials Say Operations
         are Safe," Gloucester County Times, June 8,
         1979, P. A-1.

34. Epstein, Samuel S., M.D., The Politics of Cancer,
         Anchor Books, Garden City, 1979, p. 422.

35. Hunt, Maurice, W., "Rollins Operation Environmental-
         ly Safe," Readers Opinion, Gloucester County
         Times, Spetember 9, 1980.

36. Commoner, Barry, The Closing Circle, Alfred A.
         Knopf, Inc., New York, 1972, p. 36.

37. State of New Jersey Ground-water Pollution Index,
     1975-June 1980, Department of Environmental
     Protection, Division of Water Resources.

38. Environmental Protection Agency, Survey and Sampl-
     ing for PCB's, Rollins Environmental Ser-
     vices, Inc., Logan Township, August 2-5,
     1977.

39. Letter from Kenneth A. DiMuzio, Logan Township
     Solicitor to Gloucester County Board of
     Freeholders and Solid Wastes Advisory
     Council, May 1979.

40. Personal Communication. Mrs. Esther Slusarski.

41. Memorandum from William A. Fontenot, Louisiana
     State Attorney General's Office Investiga-
     tor, March 21, 1980.

42. Letter from Itaya, Sharon, M.D., April 13, 1980.

43. Ibid.

44. Report on Governor Brendan Byrne's Hazardous Waste
     Advisory Commission, Op. Cit.

45. Letter from United States Environmental Protection
     Agency to Paul A. Giardina, Hazardous
     Management Program, New Jersey DEP,
     Trenton, May 1980.

46. Shell Environmental Impact Statement, Volumes 1-5,
     February 1973.

47. Rollins Environmental Assessment, Risk Assessment,
     draft, 1980.

48. Floral and Faunal Inventory of Land Occupied by
     Rollins Environmental Services, Inc., Logan
     Township, N.J., Prepared by Conservation
     and Environmental Studies Center, Inc.,
     Browns Mills, N.J., December 9, 1980.

49. Goldberg, Elliot, "Rollins Panel Walkout Threat
     on 'Hold'," Gloucester County Times,
     August 26, 1980.

50. Environmental Defense Fund, 1979 Annual Report,
     March/April 1980.

51. Letter from Kenneth DiMuzio, Logan Township
     Solicitor, June 23, 1980.

52. Report to Governor Brendan Byrne's Hazardous
     Waste Advisory Commission, Op. Cit.

53. Ibid.

54. New Jersey Hazardous Waste News, "N.J. Moving
     Rapidly to Site Waste Facilities," Vol. 1,
     No. 1, January, 1981.

55. Galantowitz, D., The Process of Environmental
     Assessments, Part 1, New Jersey Federation
     of Environmental Commissions.

56. Muskie, Edmund S., Senator (D-Me.), "Inter-
     ference at EPA," Guest Editorial, Environ-
     mental Science & Technology, Vol. 13,
     No. 5, May 1979, p. 501.

57. Zentner, Rene D., Shell Oil Company, Perceptions
     of Occupational Hazards in the Chemical
     Industry, Paper Presented at the AICHE 72nd
     Annual Meeting in San Francisco, Ca., in
     November 1979, p. 22.

58. Dixon, E.A., Op. Cit.

59. Muskie, Edmund, S., Senator (D-Me.), Op. Cit.

60. Kotelchuck, David, "Asbestos for Sale," Science and
     Liberation, Editors, Arditti, Rita, Brennan,
     Pat and Cavrak, Steve, South End Press,
     Boston, 1980, pp. 128-144.

61. Randall, Willard S., and Solomon, Stephen D.,
         Building G: The Tragedy at Bridesburg,
         Little, Brown, and Company, Boston, 1977.

62. Dixon, Eustace A. (Ph.D. Candidate) A Critique of
         Tobacco Industry Literature Versus the 1979
         Surgeon General's Smoking and Health Report,
         C 1980 (unpublished).

63. "President Carter to Pen Bill Creating Superfund,"
         Washington (AP), Gloucester County Times,
         December 11, 1980.

64. Ibid.

65. Editorial, Gloucester County Times, July 9, 1980,
         p. A-6.

66. Hordt, Bob, and Butcher, Dave, Explosion at Rollins
         destroys waste unit, Gloucester County Times,
         May 5, 1981.

67. Gruber, George, Rollins Presents check to Logan
         Township, Gloucester County Times, January
         21, 1982.

CHAPTER 9

SYNOPSIS

"Health is a human
  right, not a privi-
  lege to be purchased."

Congresswoman
Shirley Anita
Chisholm*
(D.-N.Y.)

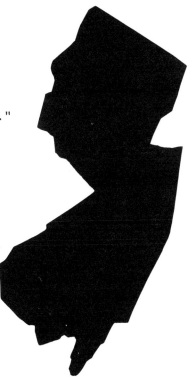

*   Congressional Record, Joint Resolution 264, 91st Congress,
    2nd Session, August 10, 1970.

CHAPTER 9

In the early 1970's, the concept of cancer as an environmentally induced disease became widely disseminated and accepted. Of all the possible etiologic factors capable of inducing cancer, chemical pollutants were widely accepted as a major cause. We began to blame industry for our cancers and since have learned that we share in the responsibility because of our life-styles. The 1973-1974 National Cancer Institute reports clearly alerted and confirmed to those concerned with health statistics, that there was a cancer problem in New Jersey. Out of the resulting state reaction came a unique and avant-garde cancer prevention and detection network. However, the benefits of those programs may not yet be reflected in current cancer statistics, because the shortest latency period for the induction of cancer is just beginning to equal the age of that detection network. So we may not display too much pride yet because New Jersey has assumed a 4th place national cancer mortality. Although there are "systematic problems" which prevent those agencies with the potential to cure and prevent cancer from being effective, organizations like the American Cancer Society and the Department of Environmental Protection, still emerge from the controversy with "white hat" images.

We have learned that cancer is a plural disease, always displaying runaway, self-centered behaviour. Further, the discussion of environmental cancer is very complex and we do not all conjure up the same image of the environment. When we assess the New Jersey environment we find that interdigitating unevenly through a varied environment and 7.3 million residents, is the chemical industry. New Jersey, the 46th state in size, once number one in the production of chemicals, has now slipped to a position of number two. Other sources of income (e.g., tourism, food processing and agriculture) indicate the diverse nature of the state's

381

economy.   Also playing an important role in discerning
the anatomy of New Jersey is resident life-style.
Hence, the two-fold environmental exploration was undertaken to demonstrate that in the former there is less
election of the exposure than in the latter.   Of course,
there are underlying reasons in each province.   Why did
industry indulge in those unsafe practises as described?
Typical responses are: that was the state of the art,
we didn't *think* it would hurt anyone, or it would cost
a lot of money to put in that many exhaust hoods.   Likewise, we individuals have underlying reasons for our
actions -- peer and advertising pressures, culture and
"the devil made me do it" philosophy.   Granted, these
are all very real behavior precursors on the part of
both industry and the individual.   However, it was the
purpose of the two-fold exploration to delineate those
areas of relative involuntary exposures versus voluntary
exposure to cancer risks and not the much more diffi-
cult-to-assay behavioral precursors.

The final impact statement on New Jersey seems
diametrically opposed to the presentation of so many
cancer risk factors.   The conclusion is that New Jersey
is a good place to live and not "Cancer Alley" any more
than a few other states.   A similar impact statement on
New Jersey yesteryear tells us that we were never free
of carcinogens, even in the "good old days".

Two models which are techniques for dealing with
major environmental problems in New Jersey are addressed.
The first simplistically attempts to accomplish detente
over those environmental problems.   Paramount over the
three typical entities in these conflicts, regulatory
agencies, the public and industry, is communication.
The individual must analyze his or her life-style and
get involved in the decision making process.   Industry
must establish believability through stewardship and
regain public trust and confidence.   Regulatory
agencies must encourage the formation of public participation groups that they intend to negotiate with in
sincerity and not as *superficial verbal fencing partners.*

The second important model will eventually emerge
from the assessment of the Rollins Environmental Ser-

vices, that is, the guidelines for the operation of a
hazardous waste treatment, storage, or disposal facility.
There will be serious data shortages in some areas.
Specifically -- how to *communicate* with the communities
where these facilities will be located. And sadly,
recent directives from state and federal government
agencies indicate that community sentiment may play no
real or apparent role in "siting." Nonetheless, the
assessment conclusions have the potential to contribute to future hazardous waste treatment, storage and
disposal facility operation.

GLOSSARY OF UNITS AND TERMS

adenocarcinoma = cancers of glandular epithelia
adenoma = benign tumor of epithelial tissue with
    glandlike structure
age - adjusted = a standardization procedure used to elim-
    inate the effects of systematic differences in the
    age composition of a population, which facilitates the
    comparison of mortalities in different areas or sub-
    groups of populations.
alpha = α
anorexia = loss of appetite
beta = β
carcinoma = malignant cellular tumors originating in
    body surface tissue and gland linings
cohort = a group under study
compare to/with = cf.
cubic meter = M^3
curie = ci, a unit of radioactivity
epidemiology = the study of the distribution and
    determination of disease frequency
gamma = γ
gram = gm, g
Hodgkin's disease = malignancies of the lymphatic system
Kilogram = Kg, 1000 gms., 2.205 lbs.
Kilometer = Km
leukemia = cancer of the blood-forming tissues
    characterized by an excess of white blood cells
lipomas = tumors composed of fat tissue, usually benign
lymphoma = any one of a group of malignant disease of
    the lymphoreticular system, typically of the lymph
    nodes
lymphosarcoma = a malignant, invasive tumor of the
    lymph node
micron = μ m
milligram = 1/1000 of a gram
myeloma = a tumor consisting of cell types normally
    found in bone marrow
nano = n=1x10^{-9}
oncogenic = causing or tending to cause tumor formation
pico = p=1x10^{-12}
ppb* = parts of vapor or gas per billion parts of air
    by volume or weight, ng/ml or ng/g

385

Glossary of Units and Terms - continued

ppm* = parts of vapor or gas per million parts of air
    by volume or weight, µg/ml or µg/g
prospective study = post-disease-occurrence monitoring
    of groups of individuals with specific characteris-
    tics
rad = a unit of absorbed radiation, 100 ergs/gm
radon daughter = a decay product of radon also
    capable of an alpha particle emission
rem = a measure of biological damage due to radiation,
    rad x quality factor
retrospective study = an after-the-fact evaluation of
    disease incidence in a group for causative factors
roentgen = a unit of gamma exposure, 90 ergs/cm^2
sarcomas = malignant tumors of the supporting body
    tissue, e.g., bone and muscle
standard mortality ratio (SMR) = a ratio of the actual
    number of cancer deaths in a given population to
    the number of deaths that would be expected had the
    population experienced the same age-- specific mor-
    tality rates as the standard population.
threshold limit value = TLV, airborne concentrations
    which persons may be exposed to daily without
    adverse effects. Established by the American
    Conference of Governmental Industrial Hygienists
watts = W

*   solids or liquids are expressed as mg/m^3,
    milligrams/cubic meter

APPENDIX A

What The American Cancer Society Does

Public Education and Information

    Breast Self Examinations
    Quit Smoking Clinics
    Early Start to Good Health materials for schools
    Regular Health Checkups
    Literature distribution
    Media Communication
    Youth Programs on Health and Science

Professional Education

    National Conferences
    Clinical Fellowships
    Clinical Scholarships
    Library of Professional Education - Films/
        Videocassettes
    Journal Publications
    Reference Center for data on unproven cancer -
        management methods

Service and Rehabilitation

    Information for cancer patients and families
    Loans of sickroom supplies, dressings
    Transportation
    Home Health Care
    Larnyx Cancer and Ostomy Task Force
    Childhood Cancer Committee
    Breast Cancer - Reach to Recovery
    Cancer Adjustment Program
    Self-Help Groups

Grants

    Research and Clinical Investigation
    Institutional Research Grants
    Research Personnel Grants
    Research Professorships
    Research Development Programs (e.g., Interferon)

Cancer Prevention Studies

    Tobacco use and Epidemiological Control data

Studies of Occupational Groups

    Asbestos workers
    Roofers
    Anesthesiologists
    Plastics Workers (vinyl chloride)
    Painters
    Rubber Plant Employees
    PCB handlers
    Photo-engravers
    Shipyard workers

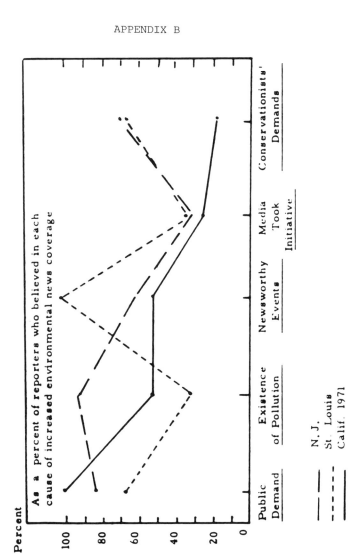

CAUSES OF INCREASED MEDIA COVERAGE AS SEEN BY REPORTERS

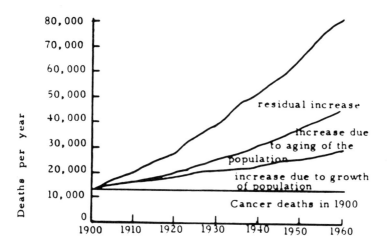

DEATHS FROM CANCER, 1900-1960 (for U.S. Death Registration Area of 1900)

Source: J.C. Bailer, H. King, and M.J. Mason, Cancer Rates and Risks, DHEW Pub. No. 1148 (Washington, D. C.: Government Printing Office, 1964), p. 6.

APPENDIX D

ALL MALIGNANT NEOPLASMS
RANGES OF RATES*, SIGNIFICANT TRENDS**, AND
ESTIMATED ANNUAL RATES OF CHANGE FOR SELECTED
CANCER SITES FOR THE MALE POPULATION
NEW JERSEY: 1949-1976

SPECIFIC ANATOMIC SITE	RANGE OF AGE-ADJUSTED RATES	SIGNIFICANT TREND	ANNUAL RATE OF CHANGE
Esophagus	4.99 - 7.86	decrease	-.068
Stomach	10.63 -29.24	decrease	-.693
Colon	20.17 -25.64	increase	.088
Rectum	5.85 -15.61	decrease	-.277
Liver and Gall-bladder	2.37 - 3.93	increase	.021
Pancreas	8.38 -12.21	increase	.077
Nose and Nasal Sinus	0.12 - 0.86	decrease	-.007
Larynx	2.80 - 4.22	decrease	-.028
Trachea, Bronchus and Lung	28.01 -66.64	increase	1.439
Prostate	16.35 -20.20	not significant	...
Testis	0.40 - 0.98	decrease	-.012
Bladder[1]	7.79 -12.08	decrease	-.089
Kidney	3.26 - 5.38	increase	.024
Hodgkin's Disease	1.31 - 2.84	decrease	-.022
Non-Hodgkin's Lymphoma	3.29 - 6.39	increase	.071
Leukemia	6.82 - 9.68	not significant	...
Malignant Melanoma of Skin	0.55 - 2.80	increase	.060
Brain[2]	3.56 - 4.55	not significant	...
Bone	0.69 - 2.30	decrease	-.049
Thyroid	0.20 - 0.70	decrease	-.007
Nasopharynx	0.21 - 0.68	not significant	...
All Malignant Neoplasms	196.31-214.37	increase	.436

APPENDIX D - continued

Note

* All rates expressed per 100,000; standard population
  is the 1960 United States population.

** Trend statistically significant at $p \leq .05$.

1 Bladder cancer mortality data analyzed for the 1949 -
  1975 period.

2 Brain cancer mortality data analyzed for the 1962 -
  1976 period.

Source: NJSDH

Annual rates of change were estimated by linear regress-
ion analysis using annual age-adjusted mortality rates
calculated by NJSDH. These estimated annual rates of
change differ from the average rates of change which
were calculated from five-year grouped data provided
by the National Cancer Institute.

APPENDIX E

ALL MALIGNANT NEOPLASMS
RANGES OF RATES*, SIGNIFICANT TRENDS**, AND
ESTIMATED ANNUAL RATES OF CHANGE FOR SELECTED
CANCER SITES FOR THE FEMALE POPULATION
NEW JERSEY: 1949-1976

SPECIFIC ANATOMIC SITE	RANGE OF AGE-ADJUSTED RATES	SIGNIFICANT TREND	ANNUAL RATE OF CHANGE
Esophagus	1.03 - 1.79	not significant	...
Stomach	4.97 -15.95	decrease	-.400
Colon	18.56 -23.77	decrease	-.186
Rectum	3.98 - 9.65	decrease	-.183
Liver and Gall-bladder	2.23 - 4.62	decrease	-.043
Pancreas	5.47 - 7.45	increase	.050
Nose and Nasal Sinus	0.08 - 0.41	not significant	...
Larynx	0.03 - 0.51	increase	.005
Trachea, Bronch-us and Lung	5.93 -17.56	increase	.377
Breast	28.07 -32.70	not significant	...
Cervix Uteri	4.11 - 9.48	decrease	-.167
Corpus Uteri	4.51 -12.32	decrease	-.269
Ovary	8.84 -10.83	not significant	...
Bladder[1]	2.35 - 4.04	decrease	-.050
Kidney	1.70 - 2.49	not significant	...
Hodgkin's Dis-ease	0.86 - 1.82	decrease	-.012
Non-Hodgkin's Lymphoma	1.89 - 4.06	increase	.055
Leukemia	4.26 - 6.33	decrease	-.033
Malignant Mela-noma of Skin	0.55 - 1.63	increase	.024
Brain[2]	2.10 - 3.17	not significant	...
Bone	0.48 - 1.59	decrease	-.025
Thyroid	0.56 - 1.14	decrease	-.013
Nasopharynx	0.03 - 0.26	not significant	...
All Malignant Neoplasms	136.95-168.03	decrease	-.933

393

APPENDIX F

INITIAL DEP AIR MONITORING PROGRAM RESULTS
OVERALL METAL CONCENTRATION BY AREA

General Area	Overall Concentrations (ug/M^3)						
	Arsenic	Cadmium	Lead	Manganese	Mercury	Nickel	Zinc
Newark	0.30	0.023	0.76	0.040	0.002	0.13	0.35
Bergen County Area	0.20	0.005	1.30	0.028	0.004	0.40	0.25
Bridgewater Township	0.68	0.003	0.57	0.024	0.004	0.07	NA
Suburban Union and Essex Counties	0.07	<0.001	0.34	0.021	0.002	0.04	0.12

NA = not included in analysis

394

APPENDIX G

1. SEX ☐1 Male ☐2 Female

2. RACE/ ORIGIN ☐1 White (non-Hispanic origin) ☐2 Black (non-Hispanic origin) ☐3 Hispanic
☐4 Asian or Pacific Islander ☐5 American Indian or Alaskan Native ☐6 Not sure

3. AGE (At Last Birthday) Years Old

4. HEIGHT (Without Shoes) Example: 5 foot, 7½ inches = ☐5 ′ ☐0☐8 ″ (No Fractions)

5. WEIGHT (Without Shoes) Pounds

6. TOBACCO ☐1 Smoker ☐2 Ex-Smoker ☐3 Never Smoked

(Smokers and Ex-smokers) Enter average number smoked per day in the last five years (ex-smokers should use the last five years before quitting.)

Cigarettes Per Day	
Pipes/Cigars Per Day (Smoke Inhaled)	
Pipes/Cigars Per Day (Smoke Not Inhaled)	

(Ex-smokers only) Enter Number of Years Stopped Smoking (Note: Enter 1 for less than one year)

7. ALCOHOL ☐1 Drinker ☐2 Ex-Drinker (Stopped) ☐3 Non-Drinker (or drinks less than one drink per week)

If you drink alcohol , enter the average number of drinks per week:

Bottles of beer per week	
Glasses of wine per week	
Mixed drinks or shots of liquor per week	

8. DRUGS/MEDICATION How often do you use drugs or medication which affect your mood or help you to relax?
☐1 Almost every day ☐2 Sometimes ☐3 Rarely or Never

9. MILES Per Year as a driver of a motor vehicle and/or passenger of an automobile (10,000 = average) Thousands of miles

10. SEAT BELT USE (percent of time used) Example: about half the time = ☐5☐0

11. PHYSICAL ACTIVITY LEVEL
☐1 Level 1 - little or no physical activity
☐2 Level 2 - occasional physical activity
☐3 Level 3 - regular physical activity at least 3 times per week

NOTE: Physical activity includes work and leisure activities that require sustained physical exertion such as walking briskly, running, lifting and carrying.

12. Did either of your parents die of a heart attack before age 60?
☐1 Yes, One of them ☐2 Yes, Both of them ☐3 No ☐4 Not sure

13. Did your mother, father, sister or brother have diabetes? ☐1 Yes ☐2 No ☐3 Not sure

14. Do YOU have diabetes? ☐1 Yes, not controlled ☐2 Yes, controlled ☐3 No ☐4 Not sure

15. Rectal problems (other than piles or hemorrhoids).
Have you had: Rectal Growth? ☐1 Yes ☐2 No ☐3 Not sure
Rectal Bleeding? ☐1 Yes ☐2 No ☐3 Not sure
Annual Rectal Exam? ☐1 Yes ☐2 No ☐3 Not sure

395

16. Has your physician ever said you have Chronic Bronchitis or Emphysema? [1] Yes [2] No [3] Not sure

17. Blood Pressure (If known — otherwise leave blank)

Systolic (High Number)

Diastolic (Low Number)

18. Fasting Cholesterol Level (If known — otherwise leave blank)

MG/DL

19. Considering your age, how would you describe your overall physical health?
[1] Excellent [2] Good [3] Fair [4] Poor

20. In general how satisfied are you with your life?
[1] Mostly Satisfied [2] Partly Satisfied [3] Mostly Disappointed [4] Not Sure

21. In general how strong are your social ties with your family and friends?
[1] Very strong [2] About Average [3] Weaker than average [4] Not sure

22. How many hours of sleep do you usually get at night?
[1] 6 hours or less [2] 7 hours [3] 8 hours [4] 9 hours or more

23. Have you suffered a serious personal loss or misfortune in the Past Year? (For example, a job loss, disability, divorce, separation, jail term, or the death of a close person)
[1] Yes, one serious loss [2] Yes, Two or More serious losses [3] No

24. How often in the Past Year did you witness or become involved in a violent or potentially violent argument?
[1] 4 or more times [2] 2 or 3 times [3] Once or never [4] Not sure

25. How many of the following things do you usually do?
- Hitch-hike or pick up hitch-hikers
- Carry a gun or knife for protection
- Keep a gun at home for protection
- Criticize or argue with strangers
- Live or work at night in a high-crime area
- Seek entertainment at night in high-crime areas or bars

[1] 3 or more [2] 1 or 2 [3] None [4] Not sure

26. Have you had a hysterectomy? (Women only) [1] Yes [2] No [3] Not sure

27. How often do you have Pap Smear? (Women only)
[1] At least once per year [2] At least once every 3 years [3] More than 3 years apart
[4] Have never had one [5] Not sure [6] Not applicable

28. Was your last Pap Smear Normal? (Women only) [1] Yes [2] No [3] Not sure [4] Not applicable

29. Did your mother, sister or daughter have breast cancer? (Women only) [1] Yes [2] No [3] Not sure

30. How often do you examine your breasts for lumps? (Women only)
[1] Monthly [2] Once every few months [3] Rarely or never

31. Have you ever completed a computerized Health Risk Appraisal Questionnaire like this one?
[1] Yes [2] No [3] Not sure

32 Current Marital Status
[1] Single (Never married) [2] Married [3] Separated
[4] Widowed [5] Divorced [6] Other

33. Schooling completed (One choice only)
[1] Did Not graduate from high school [2] High School
[3] Some College [4] College or Professional Degree

34. Employment Status
[1] Employed [2] Unemployed
[3] Homemaker, Volunteer, or Student [4] Retired, Other

35. Type of occupation (SKIP IF NOT APPLICABLE)
[1] Professional, Technical, Manager, Official or Proprietor [2] Clerical or Sales
[3] Craftsman, Foreman or Operative [4] Service or Laborer

APPENDIX H

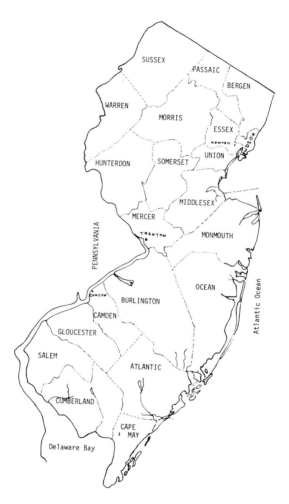

New Jersey County Map

397